JOHN F. MURRAY, M.D.

*Professor of Medicine and Member of the Senior Staff
of the Cardiovascular Research Institute,
University of California School of Medicine,
San Francisco, and Chief of Chest Division
of the Medical Service
San Francisco General Hospital, San Francisco*

The Normal Lung

The Basis for Diagnosis and
Treatment of Pulmonary Disease

W. B. SAUNDERS COMPANY
Philadelphia, London, Toronto

W. B. Saunders Company: West Washington Square
Philadelphia, PA 19105

1 St. Anne's Road
Eastbourne, East Sussex BN21 3UN, England

1 Goldthorne Avenue
Toronto, Ontario M8Z 5T9, Canada

Listed here is the latest translated edition of this book together
with the language of the translation and the publisher.

German (*1st Edition*)—F. K. Schattauer Verlag
Stuttgart, Germany

Library of Congress Cataloging in Publication Data

Murray, John Frederic, 1927–

The normal lung.

Includes index.

1. Lungs.   I. Title.
QP121.M87   612'.2   74–25480
ISBN 0–7216–6612–4

The Normal Lung   ISBN 0-7216-6612-4

Last digit is the print number: 9   8   7   6   5

To Dinny,
with love and thanks

Preface

I can remember the time, really not so long ago, when pulmonary disease consisted mainly of tuberculosis and physicians interested in the specialty were nearly always victims of the disease themselves. In striking contrast, during the past few years, large numbers of medical students, house staff, postdoctoral fellows, and physicians in practice have shown an increasing desire to learn about chest disease. Perhaps this is due to the advent of intensive care units, or to the development of fiberoptic bronchoscopy, or to the realities of the job market—or simply to the increase in pulmonary disease itself. But certainly the expansion of clinical awareness has arisen from the remarkable recent discoveries by anatomists, physiologists, biochemists, and immunologists. These and other scientists working on problems that often were not related to disease, and sometimes did not even concern the lung, are mainly responsible for the new knowledge and technical advances that have contributed to the diagnosis and management of patients with pulmonary disease.

This book represents my efforts to collate and describe as much of the new information about the lung as I could. The orientation may surprise both clinicians and basic scientists because, although a chest physician, I have stressed normality rather than disease. This is because of my firm belief that an understanding of pulmonary disease, including pathogenesis, selection of diagnostic procedures, choice of therapy, and even natural history of disease, must be based on a thorough knowledge of normal structure and function. This book attempts to provide that base.

In reading for and writing this book, I have been made deeply aware of the incompleteness of our information on many subjects. Also, as will become apparent, the acquisition of knowledge is a dynamic but capricious process. Today's data are the foundation of tomorrow's concepts. Tomorrow's concepts may become next year's principles but they also may become obsolete. Sometimes it is impossible to predict which will become which, and although I have from time to time ventured an opinion, I am equally sure that some of my opinions will turn out to have been wrong.

At least two complaints can be made about this book, as well as, I suspect, about most scientific books: the author will leave out material that others consider important, and parts of the text will be superseded before they appear in print. I hope these will be forgiven by the readers of this book. Finally, I must say that I have had considerable help in preparing the manuscript from many friends in Europe and the United States, but none of them is responsible for what I have included or omitted, or for any deficiencies in the presentation.

JOHN F. MURRAY

Acknowledgments

The Normal Lung was mostly written during a sabbatical leave from the University of California, San Francisco. Financial assistance was provided by a grant from the National Library of Medicine (LM 26,412). I was fortunate in being able to work in the library of the Brompton Institute of Diseases of the Chest in London, England; travel support and the opportunity to visit European investigators was provided by a Francis S. North Travelling Fellowship.

I was not altogether familiar at the outset with a number of particulars with which I found myself obliged to deal, so that the process of writing this book has been an educational one for me. I am indebted to many friends and colleagues for their stimulating discussions and critical review of the manuscript on any number of points. To them go my heartfelt thanks for their thoughtfulness and assistance.

Chapters in their particular field of interest were reviewed by Drs. Allen B. Cohen, Julius H. Comroe, Jr., Jon B. Glazier, James C. Hogg, Michael Hughes, H. Benfer Kaltreider, Malcolm B. McIlroy, Thomas E. Morgan, Jay A. Nadel, Lynne Reid, Daniel Simmons, and Norman C. Staub. Information for or review of certain sections was provided by Drs. A. Sonia Buist, John Clements, Geoffrey Dawes, Abraham Guz, Allison Hislop, Julien I. E. Hoffman, Joseph M. Lauweryns, Donald McDonald, Eliot A. Phillipson, Søren C. Sørensen, and John G. Widdicombe. Dr. Solly Benatar was a test reader.

Unpublished illustrations were generously supplied by Drs. Ewald R. Weibel, Nan-Sai Wang, Richard Ebert, Peter K. Jeffery, William Margaretten, Mary Williams, and Robert R. Wright. Special thanks are due to Dr. Donald McKay and Ilona Csavossy for preparing electron photomicrographs at my request. Previously published photographs of specimens were provided by Drs. Ewald R. Weibel, Joseph M. Lauweryns, Averill Liebow, Barbara Meyrick, and Una Smith Ryan. Art work and photography were done by Lindsey Pegus (Royal Marsden Hospital), Hector Escobar, Donald Longanecker, and Eugenia Kolsanoff (San Francisco General Hospital). Finally, the invaluable assistance of Susan Nutter, Phyllis McDonald, Susan Rode (Medical Service Editorial Office, San Francisco General Hospital), Aja Lipavsky, Suzanne Franks, and Nancy Wuerfel in preparing the manuscript is gratefully acknowledged.

J. F. M.

Contents

Chapter One

PRENATAL GROWTH AND DEVELOPMENT OF THE LUNG

INTRODUCTION

Venus, goddess of love, was born by rising naked from the foam of the sea. She is usually depicted as being full grown at birth, and certainly her respiratory system was completely developed because she was able to ride a scallop shell through the waves and dance on the ocean immediately after her birth. Mortal man does not leave the aquatic environment in which he develops so well equipped, because his lungs must undergo a series of complex developmental changes both during embryogenesis and after birth, culminating ultimately in the structural organization and functional capabilities of the normal adult respiratory system.

1

The purpose of this and the next two chapters is to review the growth, development, and anatomy of the normal human lung, during fetal life (Chapter 1) and from birth to maturity (Chapters 2 and 3). Although emphasis in these three chapters is on morphology and in the remainder of the book on function, both structure and function are intimately interrelated, and it is impossible to ignore one or the other completely. Therefore, a functional interpretation has been applied to morphologic evidence, and a structural basis for physiologic phenomena has been derived, whenever possible. Clinical implications are introduced when they enhance an understanding of the normal lung and its behavior.

Knowledge about the pre- and postnatal growth and development of the lung provides important insights into pulmonary function in health and disease and an explanation for developmental anomalies; it also creates a wondrous appreciation of the ability of the lung to assume, within the few minutes that it takes for the placenta to separate during birth, the complete role of providing gas exchange for the newborn baby. The heart, kidneys, liver, and other visceral organs begin functioning early in fetal life and increase their capabilities during gesta-

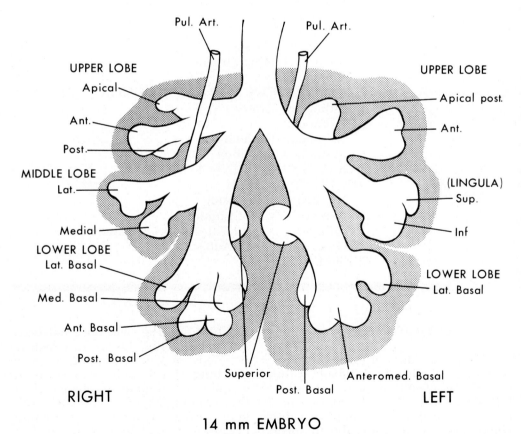

14 mm EMBRYO

Figure 1–1   Schematic drawing of the lungs of a 14 mm (six week) human embryo. The tracheobronchial tree has subdivided so that the lobar and segmental branches that characterize the adult lung can be recognized. (Adapted from Krahl.[1] Reprinted by permission from the author and publisher.)

tion. This is not so with the lungs. Because the fetus develops in a completely aquatic environment, all O_2 uptake and CO_2 elimination are provided by the placenta, and although the fetus makes breathing motions during gestation, the lung is not afforded any practice for its ultimate major role of gas exchange. Therefore, it must be carefully prepared to respond to the immediate demands of the transition from fetal to postnatal life.

EMBRYOLOGY

The entire epithelial structure of the human lung arises as a pouch from the primitive foregut and can be recognized in the third week of embryologic development (3 mm embryo). By the sixth or seventh week (14 mm embryo), through a combination of monopodial (single budding) and irregular dichotomous (dividing) branching, ten principal branches can be discerned on the right and eight on the left (Figure 1–1). The consistency of this early scheme

provides the basis for the subsequent organization of the mature lung into its familiar lobar and segmental units.[1]

The human lung develops and grows both during gestation and after birth; however, the order of maturation of the various structural components of the lung varies, as shown in Figure 1–2, and proceeds according to Reid's newly revised three "Laws of Development":

(1) The bronchial tree is developed by the sixteenth week of intrauterine life; (2) alveoli develop after birth, increasing in number until the age of eight years and in size until growth of the chest wall finishes with adulthood; and (3) the pre-acinar vessels (arteries and veins) follow the development of the airways, the intra-acinar that of the alveoli. Muscularization of the intra-acinar arteries does not keep pace with the appearance of new arteries.[3]

Thus, the growth and development of the lung follows a continuous, uninterrupted course that begins soon after conception and finishes when somatic growth ceases; however, the

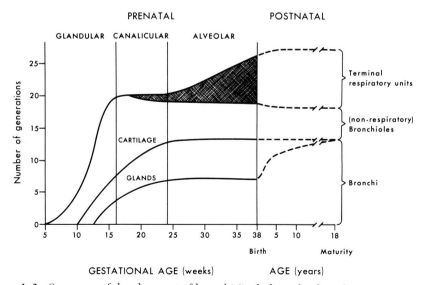

Figure 1–2 Sequence of development of bronchi (including glands and cartilage), bronchioles, and terminal respiratory units during gestation and postnatal growth. Generation number refers to an axial pathway beginning with the segmental bronchus. (Adapted from Reid.[2] Reprinted by permission from the author and publisher.)

differences in extent of development and in functional demands between intrauterine and extrauterine existence require a separation of the growth process into its prenatal and postnatal phases. This division also conveniently allows special consideration of the momentous events that occur at birth and during the first few minutes of life.

AIRWAYS AND TERMINAL RESPIRATORY UNITS

DEFINITIONS

The tracheobronchial system can be divided into two types of airways: cartilaginous airways or *bronchi* and membranous (noncartilaginous) airways or *bronchioles*. The only respiratory function of bronchi, as distinguished from their nonrespiratory role (e.g., clearance of particles), is to serve as conductors of air between the external environment and the distal sites of gas exchange. Bronchioles, however, are further subdivided to reflect their distinctive functions. *Nonrespiratory bronchioles*, including *terminal bronchioles*, serve as conductors of the gas stream, and *respiratory bronchioles* serve as sites of gas exchange. Conventionally, the definition of *conducting airways* includes the trachea, the bronchi, and the nonrespiratory bronchioles including terminal bronchioles. This omits the obvious fact that respiratory bronchioles also conduct gas to more distal respiratory bronchioles, alveolar ducts, and alveoli, but because all these structures participate in gas exchange they are designated collectively as the *terminal respiratory unit*. (The terminal respiratory unit is equivalent to the term *acinus* used in Reid's "Laws of Development.") A second important distinction between conducting airways and terminal respiratory units is that the former receive their blood supply from branches of the bronchial arteries and the latter from branches of the

pulmonary arteries. The subdivisions of airways and terminal respiratory units are shown schematically in Figure 1–3.

AIRWAYS

The primordial segmental airways undergo repeated ramifications until more than the number of generations found in the adult lung have been formed. This process is usually complete by the sixteenth week of intrauterine life, and thereafter no further formation of airways occurs.[5] In fact, the number of generations of conducting airways actually becomes reduced through the transformation of distal nonrespiratory bronchioles into respiratory bronchioles by a process of alveolarization, as shown by the cross-hatched area in Figure 1–2.

CONNECTIVE TISSUE

The cluster of proliferating bronchi invades a mass of undifferentiated mesenchymal tissue near the midline (the future mediastinum) and expands into the pleural cavities, which have become delimited from the original coelomic tube. As the mass enlarges, it becomes invested with a mesothelial lining that is continuous with the mesothelial layer of the pleural spaces (the future visceral and parietal pleuras). The progressively branching bronchi become encircled by a mass of mesenchyme that gradually differentiates into sleeves of connective tissue, layers of smooth muscle, cartilaginous rings and plates, and other supporting structures.[1] The organization of cartilage begins centrally and extends peripherally with the formation of rings that are discernible by the seventh week. Although the formation of cartilage lags behind the formation of new bronchi, spreading of cartilaginous precursors ceases at around the twenty-fifth week (Figure 1–2). Thereafter, the number of bronchial generations that contain cartilage re-

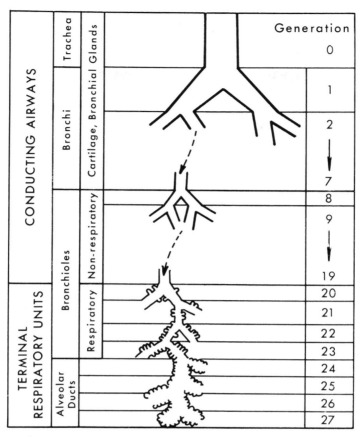

Figure 1–3 S hematic representation of the subdivisions of the conducting airways and terminal respiratory units. Note that generation number begins with the trachea. For details, see text. (Adapted from Weibel.[4] Reprinted by permission from the author and publisher.)

mains constant and is the same as that found in the adult lung.[5]

The connective tissue elements at the periphery of the proliferating lung become increasingly scanty as development proceeds. Finally, they form only a thin network of fibers. The fibrous stroma, though delicate, appears to frame and support existing alveolar ducts and alveoli and may serve to shape newly developing ones before and after birth.

MUCUS-SECRETING STRUCTURES

Goblet cells can be recognized in the epithelium of the trachea and proximal bronchi of the human fetus at the thirteenth week of intrauterine life.[6] Thereafter, they gradually appear toward the periphery, but even at term they are not found in proximal bronchioles, where they occur (though sparsely) in adults. (However, it is important to recognize that goblet cells are not normally found in terminal bronchioles in nonsmoking adults.) The first evidences of bronchial gland formation are epithelial invaginations or buds that develop at about the thirteenth week. The main growth period is between the fourteenth and twenty-eighth weeks, during which the tubuloacinar structures increase in

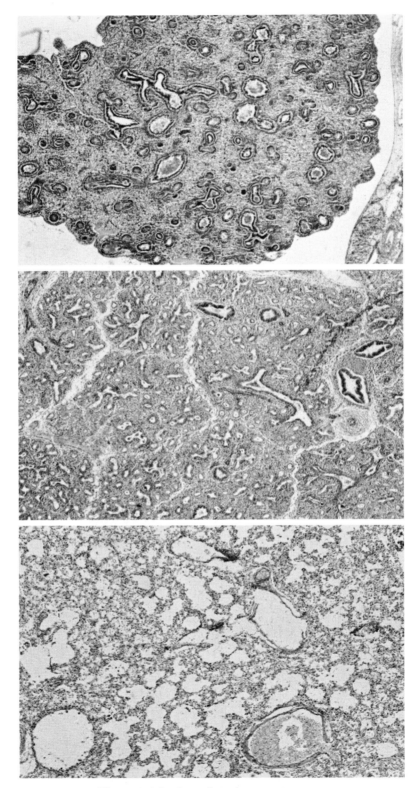

Figure 1-4 See legend on the opposite page.

complexity. Bronchial glands can be found at term in only the central half of the cartilaginous airways; the appearance of glands in the more peripheral half of the bronchi occurs after birth. Differentiation of the early cellular constituents of glands into mucus-secreting or serum-secreting cells and elaboration of secretions of characteristic chemical composition begin after the twenty-sixth week of fetal development and continue into the neonatal period.[7]

ALVEOLI

Although the pattern of formation of conducting airways is such that they are complete by birth, when they may be viewed as miniature versions of their adult counterparts, the development of alveoli follows a different course. The morphology of neonatal airspaces is sufficiently different from that of alveoli in the adult lung that some anatomists prefer to call them "saccules" and emphasize that morphologically recognizable alveoli do not develop until about two months after delivery.[8] However, there is no doubt that these saccules with their capillary lining are the sites of air-blood gas exchange in the newborn and thus serve the same respiratory function as alveoli in older persons.

The general pattern of intrauterine growth of the lung can be divided into three stages, as shown in the upper part of Figure 1–2. The *glandular period* or extended lung bud period occurs in the first sixteen weeks of gestation; during this interval the lung structures consist of a loose collection of connective tissue with an actively proliferating central bronchial mass (Figure 1–4A). The *canalicular period* occurs from 16 to 24 weeks of gestation

after all branches of the conducting airways have formed. However, by further dichotomous branching primitive bronchioles develop primitive respiratory bronchioles, the relative amount of connective tissue diminishes, a lobular pattern is recognizable, and the lung mass becomes more highly vascularized (Figure 1–4B). The *alveolar period* starts at around the twenty-fourth week and extends until term. The duct system of the canalicular period becomes more extensive, and the surface area of the spaces increases through the formation of saccules. The close contact between surface epithelium and blood vessels occurs at this stage, and capillaries line the walls and may project into the lumen (Figure 1–4C). At birth, there are about 25 million of these primitive "alveoli."[9]

The terminology of alveolar development in the human fetus is undergoing revision and the newly suggested classification includes four stages: the embryonic period (first five weeks), the pseudoglandular (instead of glandular) period, the canalicular period, and the terminal sac (instead of alveolar) period.

BLOOD VESSELS
AND CIRCULATION

PULMONARY ARTERIES

While the lung bud is forming, primitive right and left pulmonary arteries grow caudally from the aortic sac to become associated with the developing respiratory primordium. A portion of the sixth aortic arch, which originally joined the dorsal aorta to the roots of the pulmonary arteries, per-

Figure 1-4 Photomicrographs of the lungs of human fetuses showing: A, glandular period (transverse section of lung, surrounding pleural space and adjacent chest wall from about 8 weeks gestation); B, canalicular period (section of lung from about 20 weeks gestation); and C, alveolar period (section of lung from 38 week [term] fetus). For details, see text. (Hematoxylin and eosin stain; × 36. Courtesy of Dr. William Margaretten.)

See illustration on the opposite page.

sists on the left as the ductus arteri-osus.[1] Branches of the pulmonary ar-terial system assume a position next to branches of the bronchial system and maintain this partnership during sub-sequent ramifications of both airways and blood vessels, during the glandu-lar and canalicular periods. Besides the "conventional" branches of the pulmonary arterial system (i.e., those accompanying bronchi), additional arterial vessels, the so-called "super-numerary" or "accessory" arteries, are evident by the twelfth week of fetal maturation.[10] The full complement of all conventional and supernumerary arteries leading *to* the respiratory bronchioles, alveolar ducts, and sac-cules is complete in the fetus at about 16 weeks — in other words, at the same time that the adult pattern of conduct-ing airways development is com-pleted.[10] In contrast to the arteries leading *to* the future gas exchange units, the arteries *within* the struc-tures comprising the terminal units continue to proliferate, with new ones being formed up to and for several years after birth (see Chapter 2).

PULMONARY VEINS

In early embryogenesis, the blood supply to the respiratory primordium drains into a venous plexus that emp-ties into the heart through a single pulmonary vein. This vein becomes incorporated into the developing left atrium, and its principal tributaries on each side ultimately form the superior and inferior pulmonary veins.[1] The drainage pattern of the veins leading from the future gas exchange units to the hilum is complete about halfway through gestation and corresponds to the development of conducting air-ways and arteries; the fetal venous system also is similar to the arterial system because it consists of "con-ventional" and "supernumerary" veins.[11] More details about the pattern

of branching, structure, and possible function of pulmonary veins are pro-vided in the next chapter.

PULMONARY CIRCULATION

The blood flow to the lungs during fetal development is only a small pro-portion of the total cardiac output. Studies in fetal lambs have revealed that mean blood flow to the lungs through the pulmonary artery is 3.7 per cent of the cardiac output in early gestation and rises to 7.0 per cent near term; expressed in another manner, the absolute magnitude of pulmonary blood flow increases from 38 ml/100 gm (lung)/min at 60 days gestation to 126 ml/100 gm/min in late gestation (140 to 150 days).[12] These values are compared with those of other organs in Table 1–1. The increase in pulmonary blood flow after 120 days coincides with the appearance of increasing amounts of surface-active material in the lung, [13] and it is reasonable to infer that the change in blood flow is re-lated to the metabolic demands associ-ated with the production of surfactant

Table 1–1   Measurement of Cardiac Output, Distribution of Cardiac Output, and Organ Blood Flows in Fetal Lambs of Various Estimated Gestational Ages*

VARIABLE	GESTATIONAL DAYS, ESTIMATED		
	60–85	101–110	141–150
Weight, gm	80–450	901–1500	>3600
Cardiac output			
ml/min/kg	485	549	548
% to placenta	47	45	40
Blood flow, ml/100 gm organ weight/min			
Myocardium	234	208	291
Brain	30	57	132
Lung	38	53	126
Kidney	122	117	173
Gut	40	42	69
Spleen	250	265	240

*Data from Rudolph and Heymann.[12]

(see section on Intrauterine Lung Function).

Blood flow in the pulmonary circulation in experimental animals is low, but the resistance to flow is high enough to maintain pulmonary arterial pressure at or even higher than the pressure in systemic arteries. Although pulmonary vascular resistance has not been measured in human fetuses,

it is probable that pressure and resistance are similar to those in other mammals. This is believed to be true because hemodynamic conditions are reflected in the histologic appearance of blood vessels and because there is a similarity between human fetal pulmonary arteries and arteries of corresponding size in the systemic circulation. In fact, the muscle layer of

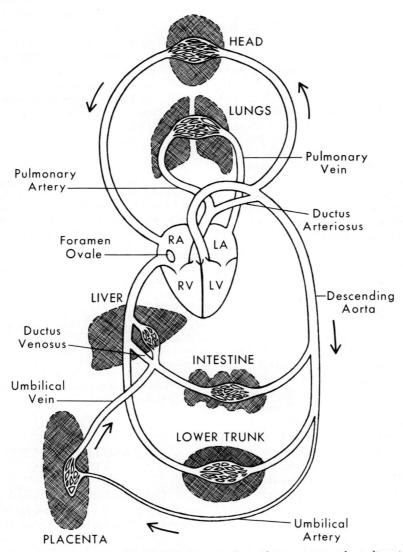

Figure 1–5   Schematic diagram of the human fetal circulation. Arrows show direction of blood flow. (Adapted from Rudolph and Heymann.[12] Reprinted by permission from the authors and The American Heart Association, Inc.)

pulmonary arteries may be even greater than that of systemic arteries.[14] The structure of fetal pulmonary arteries undoubtedly contributes to and may in part result from the high resistance and high intravascular pressure in the pulmonary circulation. The amount of smooth muscle in the vessel walls and the pulmonary arterial pressure are interrelated, and this relationship is important in the induction or failure of changes to occur in both the structure of pulmonary arteries and the pulmonary arterial pressure following birth.

We can infer from the sudden and swift drop in pulmonary arterial pressure after birth that the high pulmonary vascular resistance does not have a purely anatomic origin. Active pulmonary arterial vasoconstriction has been demonstrated in fetal lambs through the experimental use of certain vasodilator drugs and appears to be primarily a *local* vasomotor response, part of which may be induced by the hypoxic condition of the fetus. Judging from the results in experimental animals, circulating catecholamines and sympathetic nervous system stimuli do not contribute to the reaction.[15]

SYSTEMIC CIRCULATION

The major pathways of the fetal circulation are diagramed schematically in Figure 1–5. Oxygenated blood (PO_2 28 to 30 mm Hg) from the placenta is returned to the fetus through the umbilical vein and flows through the ductus venosus and inferior vena cava into the right atrium; as most of the incoming blood from the placenta flows into the right atrium it is preferentially shunted through the foramen ovale into the left atrium and left ventricle from which it is ejected into the ascending aorta for distribution to the organs supplied by the brachiocephalic vessels. Venous blood returning to the right atrium from the superior vena cava

passes into the right ventricle and is injected into the pulmonary artery; from the pulmonary artery most of the incoming blood from the head and upper extremities is shunted through the ductus arteriosus into the descending aorta for distribution to the placenta and the lower part of the body.[16] Thus, the fetal vascular system is elegantly designed for the useful purpose of distributing blood with the highest O_2 content to the heart and to the brain. The lung, it should be pointed out, mainly receives poorly oxygenated blood through the pulmonary artery, so it is among the relatively less favored (i.e., more hypoxic) fetal organs. A comparison between fetal and maternal blood gases in human beings just prior to birth is presented in Table 1–2.

Table 1–2 Systemic Blood Gases and Acid-base Values in Maternal (Arterial) and Fetal (Uterine Vein) Blood Specimens Obtained during Cesarean Section before Spontaneous Breathing by the Fetus Occurred[*][†]

VARIABLE	MATERNAL BLOOD	FETAL BLOOD
Arterial PO_2, mm Hg	97 ± 3	29 ± 3
Arterial PCO_2, mm Hg	26 ± 2	37 ± 7
Arterial pH, units	7.48 ± 0.06	7.31 ± 0.08
Buffer base, mEq/L	43 ± 5	35 ± 5
Base excess, mEq/L	-2 ± 3	-9 ± 3

[*]Data from Spackman et al.[17]

[†]Values are expressed as the mean ± standard deviation.

INTRAUTERINE LUNG FUNCTION

The fetal lung is not used as a gas exchange organ, and the question of whether it fulfills some of the nonrespiratory functions it provides in postnatal life, such as filtering, serving as a blood reservoir, providing host

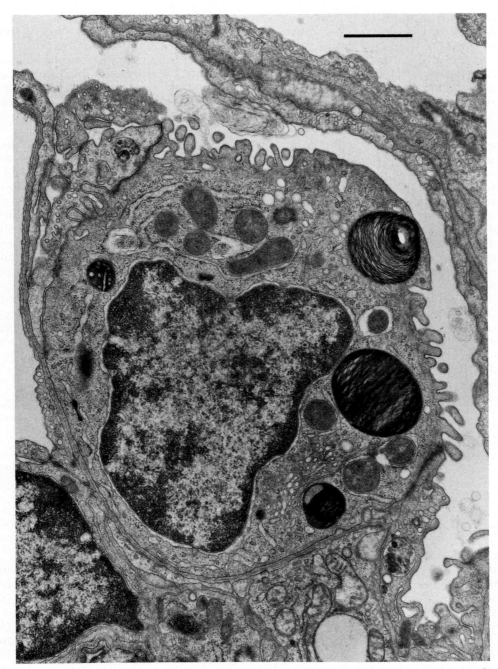

Figure 1-6   Electron photomicrograph of a type II granular pneumocyte from a rat showing three osmiophilic lamellar inclusion bodies. Horizontal bar = 1 μm. ($\times$ 18,000. Courtesy of Dr. Mary Williams.)

defenses, and activating and inactivating biologic substances, has not been examined. It seems reasonable to predict that the nonrespiratory functions of the fetal lung are quite different from those of mature lungs owing to the different requirements of intrauterine life compared with those of extrauterine life.

The fetal lung does have some well-defined special functions. Its secretory function is evident before birth because the lung is one of the main sources of amniotic fluid. The lung's glycogen stores, which increase during most of gestation and decrease toward term, may serve as a reservoir of carbohydrate to be used by the rest of the growing organism or by the lung itself to meet its own energy requirements.[18] Furthermore, the lung certainly serves as the site of production of surface-active materials (*surfactant*) that are crucial to the function of the lung, beginning with the first breath and continuing thereafter.

At about the twenty-fourth week of gestation, type II granular pneumocytes appear in the alveolar epithelium, and shortly afterward their characteristic osmiophilic lamellar inclusion bodies are detectable (Figure 1–6). These cells become more numerous until the thirtieth to thirty-second week of human fetal development and are temporally related to the appearance of surface-active substances in the lung and amniotic liquids. Figure 1–7 displays the relationship of osmiophilic inclusion bodies, surface tension (a measure of surfactant activity), and gestational age in experimental lambs[19]; it can be seen that surface tension decreases when inclusion bodies increase in number and percentage.

The biochemical processes involved in the synthesis of surface-active substances have been studied carefully owing to the disastrous consequences if the production of surfactant is faulty or delayed or if the baby is born prematurely before adequate amounts have been synthesized. Surfactant is essential not only for providing mechanical stability to the alveoli once they are air-filled but also for changing interstitial and pulmonary capillary pressures; by this means the removal of lung liquid and the lowering of pulmonary vascular resistance are enhanced during the critical first minutes after delivery.

It is generally accepted that the developmental sequence of the synthesis of surfactant in amounts sufficient to facilitate respiration after birth is mainly related to gestational age, but that certain humoral influences have been identified that will accelerate biochemical maturation and volume stability of the fetal lung.[20, 21] Surfactant is a mixture of phospholipids and protein in relatively stable proportions. The principal, but not the only, surface-active component of all mammalian lungs studied is dipalmitoyl lecithin. In mammalian lungs, lecithin may be synthesized by three pathways[22]:

(1) diacylphosphoglyceride + cytidine-diphosphocholine → lecithin + cytidine monophosphate;

(2) phosphatidyl ethanolamine + S-adenosyl methionine $\xrightarrow{\textit{sequential methylation}}$ lecithin;

(3) lysophosphatidyl choline + fatty acyl-S-coenzyme A → lecithin + coenzyme A.

The first pathway is quantitatively the most important for total lecithin synthesis in the fetus and newborn in most animal species, including man. The other pathways contribute less to total lecithin synthesis in the lung than pathway 1, and their contributions to the specific molecular species of surfactant lecithin, dipalmitoyl lecithin, remain to be determined.[22]

In the few weeks before term,

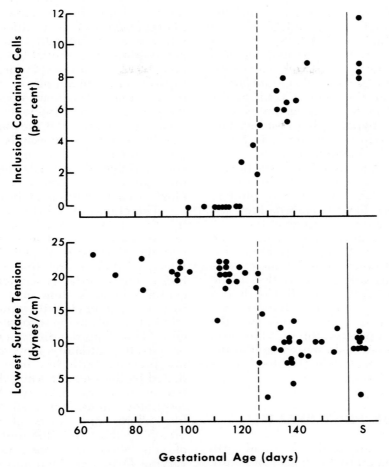

Figure 1-7   The number of alveolar cells containing osmiophilic inclusion bodies expressed as percentage of total lung tissue cells (upper panel) and the lowest surface tensions of lung extracts (lower panel) according to gestational age of fetal and spontaneously delivered (S) lambs. The interrupted vertical line at 126 days of gestation indicates the age after which surfactant is normally detectable. (Replotted from Orzalesi, Motoyama, Jacobson, Kikkawa, Reynolds, and Cook.[19] Reprinted by permission from the authors and publisher.)

there is a striking increase in volume stability of the lung that is accompanied by changes in the lipid composition of tracheal aspirates and amniotic fluid. This observation has led to the development of new screening tests to detect the presence of pulmonary surface-active material that have a high predictive value for the respiratory distress syndrome of the newborn.[23, 24] These tests should be of considerable assistance in timing elective deliveries, in applying vigorous preventive thera-

peutic maneuvers to the newborn infant, and in deciding whether or not to treat the mother prior to delivery with a substance (e.g., betamethasone) known to accelerate functional maturation of the fetal surfactant-producing system.

In view of the convincing evidence that the administration of a glucocorticoid during pregnancy will cause surfactant to appear in fetal lungs earlier than usual, the recent finding of specific cytoplasmic receptors for glucocorticoids in the lungs of fetal rabbits and lambs is of considerable interest.[25] Specific receptor activity has also been detected in human fetal lungs from specimens of 12 weeks' gestational age and later.[26]

And so, the time of birth finally arrives. The fetus, accustomed to a warm but hypoxic, hypercarbic, and acidotic medium, all alien to its future extrauterine environment, lies submerged in amniotic fluid. Its liquid-filled lungs have been virtually useless and although episodic respiratory movements have occurred, they are probably much weaker than those required after birth. Most of the blood that returns to the fetus' right heart is shunted through the foramen ovale and ductus arteriosus so that blood flow to the lungs is small. Conditions deteriorate before they improve because during contractions of the uterus and passage through the birth canal, the internal environment of the fetus as reflected in its blood gases tends to become worse.

THE FIRST BREATH

The events of delivery and birth are dominated by the legacy of nature because there is little that can be done by participating parties that will influence the multitude of changes that must occur in the first few minutes of extrauterine life. The traditional slap, aspiration of the oropharynx, and even attempts at insufflation of the lungs made to assist the newborn are minuscule external efforts compared with the extensive internal adjustments taking place. Within the few minutes required for the placenta to separate from the uterus, which removes the fetus' extracorporeal means of life, the newborn must "turn on" his central and autonomic nervous systems, replace the liquid in his lungs with air, establish a substantial pulmonary circulation, and markedly revise the direction of blood flow through his

cardiac chambers and great vessels. These should not be considered separate processes but rather as interdependent events essential to the development of a cardiorespiratory system capable of maintaining an adequate supply of O_2 to the infant's body. That these complex requirements are met seems miraculous, but they are met—usually perfectly—thousands of times a day and more often, in fact, if one considers that all mammals presumably undergo the same fundamental physiologic transformations at birth.

The climax of delivery is the first breath, an event which can also be viewed as the end of fetal existence and the beginning of postnatal life. However, before the first breath is taken, the respiratory center of the central nervous system must integrate incoming afferent impulses and initiate efferent signals to the respiratory muscles. The long-standing belief that organized ventilatory movements do not precede birth has been contradicted by the recent finding that lamb fetuses *in utero* make two types of respiratory movements: single gasp-like efforts and bursts of irregular breathing; moreover, different patterns of ventilation have been related to varying phases of sleep and wakefulness by direct inspection and by recording rapid eye movements.[27] Furthermore, episodic chest wall movements, similar to those observed in lambs, have been recorded in human fetuses using ultrasonic techniques and were found to be present about 65 per cent of the time.[28] The increase in ventilatory movements by the fetus prior to term may serve the useful purpose of exercising the respiratory muscles and readying them for sustained ventilation.

The existence of prenatal ventilation is consistent with other evidence that the various respiratory control systems known to be present in adults are functional in infants at or shortly after birth.[29] Ventilatory movements during gestation are irregular and inconstant presumably because the magnitude of the various afferent stimuli that arise from the protected fetus in its "buffered" environment is insufficient to sustain activity of the respiratory center. The additional stimulus for breathing that arises at birth is probably the result of thermal, tactile, and other *new* exteroceptive and proprioceptive stimuli, increased nerve traffic from peripheral chemoreceptors (that are actuated by sympathetic nervous system activity after cord clamping), and impulses from central chemosensitive receptors.[29] However, we must acknowledge ignorance about the relative importance of these various neurologic contributions to the first breath.

EXPANSION OF THE LUNG

Once initiated, the contractions of the respiratory muscles must generate sufficient force to (1) move air and a column of liquid (that is 100 times more viscous than air) ahead of it into the lungs, (2) overcome the forces of surface tension at the interface of the contiguous columns of air and liquid moving through small airways, and (3) distend the lung tissues.[30] Measurements made using an esophageal balloon have revealed that human infants produce extreme negative intrathoracic pressures of 40 to 80 cm H_2O during the first few breaths.[31] Figure 1–8 depicts the pressure-volume curves of the first three breaths of a normal newborn infant. High distending pressures from muscular contraction during inspiration are followed by vigorous expiratory efforts associated with positive or collapsing pressures during expiration. All the air that is taken in during the first inspiration is usually not completely exhaled, because if it were, either the lung would collapse or the liquid that had been displaced would return again. Some

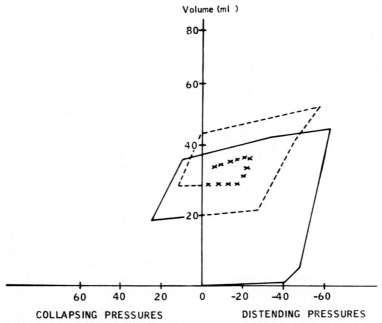

Figure 1–8 Schematic representation of the relationships between the distending and collapsing pressures and the resulting volumes during the first (———), second (-----), and third (xxxxx) breaths. (From Avery.[30] Reprinted by permission from the author and publisher.)

air is retained with each of the first few breaths so that a functional residual capacity (FRC) is gradually established. (The FRC is the amount of air left in the lungs at the end of passive expiration; normally, FRC is the lung volume at which the forces tending to expand the chest wall are balanced by the forces tending to retract the lung.)

REMOVAL OF LUNG LIQUID

Immediately before birth, the fetal lung contains about 50 ml of liquid, which is approximately equal to the volume of the air-filled lung at its resting position (FRC) a few hours after birth. Constancy of FRC in the immediate postpartum period is opposite to the expected change, if unopposed, from the addition of surface forces at the newly formed air-liquid interface of the newborn's lung. The discrepancy is probably accounted for by an increasing outward recoil (although small) of the chest wall due to progressive recruitment and "tone" of skeletal muscle fibers.

The composition of fetal lung liquid differs from that of both plasma and amniotic fluid.[32] Recent physiochemical considerations strongly suggest that lung liquid is not an ultrafiltrate of plasma but a substance actively secreted by the fetal lung itself[33]; however, the cellular source of the liquid has not been discovered. Of great significance, as will be explained subsequently, is that the lung liquid has a low protein concentration (300 mg/100 ml) and is rich in surface-active lipoproteins. The liquid is removed from the airways and alveolar spaces by two principal pathways: part of it drains externally and the remainder is removed through pulmonary capillaries or lymphatics. Drainage from the nasopharynx is facilitated by compression of the thorax during vertex delivery, which squeezes liquid out of the lungs.[34] However, removal by drainage is not an essential mechanism, because

infants born with other presentations (e.g., breech) and by cesarean section are able to dispose of their lung liquid without the assistance of thoracic compression. Expansion of the thorax by muscular contraction with its accompanying high negative intrathoracic pressure produces a negative interstitial pressure and a hydrostatic pressure difference that favors movement of the liquid from alveoli into contiguous interstitial spaces. From the interstitium, the liquid is then returned to the bloodstream by one of two possible pathways: some is reabsorbed into the alveolar capillaries — the low protein concentration of lung liquid establishes a colloid osmotic pressure difference that promotes transfer into the bloodstream; some is taken up by lymphatic channels that are located in the interstitial spaces around blood vessels and airways — the only practicable way that protein molecules in the interstitium can be returned to the bloodstream. Moreover, histologic studies performed on experimental animals within the first few hours after birth reveal distended pulmonary lymphatics,[35] and collections of the pulmonary lymphatic fluid from newborn lambs indicate that about 30 per cent of the lung liquid and virtually all of the protein from the amount of liquid originally contained in the lung is removed by lymphatic drainage.[36]

Immediately after the start of respiration in the newborn, the volume accommodated by the lung consists of both residual lung liquid and air. A few hours are required before all the liquid is displaced by air, and even though the infant no longer generates such high negative intrathoracic pressures as it did during the first few breaths, a negative interstitial pressure is maintained by the recoil characteristics of the lung, including that contributed by the deposition of surfactant as an air-liquid layer on the surface of the alveolar epithelium. Because surfactant serves to stabilize small air-spaces, it is therefore of special importance in determining the mechanical properties of the lungs of infants.[37] Moreover, the absence or shortage of surfactant can be correlated with both the incidence and the mechanical disturbances that characterize the idiopathic respiratory distress syndrome of the newborn.[38] Because lung liquid contains a large amount of surface-active lipoprotein, an advantage of removing the liquid through the lungs is not only the speed with which it can be carried out but also that a coating of essential surfactant is left behind on the alvelolar surface as removal occurs.

PULMONARY VASCULAR RESISTANCE CHANGES

An important concomitant of the first breath is the decrease in pulmonary vascular resistance and the increase in flow of blood to the lungs through the pulmonary circulation. At least three mechanisms contribute to the fall in pulmonary vascular resistance: (1) replacement of the liquid in the lungs by air and establishment of an air-liquid interface at the alveolar surface — these phenomena change the geometry of the alveolus and the newly produced surface forces "pull open" capillaries and other small vessels exposed to alveolar pressure; (2) increase of the PO_2 within the alveoli — this process alleviates alveolar hypoxia and in turn relieves a pulmonary arterial vasoconstrictor stimulus acting upon intensely reactive blood vessels; and (3) decrease of PCO_2 within the alveoli — this also decreases pulmonary arterial vasoconstriction, although it has not been established whether the response is a direct effect of changing PCO_2 or an indirect effect on pH. Judging from studies in experimental animals, these three mechanisms have effects that are additive and of similar magnitude.[15]

The effects of expansion and changing alveolar PO_2 and PCO_2 (or pH) on the pulmonary circulation are direct ones that are maintained into adult life, although to a lesser extent than in the newborn period. Experimental evidence in fetal and newborn lambs suggests that the contribution of sympathetic nervous system stimuli to pulmonary vasoconstrictor responses is not important and is a mechanism that becomes even more trivial in adult life.[15]

Distending the pulmonary blood vessels helps slightly to inflate the lung with air. However, it seems certain that this is of secondary importance compared with the beneficial effects on pulmonary vascular resistance of replacing the liquid with air.

OTHER CIRCULATORY ADJUSTMENTS

Another important consequence of the phenomena of the first breath is the alteration of the patterns of blood flow that existed during gestation. Accompanying the fall in pulmonary vascular resistance is a reversal of blood flow through the ductus arteriosus from right to left (fetal state) to left to right (newborn state); flow through the ductus arteriosus, which is labile the first few days of life, gradually ceases as the ductus closes. The shunt of blood from right atrium to left atrium through the foramen ovale, another hallmark of the fetal circulation, also ceases soon after birth. The distensibility characteristics of the left atrium do not allow it to accommodate the extra volume of blood that it must receive after pulmonary vascular resistance decreases — and essentially the entire cardiac output flows through the lungs — without a pressure increase sufficient to close the foramen.

Recent observations suggest that kinins, one of the classes of biologically active peptides, are produced in large quantities at birth and may be important mediators of neonatal cir-

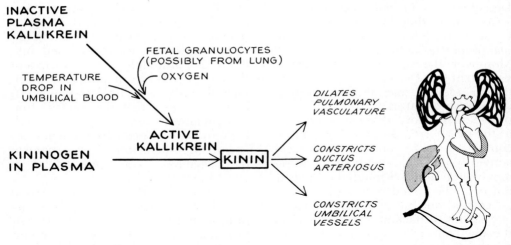

Figure 1–9   Schematic diagram of potential pathways involved in kinin activation and possible contributions of kinins to neonatal circulatory adjustments. (From Melmon, Cline, Hughes, and Nies.[39] Reprinted by permission from the authors and publisher.)

culatory changes.[39] Kinins are the most potent of all the naturally occurring vasodilator substances, and the levels found in neonatal blood samples are equal to or greater than those found in the bloodstream of patients with the carcinoid syndrome during a flush. The proposed mechanisms of kinin generation and the possible effects of kinins on the neonatal circulation are shown in Figure 1–9. Kallikrein, the enzyme that converts plasma kininogen to kinin, is believed to be activated by a drop in temperature of umbilical cord blood, the rise in arterial PO_2 that accompanies neonatal respiration, and the granulocytosis that characteristically occurs six to twelve hours after birth.[39] The pharmacologic consequences of kinin production in the newborn are dilation of the pulmonary vascular bed, constriction of the ductus arteriosus, and constriction of the umbilical vessels.

The respiratory and circulatory systems of the fetus are thus elegantly designed to adapt immediately to the strenuous requirements of neonatal life. However, once the severe tests of

the newborn period have been surmounted, the lungs must continue to grow in order to meet the demands for increased gas exchange of the adult. Postnatal growth and development of the lung will be considered in the next chapter.

REFERENCES

1. Krahl, V. E.: Anatomy of the mammalian lung. *In* Fenn, W. O., and Rahn, H. (eds.): Handbook of Physiology, Section 3. Respiration. Vol. I. Washington, D.C., American Physiological Society, 1964, pp. 213–284.
2. Reid, L.: The embryology of the lung. *In* De Reuck, A. V. S., and Porter, R. (eds.): Ciba Foundation Symposium: Development of the Lung. Boston, Little, Brown and Company, 1967, pp. 109–124.
3. Hislop, A., and Reid, L.: Growth and development of the respiratory system. *In* Davis, J. A., and Dopping, J. (eds.): Scientific Foundations of Paediatrics. London, Heineman, 1974, pp. 214–254.
4. Weibel, E. R.: Morphometry of the Human Lung. Berlin, Springer-Verlag, 1963, p. 111.
5. Bucher, U., and Reid, L.: Development of

the intrasegmental bronchial tree: the pattern of branching and development of cartilage at various stages of intra-uterine life. Thorax, 16:207–218, 1961.

6. Bucher, U., and Reid, L.: Development of the mucus-secreting elements in human lung. Thorax, 16:219–225, 1961.

7. Lamb, D., and Reid, L.: Acidic glycoproteins produced by the mucous cells of the bronchial submucosal glands in the fetus and child: a histochemical autoradiographic study. Brit. J. Dis. Chest, 66:248–253, 1972.

8. Boyden, E. A., and Tompsett, D. H.: The changing patterns in the developing lungs of infants. Acta Anat. (Basel), 61:164–192, 1965.

9. Dunnill, M. S.: Postnatal growth of the lung. Thorax, 17:329–333, 1962.

10. Hislop, A., and Reid, L.: Intra-pulmonary arterial development during fetal life — branching pattern and structure. J. Anat., 113:35–48, 1972.

11. Hislop, A., and Reid, L.: Fetal and childhood development of the intrapulmonary veins in man — branching pattern and structure. Thorax, 28:313–319, 1973.

12. Rudolph, A. M., and Heymann, M. A.: Circulatory changes during growth in the fetal lamb. Circ. Res., 26:289–299, 1970.

13. Howatt, W. F., Avery, M. E., Humphreys, P. W., Normand, I. C. S., Reid, L., and Strang, L. B.: Factors affecting pulmonary surface properties in the foetal lamb. Clin. Sci., 29:239–248, 1965.

14. Naeye, R. L.: Arterial changes during the perinatal period. Arch. Path., 71:121–128, 1961.

15. Dawes, G. S.: Pulmonary circulation in the foetus and the newborn. In De Reuck, A. V. S., and Porter, R. (eds.): Ciba Foundation Symposium: Development of the Lung. Boston, Little, Brown and Company, 1967, pp. 332–347.

16. Rudolph, A. M., and Heymann, M. A.: The circulation of the fetus in utero. Methods for studying distribution of blood flow, cardiac output and organ blood flow. Circ. Res., 21:163–184, 1967.

17. Spackman, T., Fuchs, F., and Assali, N. S.: Acid-base status of the fetus in human pregnancy. Obstet. Gynec., 22:785–791, 1963.

18. Heinemann, H. O., and Fishman, A. P.: Nonrespiratory functions of mammalian lung. Physiol. Rev., 49:1–47, 1969.

19. Orzalesi, M. A., Motoyama, E. K., Jacobson, H. N., Kikkawa, Y., Reynolds, O. R., and Cook, C. D.: The development of the lungs of lambs. Pediatrics, 35:373–381, 1965.

20. Kotas, R. V., and Avery, M. E.: Accelerated appearance of pulmonary surfactant in the fetal rabbit. J. Appl. Physiol., 30:358–361, 1971.

21. Wang, N. S., Kotas, R. V., Avery, M. E., and Thurlbeck, W. M.: Accelerated appearance of osmiophilic bodies in fetal lungs following steroid injection. J. Appl. Physiol., 30:362–365, 1971.

22. Morgan, T. E.: Pulmonary surfactant. New Eng. J. Med., 284:1185–1193, 1971.

23. Gluck, L., Kulovich, M. V., Borer, R. C., Jr., Brenner, P. H., Anderson, G. G., and Spellacy, W. N.: Diagnosis of the respiratory distress syndrome by amniocentesis. Am. J. Obstet. Gynec., 109:440–445, 1971.

24. Clements, J. A., Platzker, A. C. G., Tierney, D. F., Hobel, C. J., Creasy, R. K., Margolis, A. J., Thibeault, D. W., Tooley, W. H., and Oh, W.: Assessment of the risk of the respiratory-distress syndrome by a rapid test for surfactant in amniotic fluid. New Eng. J. Med., 286:1077–1081, 1972.

25. Ballard, P. L., and Ballard, R. A.: Glucocorticoid receptors and the role of glucocorticoids in fetal lung development. Proc. Nat. Acad. Sci. U.S.A., 69:2668–2672, 1972.

26. Ballard, P. L., and Ballard, R. A.: Cytoplasmic receptor for glucocorticoids in lung of the human fetus and neonate. J. Clin. Invest., 53:477–486, 1974.

27. Dawes, G. S., Fox, H. E., Leduc, B. M., Liggins, G. C., and Richards, R. T.: Respiratory movements and rapid eye movement sleep in the foetal lamb. J. Physiol. (Lond.), 220:119–143, 1972.

28. Boddy, K., and Mantell, C. D.: Observations of fetal breathing movements transmitted through maternal abdominal wall. Lancet, 2:1219–1220, 1972.

29. Purves, M. J.: Initiation of respiration. In De Reuck, A. V. S., and Porter, R. (eds.): Ciba Foundation Symposium: Development of the Lung. Boston, Little, Brown and Company, 1967, pp. 317–331.

30. Avery, M. E.: The J. Burns Amberson lecture — In pursuit of understanding the first breath. Am. Rev. Resp. Dis., 100:295–304, 1969.

31. Karlberg, P.: The adaptive changes in the immediate postnatal period, with particular reference to respiration. J. Pediat., 56:585–604, 1960.

32. Adams, F. H.: Functional development of the fetal lung. J. Pediat., 68:794–801, 1966.

33. Adamson, T. M., Boyd, R. D. H., Platt, H. S., and Strang, L. B.: Composition of alveolar liquid in the foetal lamb. J. Physiol. (Lond.), 204:159–168, 1969.

34. Karlberg, P., Adams, F. H., Geubelle, F., and Wallgren, G.: Alteration of the infant's thorax during vaginal delivery. Acta Obstet. Gynec. Scand., 41:223–229, 1962.

35. Lauweryns, J. M., Claessens, S., and

Boussauw, L.: The pulmonary lymphatics in neonatal hyaline membrane disease. Pediatrics, *41*:917–930, 1968.

36. Strang, L. B.: Uptake of liquid from the lungs at the start of breathing. *In* De Reuck, A. V. S., and Porter, R. (eds.): Ciba Foundation Symposium: Development of the Lung. Boston, Little, Brown and Company, 1967, pp. 348–375.

37. Clements, J. A.: Editorial: Pulmonary sur-factant. Am. Rev. Resp. Dis., *101*:984–990, 1970.

38. Avery, M. E., and Mead, J.: Surface properties in relation to atelectasis and hyaline membrane disease. Am. J. Dis. Child., *97*:517–523, 1959.

39. Melmon, K. L., Cline, M. J., Hughes, T., and Nies, A. S.: Kinins: possible mediators of neonatal circulatory changes in man. J. Clin. Invest., *47*:1295–1302, 1968.

Chapter Two

POSTNATAL GROWTH AND DEVELOPMENT OF THE LUNG

INTRODUCTION

The neonatal lung undergoes remarkable immediate functional transformations so that by the end of the first few minutes of life it is serving as an adequate organ of gas exchange. Measurements of arterial blood gases one to four hours after birth reveal a PO_2 of about 62 mm Hg and a PCO_2 of about 38 mm Hg.[1] To achieve these levels of blood gases, the newborn breathes at an average respiratory rate of 37 breaths/min and has a tidal volume of 21 ml.[2] This means that the baby has a minute ventilation of 777 ml/min (37 × 21 = 777).

Moreover, within a day or two of birth the intrathoracic pressure changes, and the ratios of wasted ventilation (i.e., physiologic dead space) to tidal volume, tidal volume to FRC, O_2 consumption to minute ventilation, and diffusing capacity to O_2 consumption are similar to those in adults. However, neonatal pulmonary function is carried out in lungs that obviously still retain their fetal structure. Although some histologic changes can be recognized in the caliber of the newborn's pulmonary blood vessels and the geometry of its alveoli (presumably related to inflation), the development of the human lung to its adult state continues long after birth. However, the rate at which the different structural components of the lung mature after birth, as well as before birth, varies considerably.

TRACHEOBRONCHIAL SYSTEM

AIRWAYS

At birth, the basic formation of cartilaginous airways is complete, and additional division does not occur. In fact, the number of generations of conducting airways actually decreases through the conversion by alveolarization of usually one to two, but at times three or more, generations of non-

respiratory bronchioles into respiratory bronchioles.[3] The process of alveolarization, which extends centrally (toward the hilum), continues until about three years of age; thereafter, the system of branches remains constant. Growth of each segment of the conducting airways appears to occur mainly in a symmetric fashion, both in length and in diameter, until growth of the thorax ceases.[4] These conclusions conflict in part with a more recent observation that in the first five years of life the growth of small airways (those distal to the twelfth to the fifteenth generation) may lag behind the growth of larger airways.[5]

The number of bronchial divisions varies markedly *within* the lungs, depending on the length of pathways from segmental bronchi to the various gas exchange units throughout the lung. For example, respiratory bronchioles near the hilum may be reached from a segmental bronchus with only ten bronchial branches, whereas more than 25 branches may be required to reach respiratory bronchioles in the most peripheral basal parts of the lung.[6]

The asymmetry in pathway lengths derives from the pattern of irregular dichotomous branching (Figure 2–1) and has important implications concerning the resistance to airflow and the transit times from mouth to gas exchange sites.[8] The engineering of the airways is also complicated by variations in the size and angulation of each pair of branches; the branch serving the longer pathway is straighter and has a larger cross-sectional area than the smaller, more angulated branch leading to the closer gas exchange units. This may serve in part to equalize slightly the distribution of resistances among the various pathways. The pattern of branching also helps to explain the location of primary tuberculosis foci that are almost invariably found within 1 cm of the pleural surface of collapsed lung specimens.[9] Inhaled (infective) droplets of

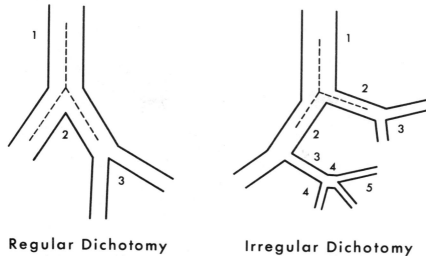

Regular Dichotomy   Irregular Dichotomy

Figure 2–1 Schematic representation of regular and irregular dichotomous patterns of airway branching. Apparent monopody shown in first and apparent trichotomy in third generation. (Adapted from Weibel.[7] Reprinted by permission from the author and publisher.)

appropriate size are more likely to escape being deposited on the airway surface if they move along the axial airstream in the straighter and larger of two possible paths through the bronchial tree; thus, particles following this route tend to be deposited near the periphery of the lung.

As seen in Figure 2–2, the diameter of each new generation of airways decreases progressively from the trachea outward. However, the change in caliber is such that the cross-sectional area of the airway lumen steadily increases at successive levels throughout the tracheobronchial system; this is especially marked distal to the origin of the bronchioles, where branching is accompanied by practically no decrease in diameter of new generations. The increases in cross-sectional area mean that the velocity of airflow must be sharply reduced as the airstream moves peripherally through the airways. This phenomenon has important implications concerning the distribution of airways resistance in both normal and diseased lungs, which are considered in Chapter 4.

The conducting airways are not merely rigid tubes through which air flows between the outside environment and the gas exchange units, but they are structures with secretory capabilities, and they dilate and contract passively in response to influences such as lung inflation and actively in response to a variety of neurohumoral and chemical stimuli. The active reactions are mediated by the elements that compose the walls of airways: epithelium, smooth muscles, glands, nerves, and cells with tiny cachets of potent pharmacologic substances—all of which contribute to bronchial reactivity under special conditions. It is teleologically appealing to speculate that bronchomotor responses operate normally in the direction of maintaining the proper balance between ventilation and blood flow in order to achieve optimum gas exchange; however, there is no evidence to support this concept. Redistribution of ventilation may occur under certain circumstances (see subsequent sections), but the mechanism appears to be smooth muscle contraction in terminal respira-

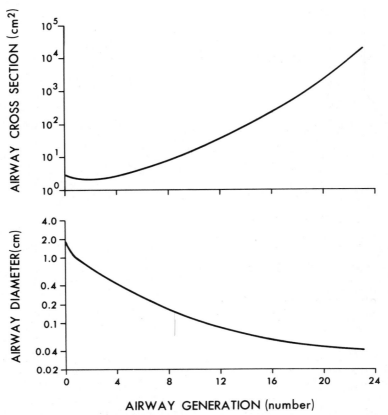

Figure 2-2   Average diameter and cross section of airway segments plotted semilogarithmically against airway generation. The trachea is generation 0, the mainstem bronchi generation 1, etc. (Adapted from Weibel.[7] Reprinted by permission from the author and publisher.)

tory units rather than in conducting airways.

BRONCHIAL EPITHELIUM

The entire system of airways, from the trachea to the respiratory bronchioles, is covered with an epithelial lining that rests on a thin basement membrane overlying the lamina propria, a loose network of fibers containing cells, a rich capillary plexus, and unmyelinated nerves.[10] In large airways, the epithelium is of the ciliated pseudostratified columnar type; however, the thickness of the lining layer gradually decreases in height as the airways become smaller so that in the terminal bronchioles, the epithelium consists of a single layer of ciliated cells that are more cuboidal than columnar, and in the respiratory bronchioles the cells are even flatter.

The pseudostratified columnar epithelium of bronchi (Figure 2–3) contains three common cell types and two cell types that are much rarer. *Ciliated cells* are the dominant cells of the epithelial layer (Figure 2–4); they are present throughout all conducting airways and extend into respiratory bronchioles. The coordinated, sweeping motion of the cilia provides the force that impels the superficial layer of secretions (the "mucus blanket") along its journey from peripheral airways into the pharynx. This so-called "ciliary escalator" is an important natural defense mechanism, since it is the chief pathway for removing inhaled particles deposited within the lung. Ciliated cells and the removal systems are considered in greater detail in Chapter 11.

Goblet cells are sandwiched be-

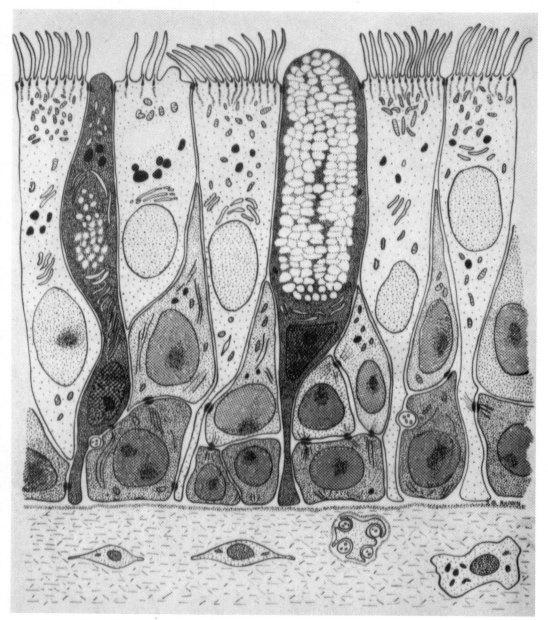

Figure 2–3 Schematic representation of the pseudostratified, ciliated epithelium of the human trachea showing ciliated cells, goblet cells, and basal cells. Compare with Figure 2–5. (From Rhodin.[10] Reprinted by permission from the author and publisher.)

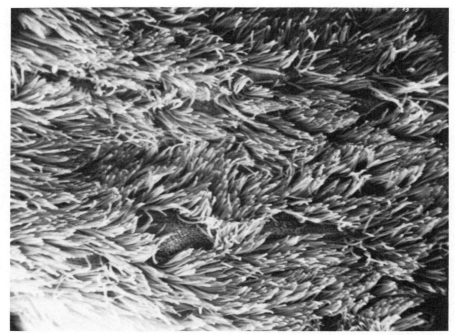

Figure 2–4 Scanning electron photomicrograph of the luminal surface of a bronchiole from a normal adult man; many cilia are evident surrounding a nonciliated cell. (× 2000. From Ebert, R. V., and Terracio, M. J.: Am. Rev. Resp. Dis., *111*:4, 1975. Reprinted by permission from the authors and publisher.)

tween adjacent ciliated cells (Figure 2–5) and contribute their secretions to the mucus layer on the surface of the epithelium. Most of the mucus is produced by glands, especially in conducting airways where glands are numerous. However, the goblet cells are normally the sole suppliers within all nonrespiratory bronchioles except terminal bronchioles. (In smokers, goblet cells are found within terminal bronchioles.)

Basal cells are not known to have a special function of their own, but they serve the important purpose of differentiating as needed to replace superficial ciliated and goblet cells. Thus, they constitute a reserve population of cells that replenishes the surface layer.

Brush cells are rare and their function remains unknown. The presence of microvilli and other similarities between brush cells of the bronchial epithelium and those in the gastrointestinal tract have suggested similar roles in liquid absorption.

Argyrophil or Kulchitsky-like cells are much more impressive in the epithelium of newborns than in that of either children or adults. Electron microscopy has demonstrated a characteristic ultrastructure and has provided suggestive evidence that the cells are innervated (Figure 2–6); histochemical studies indicate the possible presence of kinins.[12] This observation, plus the frequency with which argyrophilic cells are found in the human fetus and the newborn and their virtual absence in adults, has led Lauweryns[12] to speculate that they may be the source of some of the kinin activity that is evident in the newborn period (see Figure 1–9). These cells are also important as the precursors of bronchial carcinoids, and they may be related to the genesis of oat cell cancers.

Clumps of 10 to 30 serotonin-containing and argyrophilic cells have recently been discovered in the bronchial, bronchiolar, and even alveolar epithelium of various mammals, including man.[13] These *neuroepithelial bodies*, which are heavily innervated, are of considerable interest owing to their strategic location and the possibility that they may regulate airway and/or pulmonary blood vessel caliber. Because neuroepithelial bodies appear to have both afferent and efferent innervation, their level of activity may be modulated by stimuli from the central nervous system.[14]

The cellular components of the terminal and respiratory bronchiolar epithelium are remarkably different from those of larger airways. Ciliated cells are still present, although they are less numerous. Nonciliated *Clara cells* (Figure 2–7) are conspicuous and numerous. Some can be readily recognized by their plump protoplasmic extensions that protrude into the lumen of the air passage; the remainder do not project beyond the luminal surface. In respiratory bronchioles, the epithelium between the interstices of the outpouching alveoli consists of low cuboidal cells with diminutive cilia and nonciliated Clara cells.

It is generally believed that Clara cells have a secretory function, and they are furnished with strong-reacting oxidative enzymes.[15] Moreover, Clara cells rather than type II alveolar cells have been proposed as the chief source of surfactant[16]; although this controversy has not been completely resolved, the evidence heavily favors the type II cell as the site of production of alveolar surface-active material (see

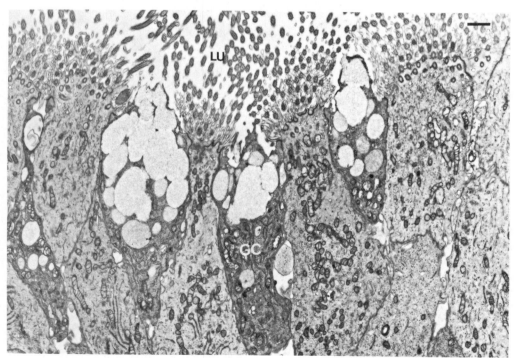

Figure 2–5 Electron photomicrograph of normal bronchial epithelium showing ciliated cells with numerous cilia projecting into the lumen (LU) of the airway and goblet cells (GC) containing mucous droplets. Horizontal bar = 1 μm. (× 6000. Courtesy of Dr. Donald McKay.)

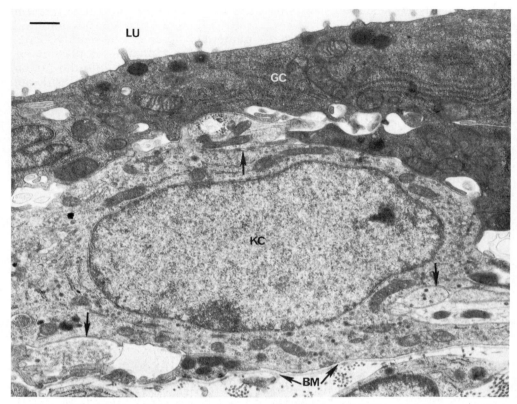

Figure 2–6   Electron photomicrograph showing a Kulchitsky cell (KC) in the tracheal epithelium of the rat. Intraepithelial nerves make contact with the cell at arrows. Horizontal bar = 1 μm; LU = tracheal lumen; GC = goblet cell; BM = epithelial basement membrane. (× 8000. From Jeffery and Reid.[11] Reprinted by permission of the authors and publishers.)

Chapter 1). Accepting this as true does not eliminate the possibility that Clara cells also have a secretory function and that they may be one of the sources of the extracellular lining of distal airways that is believed to exist in man and has been observed by electron microscopy in the terminal bronchioles of the rat.[17]

BRONCHIAL GLANDS

The bronchial glands (Figure 2–8) are one of the characteristic features of the submucosal layer beneath the lamina propria. They are simple tubuloal-veolar structures that contain many cell types: serous cells, mucous cells, collecting duct cells, clear cells (probably lymphocytes), and myoepithelial cells can be identified regularly and mast cells and Kulchitsky cells occasionally.[18] The glands are innervated by nerve fibers, which, on the basis of their ultrastructural characteristics, are believed to be efferent (cholinergic) nerves.[19] Bronchial glands are especially numerous in medium-sized bronchi, less prevalent in smaller bronchi, and absent in bronchioles.

It can be inferred from morphologic studies that mucous cells produce secretory granules continuously but release them into the glandular lumen intermittently; serous cells probably follow the same sequence but the evidence is less convincing. There are both morphologic and histochemical differences between mucous and serous cells, but the chemical composition of their respective secretions is unknown. The material that reaches the airway lumen, therefore, represents a mixture of the products of both cell types and any chemical reactions that result from the combination. (There is a possibility that secretions from serous cells may be enzymatic and alter the physical properties of secretions from mucous cells.) The factors that control the basal rate of secretion are not well understood, but studies of submucosal glands in organ culture support the clinical observations that secretory activity may be stimulated by parasympathomimetic drugs and depressed by parasympatholytic drugs.[20]

Irritants, upon reaching the mucosa, initiate a reflex via the parasympathetic nervous system that causes the submucosal glands to evacuate their contents rapidly; the discharged mucus isolates, dilutes, and may chemically alter the noxious substance. In chronic bronchitis, which may occur in response to chronic irritation of the airways from cigarette smoking or inhalation of chemicals, the submucosal glands increase markedly in their structural complexity and number of cells and constitute one of the histologic hallmarks of the disease.[21]

Mast cells closely resemble circulating basophilic leukocytes and are found in many tissues including the submucosa and connective tissues of the lung. The characteristic ultra-

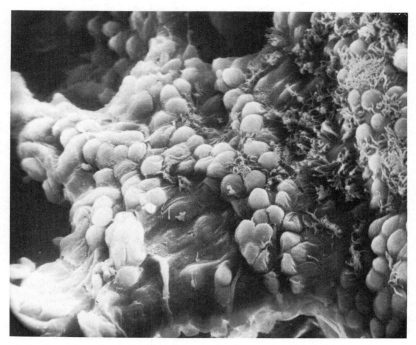

Figure 2-7 Scanning electron photomicrograph of a terminal bronchiole opening into several respiratory bronchioles. Epithelial surface is composed chiefly of Clara cells and ciliated cells. (× 900. Courtesy of Dr. Richard V. Ebert.)

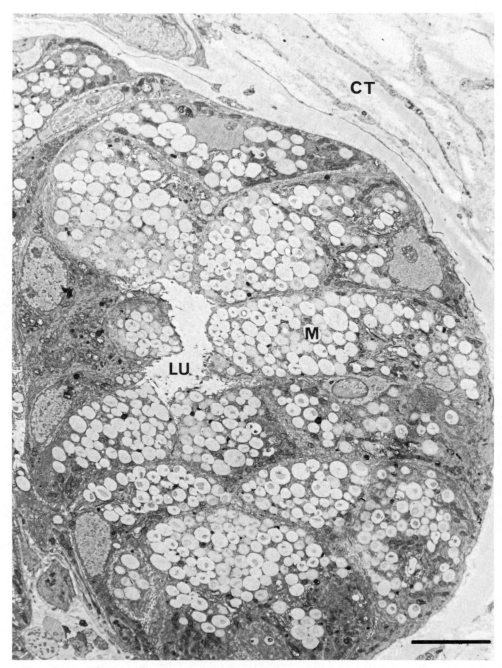

Figure 2–8 Electron photomicrograph of a transverse section through a normal bronchial gland surrounded by connective tissue (CT). Mucous droplets within mucous cells (M) are concentrated toward the lumen (LU) of the gland. Horizontal bar = 10 μm. ($\times$ 2100. Courtesy of Dr. Donald McKay.)

structural feature of mast cells is their cytoplasmic granules (Figure 2–9); however, mast cells that have degranulated are difficult to recognize in tissue preparations, a fact that complicates the use of histologic techniques to assess mast cell function. Mast cells in various mammalian species have been found to contain heparin, histamine, slow-reacting substances, eosinophil chemotactic substance, proteolytic enzymes, dopamine, and serotonin. The chemical content of human mast cells is not known, but the variety of pharmacologically active substances that have been identified in other animals has conferred upon mast cells the role of mediator of important physiologic and pathologic events. On the basis of their *in-vitro* and *in-vivo* activity, circulating basophils and mast cells have been implicated in the pathogenesis of bronchial asthma and other immediate (type I) hypersensitivity responses.[22]

SMOOTH MUSCLE

The location of smooth muscle in the walls of the tracheobronchial tree varies with the size of the airway. In the trachea and large bronchi (main and lower lobe bronchi), a band of muscle bridges the posterior opening of the U-shaped cartilages. In the next largest airways the muscle bundle connects the tips of the cartilages, but as the airway size decreases (i.e., moving peripherally in the tracheobronchial tree), the muscle attachments shift progressively along the inner surface of the cartilage until finally they are detached completely and form a separate layer between the partial rings or plates of cartilage and the epithelium.

In the trachea and mainstem bronchi, the only muscle fibers are located in the posterior muscle bundle. Medium and small bronchi have a proper muscle layer, but it does not circumscribe the airway with a band of uniform thickness. Rather, the muscles have a helical orientation with fibers spiraling in both directions and criss-crossing in the walls.[23] Thus, the effect of muscle contraction depends upon the location and density of fibers. In the large airways, muscle contraction serves to oppose or even overlap the tips of the U-shaped cartilages. In medium and small bronchi, owing to the geodesic distribution of muscle elements, contraction reduces both the caliber and length of the bronchus. Muscle contraction, therefore, leads to greater rigidity in all airways.

Smooth muscle does not end in the terminal bronchioles, but spirals of muscle form part of the walls of respiratory bronchioles, and muscle fibers have been identified in the openings of alveolar ducts[24]; contraction of these elements will affect significantly the mechanical properties of the gas exchange units. The important role of changes in airways resistance and the distensibility of terminal respiratory units in governing the partition of inspired air within the lung is discussed in Chapter 4.

CONNECTIVE TISSUE

During embryogenesis, as the developing bronchial buds penetrate the neighboring mass of undifferentiated mesenchyme, they carry with them an investment of connective tissue. By the sixteenth week of fetal life and thereafter, cartilaginous airways and large pulmonary arteries, which travel in close partnership through the substance of the lung, are surrounded by a sleeve of loose connective tissue that contains lymphatic vessels and a potential space. In contrast to bronchi, bronchioles are firmly attached to the adjacent lung parenchyma composed of the walls of the terminal respiratory units. This structural arrangement means that airways and blood vessels in central and peripheral locations within the lung are exposed to different transmural distending pressures and thus may behave differently (see Chap-

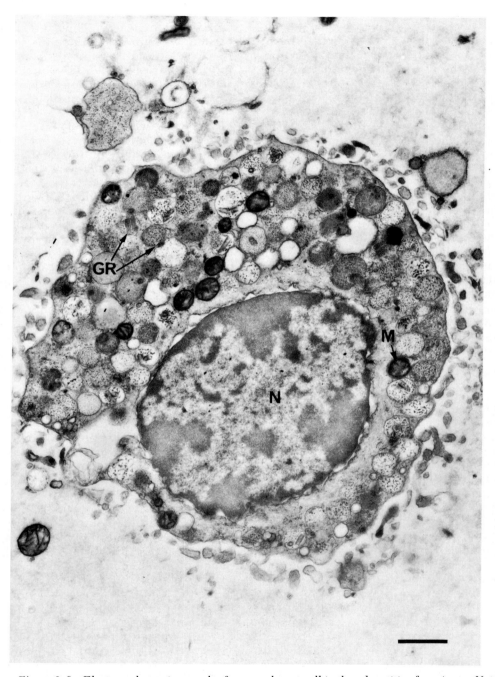

Figure 2–9   Electron photomicrograph of a normal mast cell in the adventitia of an airway. Note the numerous granules (GR) with variable staining characteristics and mitochondria (M) in the cytoplasm surrounding the nucleus (N). Horizontal bar = 1 μm. (× 12,750. Courtesy of Dr. Donald McKay.)

ters 4 and 5 for details); the connective tissue sheath around larger airways and blood vessels provides a space in which liquid and solute localize in the early stages of pulmonary edema accumulation (see Chapter 5 for details).

BLOOD VESSELS

PULMONARY ARTERIES

Generation counts have established that the number of arteries leading *to* the terminal respiratory units, both conventional and supernumerary branches, is completely formed at birth.[25] However, even at birth there are very few arteries *within* the incompletely developed gas exchange units; these arteries increase enormously in number during the first dec-

ade of life, and their development accompanies the formation of new respiratory bronchioles, alveolar ducts, and alveoli.

During gestation, all branches of the arterial system are relatively thick-walled owing to their medial layer of smooth muscle. However, after birth the vessels rapidly become thinner, so that by four months of age, as demonstrated in Figure 2–10, they show nearly the same relationship between wall thickness and external diameter that is observed in adult lungs.[26] While this change is occurring, the smooth muscle content appears to diminish in small vessels, a process that continues for several years because many new arteries without muscle are formed during the phase of rapid multiplication of alveoli. After five years of age, the multiplication of both alveoli and arteries has slowed, but new arteries

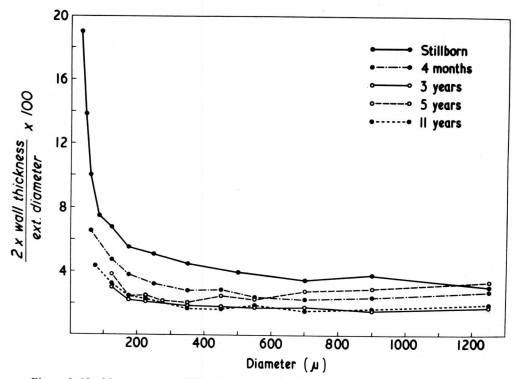

Figure 2–10 Measurements of the thickness of the pulmonary artery medial layer at birth and throughout childhood. Adult values are reached at four months of age. (From Davies and Reid.[26] Reprinted by permission from the authors and publisher.)

continue to be formed and old ones continue to grow without muscle appearing in their walls. Smooth muscle begins to extend peripherally in the medial layer of small arteries after they are formed.[26] At birth, about half the arteries accompanying terminal bronchioles are muscular, and the rest are partially muscular; by the age of five years, all have reached the adult form of completely muscular development. In contrast, less than one quarter of the arteries accompanying respiratory bronchioles are muscular at birth; furthermore, the process of muscularization is slower than with proximal larger arteries and is not complete until about the age of 19 years.[26]

It is of interest that elastic arteries extend from the hilum to nearly halfway in the bronchial tree of newborns and that this is the same level as in the adults. Moreover, the pattern of development of elastic arteries, like that of the bronchi that accompany them, is complete by the sixteenth week of gestation and is another example of adult morphology being formed in miniature well in advance of maturity.[25]

The postnatal evolution of both the abundant elastic elements in elastic arteries and the thick layer of smooth muscle in muscular arteries, from their appearance during fetal life to their final adult structure, can proceed only if pulmonary arterial pressure falls to the normal low values found in infants living near sea level. If pulmonary hypertension is maintained after birth, for example, either because of hypoxia induced by residence at high altitude or because of congenital cardiac anomalies such as a large ventricular septal defect or truncus arteriosus, then thinning and/or atrophy of the muscular and elastic elements fails to occur.

Three types of pulmonary arteries (Figure 2–11) can be identified in the normal adult human lung.[27] However, it must be recognized that this is an arbitrary classification, and because

the pulmonary arterial system is a continuous one, transitional forms must occur in regions where one type of artery gradually merges into another type. (1) The *elastic pulmonary arteries* (> 1000 μm external diameter) contain distinctive layers of elastic fibers embedded in a coat of muscle cells. The pulmonary artery trunk, its main branches, and all extralobular pulmonary arteries are of the elastic type. (2) The *muscular pulmonary arteries* (100 to 1000 μm external diameter) have a thin medial layer of muscle sandwiched between well-delimited internal and external elastic laminae. Muscular pulmonary arteries lie within lung lobules and, hence, accompany bronchioles. Although these vessels are designated by their muscular elements, the thickness of the muscle layer does not exceed about five per cent of the external diameter of the vessel; any increase above this value connotes a pathologic state and is found in well-defined conditions usually associated with pulmonary arterial hypertension. (3) The *pulmonary arterioles* (<100 μm external diameter) are the terminal branches of the pulmonary arterial system; at their origin from muscular arteries they contain a partial layer of muscle that gradually disappears (Figure 2–12) until the vessel wall consists only of endothelium and an elastic lamina. Pulmonary arterioles supply alveolar ducts and alveoli.

Functional Considerations. The different locations of pulmonary arteries mean that they, like the airways, will be exposed to different distending forces: the large arteries that travel in connective tissue spaces will be exposed to transpulmonary pressure and the small arteries and arterioles to radial traction of adjacent lung tissue. Both of these influences cause distension of the vessels during lung inflation, which increases the volume of blood that they can accommodate and lowers their resistance to blood

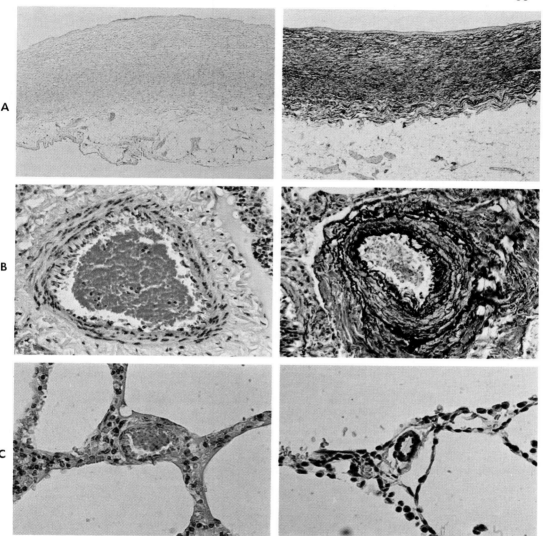

Figure 2-11 Photomicrographs of *A*, elastic (main) pulmonary artery (× 15); *B*, muscular pulmonary artery (× 60); and *C*, pulmonary arteriole (× 150). Left panels, hematoxylin and eosin stain; right panels, elastic stain. (Courtesy of Dr. Robert Wright.)

flow. However, because inflation "squeezes" pulmonary capillaries located in the alveolar septa between contiguous alveoli, resistance to blood flow through capillaries tends to increase. Thus, the effect of lung inflation on pulmonary vascular resistance is not simple, owing to the changing contributions afforded by various blood vessels to the *total* resistance. The distribution of pulmonary vascular resistance throughout the pulmonary vascular system and the effects of lung inflation, postural changes, and other influences are examined further in Chapter 5.

The partnership between branches of the bronchial and arterial systems as they course through both connective tissue boundaries and the lung paren-

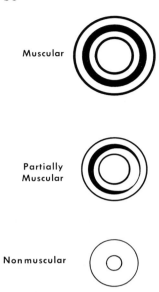

Muscular

Partially
Muscular

Nonmuscular

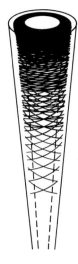

Figure 2–12 Schematic representation of the changes in the amount and thickness of the smooth muscle layer in muscular, partially muscular, and nonmuscular pulmonary arteries.

chyma, in contrast to pulmonary veins which are as far removed from the bronchoarterial pair as possible, indicates that factors that affect the regional distribution of ventilation will also affect the distribution of blood flow to the same region, and vice versa. When both ventilation and blood flow are impaired similarly, compared with disproportionate involvement of one or the other, optimum conditions for gas exchange are maintained. It is easy to appreciate how this might occur in gross pathologic conditions, such as atelectasis and tumors, but the functional implications of the anatomic arrangement can be extended to include a much more delicate control mechanism, one that confers a high degree of autonomous regulation of blood flow and ventilation to maintain optimum gas exchange. Experiments in which either blood flow or ventilation is impaired suggest that autoregulation exists, but the site of and mechanisms governing the response are unknown.[28]

The location of thin-walled mus-cular arteries and arterioles within lobules means that the vessels are exposed not only to the distending pressure in the adjacent alveolar spaces but also to the gas tensions in them as well. The intimate relationship between a pulmonary arteriole and its surrounding alveolar air spaces is evident from Figure 2–13.

Experiments have demonstrated that pulmonary arterial vasoconstriction occurs in a lung or lobe ventilated (not perfused) with low concentrations of O_2 and in addition, that the effect is mediated locally and does not require systemic neural or humoral responses.[29, 30] Anatomic studies under conditions of unilobar hypoxia in cats have shown vasoconstriction in small muscular arteries and arterioles.[31] We can surmise, therefore, that even though small pulmonary arteries contain relatively little muscle (compared with their systemic analogues), they are capable of constricting; moreover, there must be some sort of extraluminal (e.g., adventitial) receptor system that responds to alveolar hy-

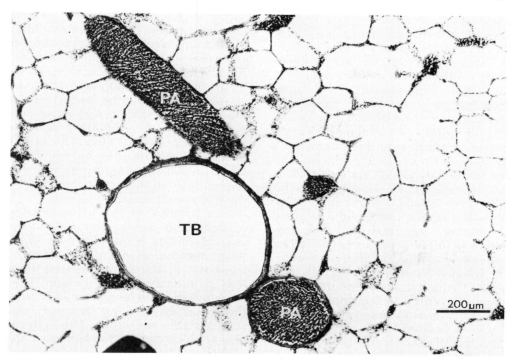

Figure 2–13 Fixed frozen section of cat lung showing terminal bronchiole (TB) and its associated pulmonary artery (PA) in a thin section. Note that the vessels and airway are completely surrounded by alveolar spaces that are usually part of the same terminal respiratory unit that the vessels and airway are supplying. Horizontal bar = 200 μm. ($\times$ 70. Courtesy of Dr. Norman Staub.)

poxia and not to pulmonary arterial hypoxemia. Obviously, it would be desirable for the lung to reduce blood flow to a gas exchange unit(s) within which the P_{O_2} is low or the P_{CO_2} is high. Because autonomous regulation has been shown to occur in whole lungs or lobes, we can infer that smaller regions are probably also capable of demonstrating similar responses. Whether or not this protective mechanism is able to modify blood flow from a slight insult, such as a collection of secretions in a small airway, is unknown. But experimental evidence indicates that in some mammals at least (the *coatimundi*), blood flow to small regions (i.e., lobules) is adjusted when inspired gas composition is altered.[32]

SUPERNUMERARY ARTERIES

Discussion in the previous section has emphasized the paired relationship between the pattern of branching of the pulmonary arteries and that of the airways. However, additional pulmonary arterial branches are present that do not accompany airways. These "supernumerary" arteries appear at the hilum and emerge from the main arterial channels as far peripherally as the end of the respiratory bronchioles.[33] The extra branches outnumber the conventional ones and provide about 25 per cent of the total cross-sectional area of the pulmonary arterial bed near the hilum and about 40 per cent of the total toward the periphery. Supernumerary arteries are present at birth but mainly leading to the terminal respiratory unit[25]; there is extensive growth of new conventional and supernumerary branches, the latter outnumbering the former, accompanying the development of alveolar ducts and alveoli during the first 18 months of childhood.[34] Supernumerary arteries continue to increase in number up to about eight years of age while new alveoli are formed.

Supernumerary vessels undoubtedly serve as an auxiliary arterial supply to the capillary beds of the terminal respiratory units, and thus they constitute an important source of collateral blood flow to the sites of gas exchange. Of interest is the observation that neither supernumerary branches nor many conventional branches fill during routine angiography[33]; whether this is a technical artifact or of functional significance is unknown.

Functional Considerations. There is no known reason to believe that the lung was accidentally equipped with "extra" pulmonary arteries. Blood undoubtedly has access to the entire arterial circulation, even though local changes in vascular resistance probably determine which pathways are utilized at any given moment. Whether or not the network was designed for filtering the bloodstream is unknown, but the extensive arterial system is well suited to carry out this important nonrespiratory function of the lung.[35]

Pulmonary blood vessels trap particles, depending on their size and physical characteristics. Some intravascular coagulation probably goes on in normal persons at all times, and the lung serves as a sieve for the aggregates of red blood cells, platelets, and fibrin. The anatomic orientation of the arterial system means that several collateral channels are available to the terminal gas exchange units in case one or more vessels become temporarily obstructed.

Besides the normal physiologic functions of trapping and removing particles that circulate in the venous bloodstream, the lung serves as a filter of materials formed in the evolution of a variety of pathologic processes. Blood clots, fat particles, tissue fragments, tumor cells, and amniotic fluid all may enter into or be formed within the venous circulation and cause pulmonary arterial embolization; collateral pathways are obviously useful in these conditions, not only to maintain gas exchange but also to preserve the viability of the lung subserved by the obstructed vessel.

In addition to sieving aggregates of cells and debris, the pulmonary circulation has been shown to affect the concentration of circulating leukocytes and platelets by releasing them into pulmonary venous blood.[36] Presumably, this can take place only after the cells have been trapped and stored within the lungs. Although no one knows where these activities are carried out within the lung, they presumably are intravascular events. The extensive arterial, venous (see next section), and capillary networks are ideal sites for the sequestration of cells followed by either their destruction or later return to the circulating bloodstream.

PULMONARY VEINS

The pulmonary veins are usually considered to be simple tubes that conduct arterialized blood from the pulmonary capillaries to the left atrium. Drainage of blood is certainly the main function of veins and the design of the system is well suited for this purpose. However, other structure-function relationships can be inferred from considerations of the extent of the venous network and the morphology of veins themselves.

There are both similarities and differences between pulmonary veins on the one hand and pulmonary arteries on the other. The development of the adult pattern of venous drainage from the terminal respiratory units to the hilum is completed, like the corresponding arteries, by about midgestation. The venous system is also similar to the arterial system because both have conventional and supernumerary branches. Both arteries and veins increase in number as new alveoli are formed, and all vessels increase in size as the volume of lung increases with age.[37]

The important differences between veins and arteries, besides the anatomy of the extrapulmonary branches leading into and away from the heart, lie chiefly in the number of vessels and the structure of their walls, both of which have important functional implications.

Functional Considerations. First, there are more veins than arteries, and because the number of conventional branches of both systems is equal, the increased density of veins per unit area of lung is accounted for by a larger number of supernumerary veins than arteries. Second, veins have thinner walls than arteries, owing to a less developed muscular layer in veins at all ages.[37] During early fetal life, pulmonary arteries are considerably more muscular than pulmonary veins; however, this discrepancy becomes less marked late in gestation as the venous muscular layer thickens. During infancy, the attrition of arterial smooth muscle makes the thickness of the layers in arteries and veins of corresponding size even more uniform. These morphologic alterations appear to be related to the intravascular pressure changes that take place within the respective vessels. Moreover, in patients with congenital or acquired heart diseases the thickness of the smooth muscle layer of pulmonary arteries and veins has been observed to vary with corresponding changes in intravascular pressures, and medial hypertrophy in the walls of veins is believed to be pathognomonic of pulmonary venous hypertension.[38]

Although no information is available on the cross-sectional area of the pulmonary venous bed, the large number of thin-walled veins implies a low resistance to blood flow, which confers the ability to accommodate large increases in cardiac output with negligible changes in pressure (see Chapter 5). The pulmonary arterial system is also a low resistance vascular bed but *not as low as* the pulmonary venous system.

Pulmonary veins serve, with the left atrium, as a reservoir of blood for the left ventricle. As shown in Figure 2–14, if pulmonary arterial inflow is suddenly interrupted, the left ventricle will continue to fill with blood from pulmonary veins and to eject a substantial stroke volume for several beats.[39] Gross disturbances in right ventricular output are ultimately reflected in left ventricular output, but minor variations, such as might occur during respiration, are probably partially "absorbed" by the pulmonary venous reservoir.

BRONCHIAL CIRCULATION

The lung receives blood from two different vascular systems, the pulmonary circulation and the bronchial circulation. There are substantial differences between the amount of blood flow, the composition of the blood, and the functional importance of these two circulations. The pulmonary circulation consists of virtually the entire cardiac output; it contains venous blood, and the "arterialization" of this blood is essential for life. In contrast, the bronchial circulation consists of only a small proportion of the cardiac output; it contains systemic arterial blood, and the normal adult lung remains viable without it. However, this statement oversimplifies the role of the bronchial circulation because it does not recognize the probable value of bronchial blood flow to the fetus and its crucial contributions to gas exchange in many varieties of congenital cardiac anomalies. Furthermore, there

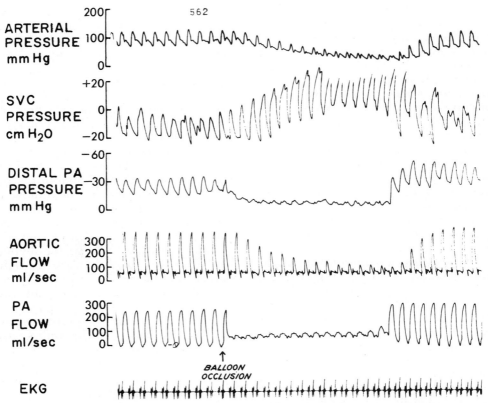

Figure 2–14 Tracing from an experiment in which sudden occlusion (arrow) of the main pulmonary artery (PA) of a dog by inflating a balloon caused an immediate cessation in pulmonary blood flow but a gradual decrease in aortic blood flow. SVC = superior vena cava. (From Hoffman, Guz, Charlier, and Wilken.[39] Reprinted by permission from the authors and publisher.)

is a striking increase in the size and number of bronchial arteries in certain kinds of lung diseases, especially chronic inflammation and neoplasms.

Morphologic studies have shown that the caliber of bronchial arteries of a human fetus is nearly the same as that of an adult.[40] This observation suggests that the lung might receive proportionately more blood flow, O_2, and nutrients from the bronchial circulation during fetal life than it does in adult life. However, studies in fetal lambs have revealed that the bronchial blood supply to the lungs is extremely low, 0.1 to 0.2 per cent of total cardiac output.[41] Moreover, low values for bronchial blood flow and its contribu-

tion to pulmonary O_2 consumption were demonstrated by other investigators who also studied fetal lambs.[42] It should be pointed out that the bronchial arteries of fetal lambs are not as large as they appear to be in human fetuses, so it is possible that there may be an important species difference in the contribution of the bronchial circulation to the metabolic needs of the developing lung.

The bronchial arteries in the human adult vary considerably in number and origin.[43] There is usually a single artery to the right lung that arises from an upper right intercostal artery or from the right subclavian or internal mammary arteries. The two arteries supplying the left lung arise as direct branches from the upper thoracic aorta. A variable number of smaller arterial branches emerge from vessels in and near the mediastinum and cross into the lung. As soon as the bronchial arteries enter the lung, they become invested in the layer of connective tissue surrounding the bronchi and begin branching. Ordinarily, two or three bronchial arterial branches, which anastomose with each other to form a peribronchial plexus with an elongated and irregular mesh, accompany each subdivision of the conducting airways.

The bronchial arteries are the principal source of nutrient blood to the bronchial tree from the mainstem bronchi to the terminal bronchioles, the pulmonary nerves and ganglia, the elastic and some muscular pulmonary arteries and veins, the lymph nodes and lymph tissue, the visceral pleura, and the connective tissue septa. Near the end of the terminal bronchioles, the bronchial arterioles terminate in a network of capillaries that anastomose extensively with the capillary plexus in the alveoli of the adjoining respiratory bronchioles. Because respiratory bronchioles are supplied by branches of the pulmonary artery, communication between the two blood supplies to the lung occurs at the junction of the conducting airways and the terminal respiratory units.

The amount of blood flow to the lung through the bronchial arterial circulation is low and, therefore, quite difficult to measure accurately in normal man. The best estimate, which is consistent with data obtained from animal studies, is that flow through the bronchial circulation in adults is less than 1 to 2 per cent of the total cardiac output.[44]

Effluent blood from capillaries supplied by bronchial arteries returns to the heart in two different venous pathways (Figure 2–15). True *bronchial veins* are found only at the hilum; they are formed from tributaries that originate around the lobar and segmental bronchi and from branches from the pleura in the neighborhood of the hilum. Bronchial venous blood empties into the azygos, hemiazygos, or intercostal veins and then flows into the right atrium. Veins that originate from bronchial capillaries within the lung unite to form venous tributaries that join the pulmonary vein; these communicating vessels are sometimes called *bronchopulmonary veins*. Blood leaving the capillary bed around terminal bronchioles flows through anastomoses with the alveolar capillaries, and the mixture of blood returns to the left atrium through pulmonary veins.

The distribution of bronchial arterial inflow between the two available venous outflow pathways has never been determined in man, and only tentative conclusions can be drawn from the technically difficult studies in experimental animals. These indicate that about 25 to 33 per cent of the bronchial arterial supply returns ultimately to the right atrium via bronchial veins, and 67 to 75 per cent flows into the left atrium via pulmonary veins.[46]

A controversy has raged for many years over the presence and significance of *bronchopulmonary arterial anastomoses*, direct vascular connections between pulmonary arteries and bronchial arteries. Dispassionate conclusions, based on the evidence available, are that bronchopulmonary arterial anastomoses do exist, that they occur sporadically and infrequently in normal lungs, that they are more easily demonstrable in the lungs of infants than of adults, and that they may increase considerably in number in certain pathologic disorders.

Although the magnitude of the bronchial arterial inflow, the partition of its venous outflow, and the identity of bronchopulmonary arterial anastomoses all are uncertain, reliable experimental data are available concerning the physiology of the bronchial circu-

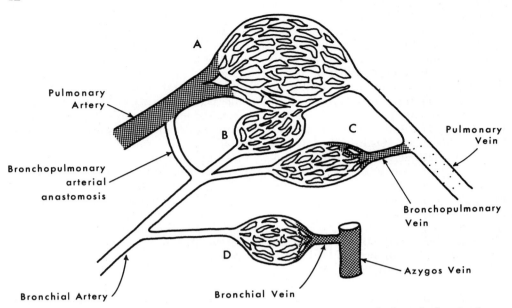

Figure 2-15 Schematic representation of the relationships between the bronchial and pulmonary circulations. The pulmonary artery supplies the pulmonary capillary network A. The bronchial artery supplies capillary networks B, C, and D. Network B represents the bronchial capillary supply to bronchioles that anastomoses with pulmonary capillaries and drains through pulmonary veins. Network C represents the bronchial capillary supply to most bronchi; these vessels form bronchopulmonary veins that empty into pulmonary veins. Network D represents the bronchial capillary supply to lobar and segmental bronchi; these vessels form true bronchial veins that drain into the azygos, hemiazygos, or intercostal veins. Shaded areas represent blood of low O_2 content.

lation, especially the functional interrelationships between the bronchial and the pulmonary circulations. Blood flow to the lung through its two circulations, even though the amount supplied by each differs markedly, is balanced so that if the perfusing pressure in one system increases or decreases, there is a change in the opposite direction in the amount of blood supplied by the other system.[47] This means that if pressure falls in part of the pulmonary arterial circulation (e.g., distal to the site of a pulmonary embolus), blood flow to that part of the lung through the bronchial circulation will increase. And conversely, if pressure in the bronchial system falls (e.g., in autotransplantation, which deprives the lung of all its bronchial blood flow), blood flow in the pulmonary circulation will increase and supply those tissues that formerly received blood through the bronchial circulation.

This reciprocal relationship is obviously of great benefit in preserving viability of pulmonary structures when one or the other circulation is impaired. The adequacy of the mechanism depends on the presence of functioning anastomoses between the two circulations that are capable of accommodating an increase in blood flow. When circumstances prevent the increase in collateral flow from occurring, lung damage develops: pulmonary infarction will follow pulmonary embolism when the bronchial circulation is compromised, or necrosis of the airways will follow lung transplantation when the pulmonary circulation is affected.[48]

TERMINAL RESPIRATORY UNIT

DEFINITION

A terminal respiratory unit consists of the structures distal to the end of a terminal bronchiole. A typical unit, shown schematically in Figure 2–16, contains a characteristically variable branching pattern. There are usually two to five orders of respiratory bronchioles (indicated by Roman numerals in Figure 2–16), the last of which leads into the first of two to five orders of alveolar ducts (indicated by Arabic numerals). Alveolar ducts are relatively short (with lengths only one to one and one-half times the diameter) and they branch in rapid

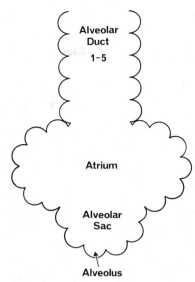

Figure 2–17 Schematic representation of the last alveolar duct (order 1–5) terminating in an atrium that communicates directly with three alveolar sacs from which alveoli project.

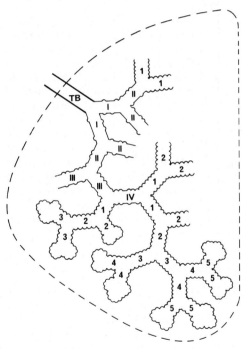

Figure 2–16 Schematic representation of the anatomic subdivisions in a single plane through a terminal respiratory unit (i.e., those structures distal to a terminal bronchiole, TB). Roman numerals indicate respiratory bronchioles, arabic numerals indicate alveolar ducts. The entire unit can be visualized by rotating the structures within the hatched boundary through 360 degrees.

sequence; each duct has openings for 10 to 16 alveoli.[49] The last in the series of alveolar ducts empties through the atrium (practically an obsolete term) into one to three dome-shaped alveolar sacs from which the terminal alveoli project (Figure 2–17).

As indicated in Figure 2–16, the extent of alveolarization of respiratory bronchioles increases, proceeding from the terminal bronchiole toward the periphery. The chief difference between alveolar ducts and respiratory bronchioles is that the ducts are completely alveolarized and ciliated respiratory epithelium is absent. Alveolar ducts can be viewed mainly as a supporting framework of delicate connective tissue fibers and slender smooth muscle cells interspersed between a continuous succession of alveoli. The three-dimensional lacework of connective tissue fibers that support alveoli is continuous throughout the lung parenchyma and is anchored peripherally and centrally, the former through a system of fibers connected to the visceral pleura and the latter through an axial fiber system that is a continuation of the fibrous sheath of conducting airways.[49]

The terminal respiratory unit shown in Figure 2–16 is displayed in only one plane; a "complete" unit can be visualized by rotating the structures within the hatched line through 360 degrees. Furthermore, it should be emphasized that adjacent terminal respiratory units are not separated by spaces or by well-defined anatomic boundaries and that they interdigitate with each other like a three-dimensional jigsaw puzzle.

A cluster of three to five terminal bronchioles, each with its appended terminal respiratory unit, is usually referred to as a *lobule*; a typical lobule is shown schematically in Figure 2–18. Contiguous lobules in human lungs are partly but incompletely delimited by connective tissue septa; in other mammals, such as the cow, the septal barriers between adjacent lobules are structurally complete. The lobular architecture of the lung is important in determining whether or not collateral

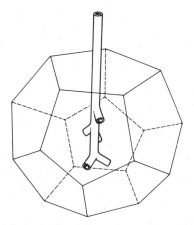

Figure 2–18 Schematic representation of a pulmonary lobule, in this instance composed of five terminal bronchioles. The five terminal respiratory units (not shown) occupy the space within the boundaries of the lobule.

ventilation occurs (see next section) and also serves as the anatomic basis for differentiating emphysema into either "centrilobular" or "panlobular" varieties.

The blood supply of several adjacent lobules is shown in Figure 2–19. The upper panel demonstrates the lobular architecture in a lung specimen of a dog in which the pulmonary artery was injected with opaque material; branches of both pulmonary arterial and bronchial systems travel together and supply the terminal respiratory units within a *single* lobule. In contrast, as shown in the lower panel (Figure 2–19), a pulmonary vein drains blood from *many* lobules that can be identified by their parent bronchioles.

The modern terminology used by various authors to describe the gas exchange regions of the lung differs from that advocated by the great lung anatomist Miller[23] and needs to be standardized. Equivalent terms are listed in Table 2–1. The terminal unit as just defined is equivalent to the *acinus* used by many authors; the term acinus literally means grape and is preferred by morphologists in view of its obvious descriptive connotation. As shown in Table 2–1, the term "terminal respiratory unit" will be used throughout this text in recognition of its role as the anatomic site of gas exchange.

ALVEOLI

Alveoli in newborns are fewer in number and less complex in anatomic detail than their counterparts in adults; this dissimilarity has led some morphologists to call them "saccules" rather than alveoli.[51] However, neonatal alveoli, even though primitive, correspond to Macklin's definition of alveoli as "the ultimate respiratory chamber."[52] They contain numerous capillaries in their walls and thus serve as the site of gas exchange.

Evidence from several sources

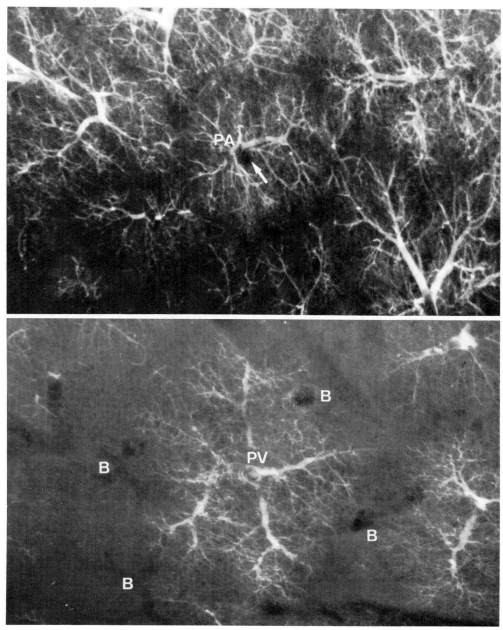

Figure 2–19 *Upper panel*, section of a dog lung showing pulmonary arteries injected with a barium sulfate suspension. A branch of the pulmonary artery (PA) lies next to a radiolucent bronchiole (arrow). The architecture of several adjacent lobules is distinctly outlined. *Lower panel*, injected specimen of dog lung showing how pulmonary veins (PV) receive blood from several lobules that can be identified by the location of their parent bronchioles (B). (× 7.0 upper, × 6.3 lower. From Lauweryns.[50] Reprinted by permission from the author and Sommers. Pathology Annual, 1971. Courtesy of Appleton-Century-Crofts, Publishing Division of Prentice-Hall, Inc.)

Table 2–1 Partial List of Common Synonyms and Their Definitions Used To Describe the Gas Exchange Regions of the Lung*

SYNONYMS	DEFINITION
Terminal respiratory unit Acinus[50] Primary lobule[23]	Those structures distal to the end of a terminal bronchiole
Lobule Secondary lobule[23]	A cluster of a variable number of terminal respiratory units that are separated from adjacent clusters by connective tissue septa

*The terms employed in this text are *italicized.*

has established that alveoli increase in number from about 25 million at birth to several hundred million when the lung is fully grown.[26, 51, 53] New alveoli are formed by multiplication of old ones and by alveolarization of (originally) nonrespiratory bronchioles; the latter process is complete by three years of age, but the former process continues much longer.[3] Alveoli multiply during the first three to four years of life more rapidly than afterward. Precisely when multiplication ceases is unknown and is probably variable, but it is clear that the process stops before somatic growth is complete. Thereafter, while growth of the thorax continues, alveoli must increase in size. Alveoli of a human adult are about 250 μm in diameter and relatively uniform in size ($\pm$10 per cent of the mean).[49] The number of alveoli is not as constant among persons as customarily taught (300,000,000 is the conventional figure), but varies with body length.[53] Because the number of terminal bronchioles does not differ among individuals and the number of alveoli does,[54] it follows that a tall person must have more alveoli in a terminal gas exchange unit than a short person. The implications of this variable architecture—for example, the consequences of small airways involvement, tendency to emphysema, and effects on gas exchange (the dis-

tance for gas-phase diffusion would be lengthened)—need to be examined.

Not only do alveoli increase in number by multiplication and alveolarization of bronchioles, but also alveolar surface area increases more rapidly than can be accounted for by the addition of new alveoli *per se.* This suggests that alveoli become more complex in shape as they grow, and thus present more alveolar surface area for a given proportion of lung volume. Enlargement of alveolar surface area during growth from infancy to adulthood is closely related to increasing O_2 requirements.

The lessons from studies of comparative morphology are clear concerning lung volume on the one hand and alveolar surface area on the other. Lung volume correlates with body weight, but alveolar surface area correlates with metabolic activity, regardless of body size.[55] This is illustrated by comparing two animals who are similar in size but have different metabolic rates; the lungs of both will be equal in volume, but the alveolar surface area of the one with the higher metabolism will be greater than that of the other. The difference in area can only be attained by increased compartmentalization, which is evidenced by a change in size and number of alveoli. These features are another example of the interdependence of structure and function based upon an optimum design for functional requirements. Although the basic structure of the lung is undoubtedly fixed genetically, evidence is accumulating that morphologic adaptations may in fact take place in response to changing physiologic conditions (see section on Adaptation).

The total alveolar surface area of a normal human adult is about 80 m², of which nearly 85 to 95 per cent is covered with pulmonary capillaries[7, 49]; thus, the alveolar capillary interface has a surface area of approximately 70 m² and provides an area of contact between the body and its external en-

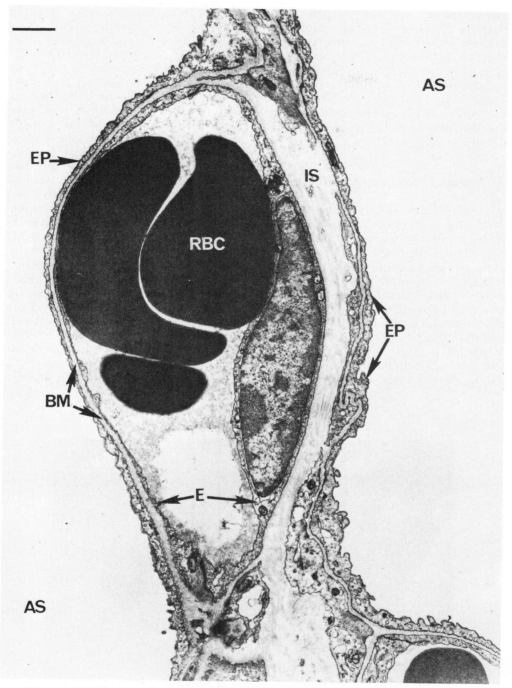

Figure 2–20   Electron photomicrograph of a transverse section through capillaries in the inter-alveolar septum. The surface of the septum facing the alveolar spaces (AS) is lined by continuous epithelium (EP). The capillary containing red blood cells (RBC) is lined by endothelium (E). Both layers rest on basement membranes (BM) that appear fused over the "thin" portion of the membrane and that are separated by an interstitial space (IS) over the "thick" portion of the membrane. Horizontal bar = 1 μm. ($\times$ 11,500. Courtesy of Dr. Ewald R. Weibel.)

vironment that is 40 times greater than that via the skin. To protect itself and the rest of the body from the numerous potentially noxious substances and infectious agents that are inhaled and may be deposited within the lung, the airways and alveolar surfaces are equipped with elaborate defense mechanisms that are considered in detail in Chapter 11.

ALVEOLAR-CAPILLARY MEMBRANE

The old controversy regarding how many tissue layers compose the interalveolar septum was indubitably settled shortly after the introduction of electron microscopic techniques for histologic examination in the 1950s. It is now agreed that the alveolar-capillary membrane (Figure 2–20) consists of (1) alveolar epithelium, (2) capillary endothelium, (3) contiguous tissue elements in the intercalated interstitial space, and (4) surfactant lining.

1. The alveolar epithelium consists of a continuous layer of tissue made up of two principal cell types: type I cells, or *squamous pneumocytes*, have broad, thin extensions, 0.1 to 0.3 μm thick, which contain mainly cytoplasmic ground substance and cover 95 per cent of the alveolar surface. Cytoplasmic organelles, such as mitochondria, are rare and are usually located in the cytoplasm surrounding the nucleus. Type II cells, or *granular pneumocytes*, are more numerous than type I cells, but owing to their cuboidal shape they occupy less than five per cent of the alveolar surface. The electron microscopic hallmarks of type II cells are their microvilli (Figure 2–21) and their osmiophilic lamellated inclusion bodies (Figure 1–6); the convincing data linking the osmiophilic bodies of type II cells with surfactant are reviewed in Chapter 1. Type II cells have also been shown to be the chief cell type involved in the repair of the alveolar epithelium following experimentally induced pulmonary O_2 toxicity in monkeys. The similarity of this process

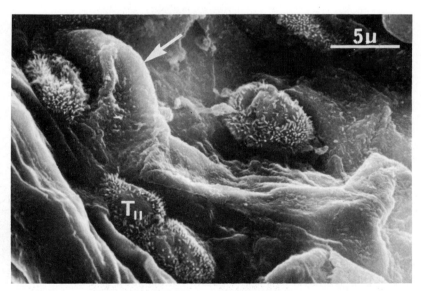

Figure 2–21 Scanning electron photomicrograph of the surface of a human alveolus showing several type II cells with characteristic microvilli; the rest of the surface is covered by the cytoplasmic extensions of type I cells. A red blood cell can be seen bulging in a pulmonary capillary (arrow). (× 3500. Courtesy of Dr. N. S. Wang.)

to that seen in man and in other mammals suggests that type II cell hyperplasia may be a basic mechanism of repair after destruction of type I cells in numerous other conditions.[56] Furthermore, evidence is accumulating that regenerated type II cells may differentiate into type I cells. Type III cells, *alveolar brush cells*, were originally discovered in rat lung,[57] but they also occur, though very rarely, in the human lung.[49] Alveolar brush cells bear a striking resemblance to brush cells found in the epithelium of large airways.

2. The capillary endothelium is composed chiefly of the cytoplasmic extension of the endothelial cells, which by their contiguous arrangement form a thin capillary tube. These extensions, like those of the squamous epithelial cells lining alveoli, rarely contain organelles. Besides its important but passive role in gas and liquid exchange, the capillary endothelium is now known to be the site of active biochemical events, such as the conversion and inactivation of polypeptides, prostaglandins, nucleotides, and amines, that have important physiologic functions.[58] The endothelium of other pulmonary blood vessels may also perform similar biochemical transformations, but the large surface area of the capillary bed makes it the predominant locus of these activities, which are discussed in Chapter 5.

3. The alveolar epithelium and the capillary endothelium both rest on separate basement membranes, but owing to the presence of structural differences that have important functional implications, the alveolar-capillary membrane has been subdivided into two separate regions: (1) The "thin portion" of the septum, or *air-blood barrier*, occurs over the convex half of the capillary surface that bulges into the alveolus (Figure 2–20) and over which the two basement membranes appear to be fused. (2) The "thick portion" is found where the basement membranes are separated by an interstitial space containing fine elastic fibers, small bundles of collagen fibrils, and a few fibroblasts. Pulmonary capillaries weave their way back and forth through the interstitial space of the interalveolar septum, first bulging into one alveolus and then the other. Thus, the interstitial space is perforated by capillaries and should be viewed as a communicating meshwork, not as a continuous sheet. The interstitial space of the interalveolar septum extends directly into the connective tissue sheath and the interstitial space surrounding airways and blood vessels.[49] Diffusion of gases (Chapter 6) takes place mainly across the thin portion, and liquid and solute exchange (Chapter 5), mainly across the thick portion.

4. Surfactant can be recovered easily in lung extracts and washes, but definition of its anatomic location has proved to be more elusive. Originally, surfactant was believed to be situated at the air-liquid interface of alveoli in order to explain the mechanical behavior of the lung. Recently, an extraepithelial lining layer has been demonstrated in experimental animals through the use of special techniques of fixation and preparation.[59] This layer is continuous over the alveolar surface, but irregular in its thickness (Figure 2–22). The extraepithelial layer is thickest where there are clefts or pits between adjacent cells, giving an appearance that it is smoothing out irregularities in the surface extension of alveolar cells. At the top of this layer is a very thin, osmiophilic surface film. The location and some of the staining characteristics of this material suggest strongly that it is surfactant, and although the temptation to link the electron microscopic evidence with what is known about surfactant is nearly irresistible, further chemical analysis of the film must be performed before its identity can be established.

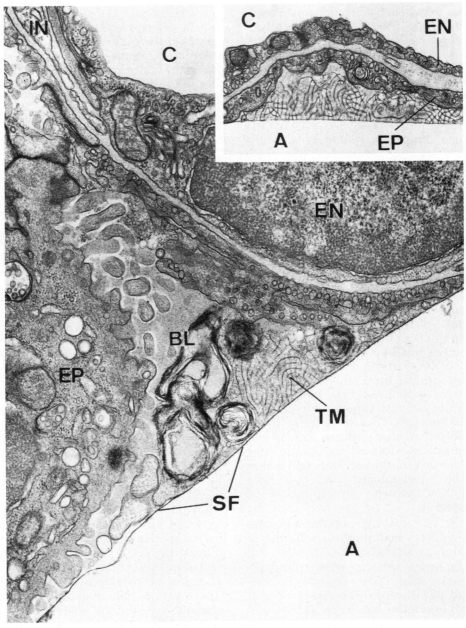

Figure 2-22 Electron photomicrograph of a thin section of rat lung fixed by vascular perfusion. The depression in the surface of the alveolar epithelium (EP) is smoothed out with extracellular material. Its base layer (BL) contains globular and tubular myelin figures (TM) with some of the osmiophilic lamellae reaching and connecting with the surface film (SF). ($\times$ 26,400). The inset shows similar structures in a region where the alveolar-capillary tissue barrier is thin ($\times$ 23,010). A = alveolar space; C = capillary; EN = endothelium; IN = interstitial space. (From Untersee, Gil, and Weibel.[59] Reprinted by permission from the authors and publisher.)

OTHER CELLS

Alveolar macrophages are phagocytic cells that are found in varying numbers lying submerged in the extracellular lining of the alveolar surface. There is general agreement that alveolar macrophages originate from stem cell precursors in the bone marrow and reach the lung through the bloodstream, presumably as circulating monocytes. However, since the enzyme profile of alveolar macrophages differs considerably from that of monocytes, direct transcapillary migration from blood to alveolus is untenable. Transformation of blood monocytes to alveolar macrophages is believed to occur within a population of proliferating interstitial cells.[60] Additional experimental evidence suggests that alveolar macrophages may also reproduce themselves by division within the lung.[61] Alveolar macrophages are of considerable interest because they constitute the chief mechanism of clearance of bacteria and other particles that are deposited in the terminal respiratory units, and deficiencies in their function undoubtedly contribute to the pathogenesis of pulmonary infections (Chapter 11). Furthermore, they can be obtained from man in relatively large numbers by lung lavage, separated from other cells, and grown in tissue culture so that their metabolic and functional characteristics can be studied.[62]

INTERCOMMUNICATING CHANNELS

One of the important developments in pulmonary physiology during the last few years is the resurgence of experimental activity concerning the structural basis and functional consequences of collateral ventilation. The increased interest is related to observations that the physiologic effects of airways obstruction, both in patients with various forms of obstructive lung disease and in laboratory animals, are critically dependent upon the magnitude of collateral ventilation.[63] Despite the compelling physiologic evidence that has underscored the importance of intercommunicating channels to normal respiratory function and to the pathogenesis of common lung diseases, only limited descriptive anatomic information is available about the possible pathways involved, and detailed morphometric data are needed before a complete understanding of the subject is possible.

ALVEOLAR PORES OF KOHN

Originally, considerable doubt existed whether the alveolar pores of Kohn were normal structures or fixation artifacts. Now, however, there is general agreement that pores are anatomic entities and that they occur in the interalveolar septa of nearly all mammalian species, including man. Alveolar pores (Figure 2–23) are openings in alveolar walls that provide channels for gas movement between contiguous alveoli. The pores are located in intercapillary spaces and are often bordered by a capillary loop. They are lined with alveolar epithelial cells that usually abut adjacent cells in the alveolar wall on each side of the opening.[63]

Alveolar pores can be viewed as short cylinders whose dimensions, although they have not been measured directly, probably vary with lung volume. This conclusion is based on the response to lung inflation of microholes that were punctured in the alveolar walls of experimental animals.[64] The diameter of alveolar pores varies from 3 to 13 μm, and their width, which is the thickness of the alveolar septum (between capillaries), is about 2 μm. During inflation of the lung, the diameter presumably increases and the width decreases as the alveolar wall stretches.

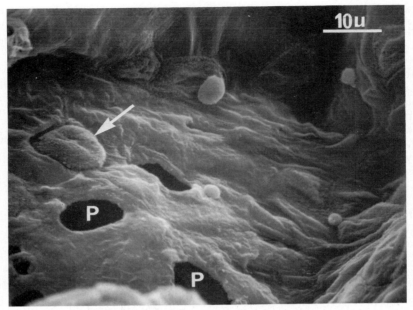

Figure 2-23 Scanning electron photomicrograph of the surface of a human alveolus showing pores of Kohn (P) and a macrophage (arrow). (× 1500. Courtesy of Dr. N. S. Wang.)

Although quantitative estimates are lacking, alveolar pores are absent during prenatal development and in the newborn period; thereafter and throughout life, both the number and size of pores appear to increase gradually. The mechanism of formation of pores is completely unknown. Theories about their development consider that they might be related to one or more of the following: a pathologic process causing desquamation of epithelial cells, the "normal" degeneration of tissues and other structures with advancing age, and the behavior of previously fixed alveolar macrophages that, following activation, migrate away leaving a gap in their original location.[63] Regardless of uncertainties about how pores are "normally" formed during aging, it is evident that the process is accelerated by the presence of many diseases that involve the lung parenchyma, a structural modification that undoubtedly con-tributes to the increased collateral ventilation found in these conditions.

CANALS OF LAMBERT

Lambert and her co-workers[65, 66] have demonstrated the presence of accessory pathways from respiratory bronchioles, terminal bronchioles, or even larger airways to airspaces supplied by other airways — in other words alternate channels for gas movement to distal respiratory units. Details about the number, location, and extent of Lambert's canals are lacking; although they have been identified in infants, virtually nothing is known about the factors that influence the development of the communications other than that they appear to be increased in the lungs of patients with emphysema and honeycombing.[67] Lambert's canals may well prove to be important pathways for collateral ventilation in normal subjects and patients with lung diseases.

It is regrettable that so little is known about them.

OTHER PATHWAYS

Physiologic studies have revealed that polystyrene spheres 64 μm in diameter can pass through collateral pathways in excised human lung.[68] Even larger spheres (120 μm in diameter) can traverse collateral channels in dog lungs.[69] Neither the pores of Kohn nor the canals of Lambert, unless the latter are remarkably distensible, are large enough to permit passage of a 64 μm diameter particle; thus, the inference can be made that there must be other—and larger—interconnections between airspaces. Accessory communications between respiratory bronchioles and alveolar ducts have, in fact, been observed in dog lungs, but similar structures have not been demonstrated in human lungs, although they have been looked for, except when the parenchymal architecture is distorted by certain diseases.[63]

Thus, it is uncertain how collateral ventilation is partitioned among the pathways that have been identified conclusively in man; also, it is possible that important interconnections remain to be discovered. There are more questions than answers at present about the structural and functional interrelationships of collateral ventilation in normal subjects and how these factors are changed by diseases of the lung.

ADAPTATION AND AGING

ADAPTATION

Most organs of the body thrive on work and languish without it; the prototype is skeletal muscle but included also is the brain (especially the mind). The lung, however, exhibits a limited capacity to adapt to additional functional demands even though other continuously working organs, such as the heart and the kidney, increase their functioning mass when a chronic work load must be dealt with. The lung may, in fact, demonstrate adaptive capabilities, but the question can still be asked why is it so large to begin with? The human body's maximum O_2 utilization depends much more upon the cardiovascular system and skeletal muscles than upon the lungs. World records are set by highly motivated athletes with large hearts and blood volumes and extremely well-trained muscles, not by persons with huge lungs. The large reserve of gas exchange capacity that is seldom exhausted by normal persons may be a genetic reminder of prehistoric days when survival depended upon "extra" lung function. This situation could have occurred either if lung diseases were prevalent in the population or if the physical demands of our ancestors' terrestrial or semiaquatic life were more rigorous than they are today.

In order to determine whether adaptation of the lung occurs, unusual conditions must be examined in which continuous "excess" pulmonary function is essential to survival. Probably the greatest natural stress that human lungs have to endure is to maintain O_2 transport in the hypoxic environment of high altitude. It is well known that long-term residents of high altitude, especially natives, are capable of astonishing physical feats that require large amounts of O_2. But it is less well known how this work capacity is achieved and, in particular, what the contributions of the lung are to the total responses.

Although the lungs of natives of high altitude are slightly larger than those of residents at sea level or acclimatized sojourners, the most striking difference in respiratory performance between these groups of subjects is in their pulmonary diffusing capacities.[70] Natives of high altitude are favored with a diffusing capacity 20 to 30 per cent higher than their counterparts at sea level. This difference cannot be explained on the basis of the elevated pulmonary arterial pressure and polycythemia found in natives of high altitude, which increase the diffusing capacity by increasing the number of red blood cells in pulmonary capillaries. This is because natives have a higher diffusing capacity than acclimatized sojourners, despite both groups having nearly comparable pulmonary artery pressures and hematocrit ratios. These observations raise the possibility that either adaptive responses or genetic factors account for the fact that natives have an increased ability to transfer O_2.

Morphometric studies performed on lungs of five natives of high altitude who died accidentally revealed an increase in number and size of alveoli, both of which contributed to an increase in alveolar surface area compared with matched control subjects who lived at sea level.[71] Whether these differences represent adaptation or whether they are genetically determined is not known; however, evidence from experimental animals may be useful in this context. Meticulous examination by quantitative morphometric techniques has established beyond dispute that the lungs of young mice reared at high altitude are larger and have a greater surface area for diffusion than the lungs of mice of equal body weight reared near sea level. The thickness of the air-blood barrier through which diffusion takes place did not differ between high altitude-raised mice and those that lived at sea level. Japanese waltzing mice, which have a genetic abnormality that results in their having a greatly increased O_2 consumption in keeping with their metabolic needs, also increased their morphometrically measured diffusing capacity; these mice have both an increase in lung volume and a proportionately greater increase in surface

area due to the proliferation of small-sized alveoli.[73]

It is always dangerous to extrapolate from the results of animal experiments to pronouncements about human biology. The studies of the influence of different O_2 environments certainly demonstrate adaptation by the lungs of growing mice, and the changes are consistent with those observed in natives of high altitude. The experiments with waltzing mice suggest that the responses may be governed by the O_2 needs of the animal, although the role of genetic factors cannot be excluded. The changes described all appeared during the growth phase of the animals, and whether or not lung structure can change after epiphyses fuse is uncertain. Studies of male acromegalic patients suggest, at least, that some functional differentiation is possible.[74]

Clearly, more studies concerning the capability of the human lung to adapt to changing physiologic requirements are needed. The uncertain state of knowledge can be summarized by saying that some mammalian lungs are able to adapt to a reduction in environmental O_2 tension; moreover, this response is more completely expressed if the stimulus occurs during the growth phase of the animal. Whether or not man manifests similar behavior remains to be determined.

AGING

The growth and development of the lung cease in normal human beings when somatic growth stops. As indicated in extreme pathologic conditions (e.g., excess growth hormone), functional modifications may occur, but these are rare. The lung shares with the rest of the body the consequences of advancing years, and as in other organs aging causes changes in the lung's morphometry and chemical composition as well as in its function. Because the effects of aging are expressed in deterioration of specific aspects of lung function that have not yet been explained, complete discussion of age-related changes is deferred until the last chapter of this book.

REFERENCES

1. Polgar, G., and Promadhat, V.: Pulmonary Function Testing in Children: Techniques and Standards. Philadelphia, W. B. Saunders Company, 1971, p. 207.
2. Swyer, P. R., Reiman, R. C., and Wright, J. J.: Ventilation and ventilatory mechanics in the newborn. J. Pediat., 56:612–622, 1960.
3. Boyden, E. A., and Tompsett, D. H.: The changing patterns in the developing lungs of infants. Acta Anat. (Basel), 61:164–192, 1965.
4. Hislop, A., Muir, D. C. F., Jacobsen, M., Simon, G., and Reid, L.: Postnatal growth and function of the pre-acinar airways. Thorax, 27:265–274, 1972.
5. Hogg, J. C., Williams, J., Richardson, J. B., Macklem, P. T., and Thurlbeck, W. M.: Age as a factor in the distribution of lower-airway conductance and in the pathologic anatomy of obstructive lung disease. New Eng. J. Med., 282:1283–1287, 1970.
6. Horsfield, K., and Cumming, G.: Morphology of the bronchial tree in man. J. Appl. Physiol., 24:373–383, 1968.
7. Weibel, E. R.: Morphometry of the Human Lung. Berlin, Springer-Verlag, 1963, p. 111.
8. Horsfield, K., and Cumming, G.: Functional consequences of airway morphology. J. Appl. Physiol., 24:384–390, 1968.
9. Medlar, E. M.: Behavior of pulmonary tuberculous lesions; pathological study. Am. Rev. Tuberc., 71(Mar. suppl.):1–244, 1955.
10. Rhodin, J. A. G.: Ultrastructure and function of the human tracheal mucosa. Am. Rev. Resp. Dis., 93 (suppl.):1–15, 1966.
11. Jeffery, P. and Reid, L.: Intra-epithelial nerves in normal rat airways: a quantitative electron microscope study. J. Anat., 114:35–45, 1973.
12. Lauweryns, J. M., Peuskens, J. C., and Cokelaere, M.: Argyrophil, fluorescent and granulated (peptide and amine producing?) AFG cells in human infant bronchial epithelium. Light and electron microscope studies. Life Sci., 9:1417–1429, 1970.
13. Lauweryns, J. M., and Peuskens, J. C.: Neuro-epithelial bodies (neuroreceptor or secretory organs?) in human infant bronchial and bronchiolar epithelium. Anat. Rec., 172:471–482, 1972.
14. Lauweryns, J. M., Cokelaere, M.: Hypoxia-sensitive neuro-epithelial bodies: intra-pulmonary secretory neuroreceptors, modulated by the CNS. Z. Zellforsch., 145:521–540, 1973.
15. Azzopardi, A., and Thurlbeck, W. M.: The histochemistry of the nonciliated bronchiolar epithelial cell. Am. Rev. Resp. Dis., 99:516–525, 1969.
16. Niden, A. H.: Bronchiolar and large alveolar cell in pulmonary phospholipid metabolism. Science, 158:1323–1324, 1967.
17. Gil, J., and Weibel, E. R.: Extracellular lining of bronchioles after perfusion-fixation of rat lungs for electron microscopy. Anat. Rec., 169:185–200, 1971.
18. Meyrick, B., and Reid, L.: Ultrastructure of cells in the human bronchial submucosal glands. J. Anat. 107:281–299, 1970.
19. Bensch, K. G., Gordon, G. B., and Miller, L. R.: Studies on the bronchial counterpart of the Kultschitzky (argentaffin) cell and innervation of bronchial glands. J. Ultrastruct. Res., 12:668–686, 1965.
20. Sturgess, J., and Reid, L.: An organ culture study of the effect of drugs on the secretory activity of the human bronchial submucosal gland. Clin. Sci., 43:533–543, 1972.
21. Reid, L.: Measurement of the bronchial mucous gland layer: A diagnostic yardstick in chronic bronchitis. Thorax, 15:132–141, 1960.
22. Ishizaka, K., and Ishizaka, T.: IgE and reaginic hypersensitivity. Ann. N.Y. Acad. Sci., 190:443–456, 1971.
23. Miller, W. S.: The Lung. Baltimore, Charles C Thomas, 1937, pp. 27–36.
24. von Hayek, H.: The Human Lung. New York, Hafner Publishing Company, Inc., 1960, pp. 206–212.
25. Hislop, A., and Reid, L.: Intra-pulmonary arterial development during fetal life—branching pattern and structure. J. Anat., 113:35–48, 1972.
26. Davies, G., and Reid, L.: Growth of the alveoli and pulmonary arteries in childhood. Thorax, 25:669–681, 1970.
27. Heath, D.: Pulmonary vasculature in postnatal life and pulmonary hemodynamics. In Emery, J. (ed.): The Anatomy of the Developing Lung. Suffolk, W. Heinmann Ltd., 1969, pp. 147–169.
28. Staub, N. C.: The interdependence of pulmonary structure and function. Anesthesiology, 24:831–854, 1963.
29. Fishman, A. P.: Respiratory gases in the regulation of the pulmonary circulation. Physiol. Rev., 41:214–280, 1961.
30. Glazier, J. B., and Murray, J. F.: Sites of pulmonary vasomotor reactivity in the dog during alveolar hypoxia and serotonin and histamine infusion. J. Clin. Invest., 50:2550–2558, 1971.
31. Kato, M., and Staub, N. C.: Response of small pulmonary arteries to unilobar hypoxia

and hypercapnia. Circ. Res., *19*:426–440, 1966.

32. Hughes, J. M. B., Grant, B. J. B., Jones, H. A., and Davies, E. E.: Relationship between blood flow and alveolar gas tensions in lung lobules. Scand. J. Resp. Dis. 1975 (in press).

33. Elliott, F. M., and Reid, L.: Some new facts about the pulmonary artery and its branching pattern. Clin. Radiol., *16*:193–198, 1965.

34. Hislop, A., and Reid, L.: Pulmonary arterial development during childhood: Branching pattern and structure. Thorax, 28:129–135, 1973.

35. Heinemann, H. O., and Fishman, A. P.: Nonrespiratory functions of mammalian lung. Physiol. Rev., 49:1–47, 1969.

36. Bierman, H. R., Kelly, K. H., Cordes, F. L., Byron, R. L., Jr., Polhemus, J. A., and Rappoport, S.: The release of leukocytes and platelets from the pulmonary circulation by epinephrine. Blood, 7:683–692, 1952.

37. Hislop, A., and Reid, L.: Fetal and childhood development of the intrapulmonary veins in man—branching pattern and structure. Thorax, 28:313–319, 1973.

38. Heath, D., and Edwards, J. E.: Histological changes in the lung in diseases associated with pulmonary venous hypertension. Brit. J. Dis. Chest., 53:8–18, 1959.

39. Hoffman, J. I. E., Guz, A., Charlier, A. A., and Wilken, D. E. L.: Stroke volume in conscious dogs; effect of respiration, posture, and vascular occlusion. J. Appl. Physiol., *20*:865–877, 1965.

40. Marchand, P., Gilroy, J. C., and Wilson, V. H.: An anatomical study of the bronchial vascular system and its variations in disease. Thorax, 5:207–221, 1950.

41. Heymann, M. A. Unpublished observations, 1973.

42. Campbell, A. G. M., Cockburn, F., Dawes, G. S., and Milligan, J. E.: Pulmonary vasoconstriction in asphyxia during cross-circulation between twin foetal lambs. J. Physiol. (Lond.), *192*:111–121, 1967.

43. Miller, W. S.: The vascular supply of the bronchial tree. Am. Rev. Tuberc., *12*:87–94, 1925.

44. Cudkowicz, L., Abelmann, W. H., Levinson, G. E., Katznelson, G., and Jreissaty, R. M.: Bronchial arterial blood flow. Clin. Sci., *19*:1–15, 1960.

45. Ellis, F. H., Jr., Grindlay, J. H., and Edwards, J. E.: The bronchial arteries. I. Experimental occlusion. Surgery, *30*:810–826, 1951.

46. Aviado, D. M.: The Lung Circulation. Vol. 1. Oxford, Pergamon Press Ltd., 1965, pp. 185–254.

47. Auld, P. A., Rudolph, A. M., and Golinko,

R. J.: Factors affecting bronchial collateral flow in the dog. Am. J. Physiol., *198*: 1166–1170, 1960.

48. Fisher, A. B., Kollmeier, H., Brody, J. S., Hyde, R. W., Hansell, J., Friedman, J. N., and Waldhausen, J. A.: Restoration of systemic blood flow to the lung after division of bronchial arteries. J. Appl. Physiol., *29*:839–846, 1970.

49. Weibel, E. R.: Morphological basis of alveolar-capillary gas exchange. Physiol. Rev., 53:419–495, 1973.

50. Lauweryns, J. M.: The blood and lymphatic microcirculation of the lung. *In* Sommers, S. C. (ed.): Pathology Annual 1971. New York, Appleton-Century-Crofts, 1971, pp. 365–415.

51. Dunnill, M. S.: Postnatal growth of the lung. Thorax, 17:329–333, 1962.

52. Macklin, C. C.: Musculature of bronchi and lungs. Physiol. Rev., 9:1–60, 1929.

53. Angus, G. E., and Thurlbeck, W. M.: Number of alveoli in the human lung. J. Appl. Physiol., *32*:483–485, 1972.

54. Matsuba, K., and Thurlbeck, W. M.: The number and dimensions of small airways in nonemphysematous lungs. Am. Rev. Resp. Dis., *104*:516–524, 1971.

55. Tenney, S. M., and Remmers, J. E.: Comparative quantitative morphology of the mammalian lung: diffusing area. Nature, *197*:54–56, 1963.

56. Kapanci, Y., Weibel, E. R., Kaplan, H. P., and Robinson, F. R.: Pathogenesis and reversibility of the pulmonary lesions of oxygen toxicity in monkeys. II. Ultrastructural and morphometric studies. Lab. Invest., *20*:101–118, 1969.

57. Meyrick, B., and Reid, L.: The alveolar brush cell in rat lung—a third pneumonocyte. J. Ultrastruct. Res., *23*:71–80, 1968.

58. Vane, J. R.: The release and fate of vasoactive hormones in the circulation. Brit. J. Pharmacol., 35:202–242, 1969.

59. Untersee, P., Gil, J., and Weibel, E. R.: Visualization of extracellular lining layer of lung alveoli by freeze-etching. Resp. Physiol., *13*:171–185, 1971.

60. Bowden, D. H., and Adamson, I. Y. R.: The pulmonary interstitial cell as immediate precursor of the alveolar macrophage. Am. J. Pathol., 68:521–535, 1972.

61. Evans, M. J., Cabral, L. J., Stephens, R. J., and Freeman, G.: Cell division of alveolar macrophages in rat lung following exposure to NO_2. Am. J. Pathol., 70:199–207, 1973.

62. Cohen, A. B., and Cline, M. J.: The human alveolar macrophage: Isolation, cultivation in vitro, and studies of morphologic and functional characteristics. J. Clin. Invest., 50:1390–1398, 1971.

63. Macklem, P. T.: Airway obstruction and col-

lateral ventilation. Physiol. Rev., *51*:368–436, 1971.

64. Kuno, K., and Staub, N. C.: Acute mechanical effects of lung volume changes on artificial microholes in alveolar walls. J. Appl. Physiol., *24*:83–92, 1968.

65. Lambert, M. W.: Accessory bronchiole-alveolar communications. J. Path. Bact., *70*:311–314, 1955.

66. Duguid, J. B., and Lambert, M. W.: The pathogenesis of coal miner's pneumoconiosis. J. Path. Bact., *88*:389–403, 1964.

67. Liebow, A. A.: Recent advances in pulmonary anatomy. *In* De Reuck, A. V. S., and O'Conner, M. (eds.): Ciba Foundation. Boston, Little, Brown and Company, 1962, pp. 2–28.

68. Henderson, R., Horsfield, K., and Cumming, G.: Intersegmental collateral ventilation in the human lung. Resp. Physiol., *6*:128–134, 1968.

69. Martin, H. B.: Respiratory bronchioles as the pathway for collateral ventilation. J. Appl. Physiol., *21*:1443–1447, 1966.

70. Lenfant, C., and Sullivan, K.: Adaptation to high altitude. New Eng. J. Med., *284*:1298–1309, 1971.

71. Saldana, M., and Garcia-Oyola, E.: Morphometry of the high altitude lung. Lab. Invest., *22*:509, 1970.

72. Burri, P. H., and Weibel, E. R.: Morphometric estimation of pulmonary diffusion capacity. II. Effect of Po_2 on the growing lung. Resp. Physiol., *11*:247–267, 1971.

73. Geelhaar, A., and Weibel, E. R.: Morphometric estimation of pulmonary diffusion capacity. III. The effects of increased oxygen consumption in Japanese waltzing mice. Resp. Physiol., *11*:354–366, 1971.

74. Brody, J. S., Fisher, A. B., Gocmen, A., and DuBois, A. B.: Acromegalic pneumonomegaly: lung growth in the adult. J. Clin. Invest., *49*:1051–1060, 1970.

Chapter Three

LYMPHATIC AND NERVOUS SYSTEMS

INTRODUCTION

More is known about the pre- and postnatal growth and the development and function of airways, blood vessels, and components of the terminal respiratory units in man than about the structure and function of pulmonary lymphatic vessels, lymph nodes, and nerves. The lack of information is not because the lymphatic and nervous systems are unimportant, but because they are extremely difficult to examine, especially in human beings. However, investigations using new histologic and physiologic techniques have demonstrated that both the lymphatic supply and the innervation of the lung are essential to the maintenance of homeostasis. Furthermore, the results of these and other recent studies have begun to clarify the contributions of lymphatics and nerves to such common clinical problems as pulmonary edema and the sensation of breathlessness. The purpose of this chapter is to review the structure-function rela-

tionships of the lymphatic drainage pathways and the innervation of the lung. Additional details are provided about the role of lymph vessels in liquid and solute movement in Chapter 5, and pulmonary defense mechanisms in Chapter 11, and about the role of the nervous system in controlling breathing in Chapter 9.

LYMPHATIC VESSELS AND LYMPH NODES

LYMPHATIC VESSELS

The lack of concern until recently about pulmonary lymphatics was undoubtedly due to the mistaken belief that the lung was a "dry organ" with little transcapillary movement of liquid and protein and therefore that lymphatic vessels were not needed under ordinary conditions of function. Now it is known that the rate of formation of interstitial liquid in the lung is at least as great as that in other organs, and, as is also the case in other organs, lym-

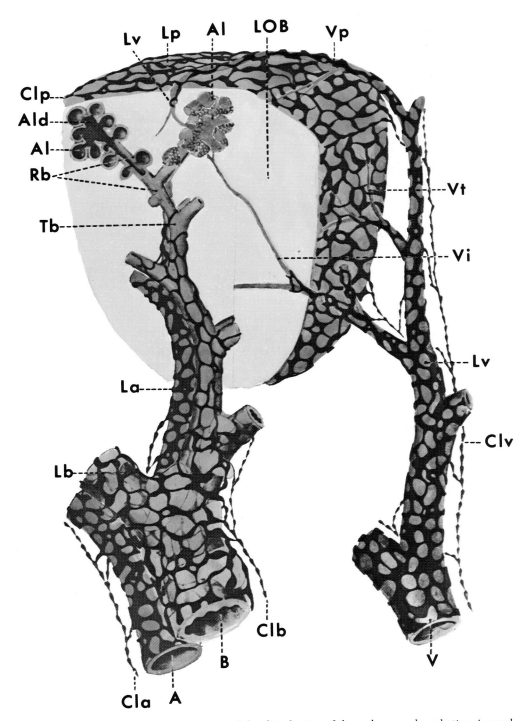

Figure 3-1 Schematic representation of the distribution of the pulmonary lymphatics. A = pulmonary artery; Al = alveolus; Ald = alveolar duct; B = bronchus; Cla = collecting lymph vessel accompanying pulmonary artery; Clb = collecting lymph vessel accompanying bronchus; Clp = subpleural collecting lymph vessel; Clv = collecting lymph vessel accompanying pulmonary vein; La = periarterial lymphatic plexus; Lb = peribronchial lymphatic plexus; LOB = lobule; Lp = subpleural lymph vessel; Lv = perivenous lymphatic plexus; Rb = respiratory bronchiole; Tb = terminal bronchiole; V = pulmonary vein; Vi = intralobular branch of pulmonary vein; Vp = subpleural branch of pulmonary vein; Vt = interlobular branch of pulmonary vein. (From Nagaishi.[2] Reprinted by permission from the author and publisher.)

phatic channels are essential for the removal of excess liquid and virtually all of the protein molecules that "leak" out of blood vessels.

Attention was directed in Chapter 1 to the role of the pulmonary lymphatics in removing lung liquid in the newborn period. The histologic demonstration that pulmonary lymphatic capillaries are markedly, but transiently, distended during the first few hours after birth, in conjunction with the decrease in water content of the lung during the same period, implies that the lymphatic vessels not only are well developed at birth but also are capable of participating in the removal of liquid immediately afterward.[1]

Studies of the pulmonary lymphatic system in adults have established the presence of two sets of vessels (Figure 3-1): the superficial or pleural network and the deep or parenchymatous (peribronchovascular) lymphatic plexus.[3] Valves are numerous in all lymph channels and are usually 1 to 2 mm apart. The unicuspid funnel-shaped valves (Figure 3-2) are placed to direct flow for variable distances on the surface of the lung in pleural lymphatics, but ultimately most branches enter the lung, and flow is toward the hilum through interlobular and peribronchovascular vessels. Although the principal routes of lymph flow to the hilum are through the lung, the superficial network is a continuous one; thus, it is possible for lymph to flow around the surface of the lung and reach the hilum.

More pleural lymphatic vessels have been identified on the surface of both lower lobes than on the surface of the upper or middle lobes, and the superficial lymphatic pathways over the left lower lobe were reported to be considerably more numerous and larger compared with those over the right lower lobe.[5] * Thus, the anatomy

---

*This interesting finding needs to be confirmed.

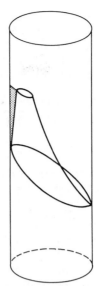

Figure 3-2 Schematic representation of a funnel-shaped, monocuspid valve from a lymphatic vessel. (Adapted from Lauweryns.[4] Reprinted by permission from the author and publisher.)

of intrathoracic lymphatics affords two possible explanations for a common clinical observation that patients with bilateral pleural effusions nearly always have more liquid on the right side than on the left. This discrepancy might be caused either by increased removal of liquid from the left pleural space through the dense network of lymphatics over the left lower lobe or by increased leakage from the conducting lymph channels that drain the abdomen and lower extremities and pass mainly along the right mediastinal pleura in their journey through the thorax.

When distended and thickened by pathologic processes, anastomotic connections between perivenous and peribronchoarterial vessels become a useful roentgenographic landmark, Kerley "A" lines. Similarly, thickening of the whole interlobular septum around subpleural interlobular lymphatic vessels produces another distinctive condition that can be identified radiologically, Kerley "B" lines.[6]

The forces that propel pulmonary lymph centrally were believed originally to include the massaging effects of inflation and deflation of the lung, cardiovascular pulsations, and movements of the thorax and abdomen. Now it is known that lymph flow in awake healthy sheep is predominantly due to active contraction of smooth muscles in the walls of the lymphatic vessels.[7] Because the pulsatile pressures (1 to 25 mm Hg) and pulse frequencies (1 to 30/min) were related to the rate of lymph formation in various organs, it was concluded that the contractile mechanism serves to cause removal of lymph in proportion to its rate of formation. It is likely that this process operates in man as well.

Lymphatic capillaries have not been demonstrated convincingly to exist at the level of the air-blood barrier or within the interalveolar septum. However, typical lymphatic channels have been observed *between* adjacent terminal respiratory units where there is connective tissue and within the interlobular, pleural, and peribronchovascular connective tissue sheaths; these vessels have been called by Lauweryns[3] the *juxta-alveolar lymphatics* (Figure 3–3). Judging from the dimensions of the terminal respiratory unit, all pulmonary capillaries within the interalveolar septum are probably within a few 100 μm or, at most, 1 mm of the nearest juxta-alveolar lymphatic. Electron microscopic studies of lymphatic capillaries have revealed that the endothelium is interrupted by open junctions and intercellular gaps (pores) and that the basement membrane is discontinuous.[8] This allows the contents of the perilymphatic interstitial space to flow directly into the lumen of lymphatic channels and indicates that the composition of lymph must be virtually identical with that of interstitial liquid.

Thus, although lymphatic capil-

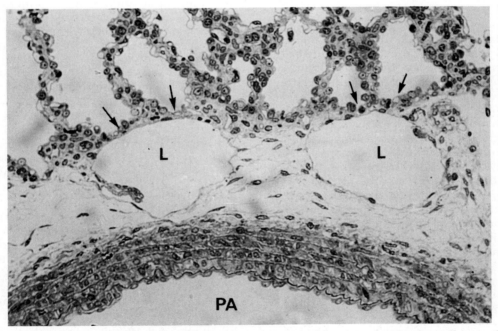

Figure 3–3 Juxta-alveolar lymphatic capillaries (L) located between the alveolar wall (arrows) and the adventitial connective tissue of a large pulmonary artery (PA) in a newborn rabbit. (× 634. From Lauweryns.[4] Reprinted by permission from the author and publisher.)

laries are not an integral part of the interalveolar septum, they are strategically located and well designed to participate in the removal of liquid (exudates and transudates) and other substances (e.g., inhaled particles or microorganisms) that gain entrance into the interstitial space of the lung parenchyma.

LYMPHOID TISSUE

Scattered lymphocytes and plasma cells are found in the wall of the entire tracheobronchial tree, and to a lesser extent surrounding blood vessels. Lymphocytes are particularly noticeable in the lamina propria of the mucosa and are more numerous and appear to form small clusters at the points of airways branching. Collections of lymphoid tissue have been described by von Hayek[9] in intimate relationship with the mucous membrane of bronchi and bronchioles. Lymphoid tissue has also been identified at the junction of terminal bronchioles and respiratory bronchioles. It is believed that the tracheobronchial lymph tissue probably makes an important contribution to both antibody-mediated and cell-mediated pulmonary immune responses; furthermore, the lymphatic aggregations in bronchioles are situated where they appear to favor the traffic of alveolar macrophages during their journey from interstitial tissue to airway lumen. The roles of lymphoid structures in pulmonary defense mechanisms are considered in greater detail in Chapter 11.

Bronchopulmonary lymphoid tissue is sparse at birth and increases afterward. The proliferation is likely to represent an adaptive response to

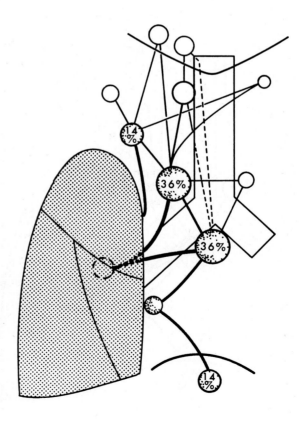

Figure 3–4 Schematic representation of the primary (heavy lines and shaded circles) and secondary (thin lines and open circles) lymphatic drainage pathways of the right lung following injection of the lobar lymph node complex shown. (From Dyon.[10] Reprinted by permission from the author.)

cumulative antigenic challenge during the person's lifetime.

LYMPH NODES

Formed lymph nodes with germinal centers and a definite sinusoidal structure appear in the lung at birth or during infancy. Because they usually contain only a small number of cells, they are difficult to identify within the lung except when they are enlarged owing to a pathologic process.

According to Dyon,[10] the extrapulmonary lymph drainage of the human lungs occurs through a maze of interconnecting mediastinal, paratracheal, and subdiaphragmatic lymph nodes and channels. The principal and secondary drainage pathways of the right and left lungs are depicted schematically in Figures 3–4 and 3–5. The main right lymphatic ducts follow the right side of the trachea and join the venous system at the junction of the right jugular and subclavian veins; the left lymphatic ducts, which usually are smaller than those on the right, lie along the left side of the trachea until they empty into the thoracic duct as it terminates in the confluence of veins in the left side of the neck. It no longer is believed that the right lymphatic duct drains about 80 per cent of the total pulmonary lymph and that the remaining 20 per cent, mainly from the left upper lobe, drains through the left lymphatic duct; it is now agreed that pulmonary lymph drainage patterns are complex and variable, a fact that has important clinical implications concerning the diagnosis and prognosis of bronchogenic cancer.

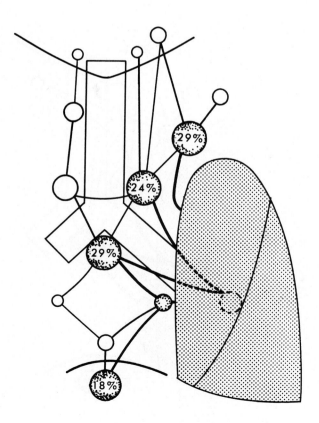

Figure 3–5 Schematic representation of the primary (heavy lines and shaded circles) and secondary (thin lines and open circles) lymphatic drainage pathways of the left lung following injection of the lobar lymph node complex shown. (From Dyon.[10] Reprinted by permission from the author.)

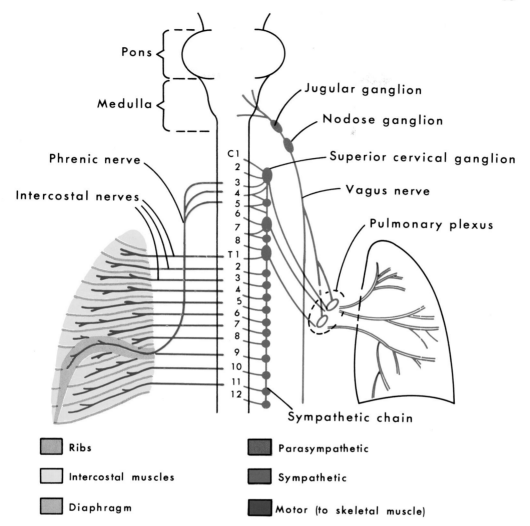

Figure 3-6 Schematic depiction of the autonomic innervation (motor and sensory) of the lung and the somatic (motor) nerve supply to the intercostal muscles and diaphragm.

NERVE SUPPLY OF THE LUNG

AFFERENT AND EFFERENT PATHWAYS

The lung is innervated by branches from the vagus nerve and thoracic sympathetic ganglia (Figure 3–6). The vagus nerves and the upper four or five thoracic sympathetic ganglia contribute fibers to the anterior and pos-terior pulmonary plexuses at the roots of the lungs. As the bronchi, arteries, and veins enter the lung at the hilum, they carry with them extensions of the plexus, the largest branches accompanying the bronchi and the smallest accompanying the veins. Ramifying nerve fibers continue to invest airways and blood vessels as they subdivide within the lung.[11]

Unmyelinated efferent fibers (Figure 3–7) have been followed to the smooth musculature of all divisions of conducting airways, respiratory bronchioles, and alveolar ducts. Although the distribution of postganglionic autonomic fibers in the walls of airways is extensive, these fibers have not been identified in the epithelial layer of the experimental animals studied (rabbits and dogs). Physiologic observations have demonstrated that the efferent fibers innervating smooth muscles along conducting airways are of both vagal (bronchoconstrictor) and sympathetic (bronchodilator) origin.[12] Similarly, efferent fibers from both systems innervate bronchial glands. Stimulation of the vagus causes immediate discharge of the contents of the glands, but the response to sympathetic stimulation is more difficult to discern. In general, both from anatomic and physiologic examinations, parasympathetic innervation of the airways predominates over that of the sympathetic system.

As indicated previously, the ultrastructure of the argyrophil cells and the neuroepithelial bodies of the epithelium suggest that they are also innervated. The motor innervation of pulmonary blood vessels and the functional consequences of stimulation of the components of the autonomic nervous system need to be clarified further. In the dog, nerve fibers that appear to be of sympathetic origin have been demonstrated by various histologic techniques to lie within the walls of pulmonary artery branches, including arterioles as small as 30 μm[13]; a similar distribution of motor fibers has been observed in human lungs.[11] The arrangement of parasympathetic nerves within the pulmonary circulation is less certain and probably less extensive. Sympathetic vasoconstrictor activity has been observed in the pulmonary circulation of dogs,[14] but has not been demonstrated in man. The effect of vagal stimulation on pulmonary blood vessels is difficult to document, and although vasodilator

responses have been reported, they are too feeble to be of physiologic importance. Certainly, it has not been possible to demonstrate any influences mediated by the autonomic nervous system on the pulmonary circulation of spontaneously breathing, normal human adults.[15]

More is known about the neuroanatomy of the sympathetic and parasympathetic efferent pathways within the lung than about their physiologic contributions to homeostasis. Efferent nerves control the caliber of the conducting airways, the volume of terminal respiratory units, the activity of bronchial glands, and the tone and diameter of pulmonary blood vessels. Thus, pulmonary motor fibers mediate vital responses which may affect the adequacy of gas exchange by regulating the distribution of ventilation and perfusion and which contribute to the defense of the lung and body against injury from inhaled substances.

It is generally accepted that virtually all afferent nerve fibers to the central nervous system from the lung travel in the vagus nerve. Controversy exists concerning the presence in some experimental animals of sympathetic afferent nerves, and certainly they have not been demonstrated convincingly in man.

Numerous other signals that affect respiration are transmitted to the central nervous system via afferent nerves that serve receptors located in parts of the body other than the lungs. The structure and function of the most important of these, the chemoreceptors and skeletal muscle proprioceptors, are considered in Chapter 9.

RECEPTORS

There are three well-defined vagal sensory receptors in the lungs[16]: the bronchopulmonary stretch receptors, the irritant receptors, and the J receptors. These receptors and their reflex effects have been differentiated by neurophysiologic studies in experi-

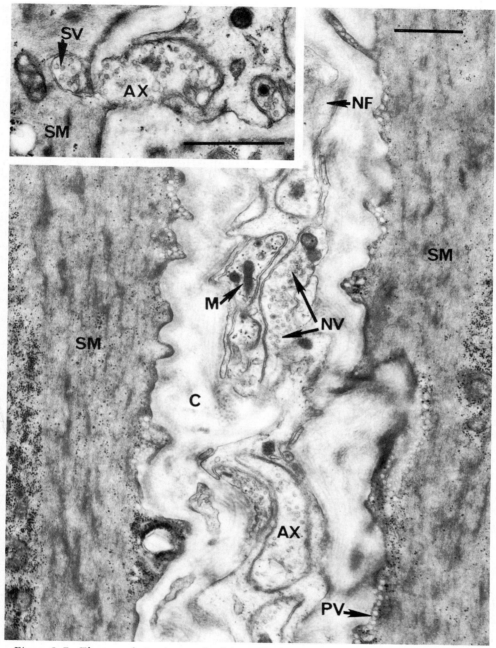

Figure 3-7 Electron photomicrograph of the wall of a bronchus from an adult woman showing unmyelinated axons (AX) (probably motor) lying in a connective tissue space containing collagen (C) between two smooth muscle cells (SM). Within the axons are mitochondria (M), neurovesicles (NV), and neurofilaments (NF). Pinocytotic vesicles (PV) are evident in the cytoplasmic membrane of the muscle cell. The inset shows a nerve terminal containing synaptic vesicles (SV) located at the junction between an axon and muscle cell. Horizontal bar = 1 μm. ($\times$ 18,225 and 26,000 [inset]. Courtesy of Dr. Donald McKay.)

mental animals and are characterized by the features listed in Table 3–1. Although the neural pathways and the effector responses are well established, there is still uncertainty about the precise location and morphology of the receptors that detect the appropriate stimuli. There is, however, anatomic and physiologic evidence in support of the receptors included in Table 3–1. In addition, chemoreceptors have been proposed as a fourth set of intrapulmonary sensory elements, but convincing demonstration of their presence and physiologic function is lacking.

1. Slowly adapting pulmonary *stretch receptors* are believed to be the nerve filaments that are closely associated with smooth muscles throughout the intrapulmonary conducting airways. The receptors appear to be stimulated by deformation of the endings when changes occur in the caliber of the bronchial wall; therefore, changes in the distending pressure "across" the airways, as well as the actual volume of air entering the lung, should be appropriate stimuli.

Pulmonary stretch receptors respond phasically during breathing to terminate inspiration; impulses from the receptors progressively increase during inflation of the lung until the activity signals the end of inspiration and expiration ensues.[17] However, recent work in conscious dogs has demonstrated that the effect of the inflation reflex may not be to regulate the depth of inspiration, as customarily taught, but to influence the duration of the expiratory pause between breaths.[18] The inhibitory effect of lung inflation on respiratory rate is one component of the Hering-Breuer reflex; the other mediates, in part, the adjustments of respiratory muscles to transient mechanical loads. However, it is now known that the contribution of vagal reflexes to respiratory load-compensation, which is important in some experimental animals, is weak or absent in man.[19] Additional reflex effects from stimulating stretch receptors are bronchodilatation, an increase in heart rate, and a fall in peripheral vascular resistance.

Recordings from afferent nerves subserving stretch receptors in experimental animals reveal that about 60 per cent of the fibers have detectable activity during the pause between breaths; the remainder of the nerves are progressively recruited as inflation

Table 3–1 Characteristics of the Three Pulmonary Vagal Sensory Reflexes

RECEPTOR	LOCATION	FIBER TYPE	STIMULUS	RESPONSES
Pulmonary stretch, slowly adapting	Associated with smooth muscle of intrapulmonary airways	Medullated	1. Lung inflation 2. Increased trans-pulmonary pressure	1. Hering-Breuer inflation reflex 2. Bronchodilatation 3. Increased heart rate 4. Decreased peripheral vascular resistance
Irritant, rapidly adapting	Epithelium of (mainly) extra-pulmonary airways	Medullated	1. Irritants 2. Mechanical stimulation 3. Anaphylaxis 4. Pneumothorax 5. Hyperpnea 6. Pulmonary congestion	1. Bronchoconstriction 2. Hyperpnea 3. Expiratory constriction of larynx 4. Cough
Type J	Alveolar wall	Nonmedullated	1. Increased interstitial volume (congestion) 2. Chemical injury 3. Microembolism	1. Rapid shallow breathing 2. Severe expiratory constriction of larynx 3. Hypotension, bradycardia 4. Spinal reflex inhibition

proceeds. Section or blockade of the vagus in most mammalian species causes a slow frequency large tidal volume pattern of breathing without changing the level of arterial CO_2 tension. These observations led to speculation that pulmonary stretch receptors may regulate the rate and depth of breathing and that they adjust the pattern to achieve the optimal combination at which mechanical work and/or inspiratory force is minimal.[20] But this attractive hypothesis does not appear to apply to man, because the Hering-Breuer reflex is very weak or absent during normal quiet breathing in healthy adults.[21] At large tidal volumes, however, an inflation reflex can be demonstrated in anesthetized man and a brisk inflation reflex has been reported in newborn babies.[22]

2. Rapidly adapting *irritant receptors* are not active in normal breathing but respond to a variety of stimuli: inhalation of gaseous irritants, mechanical stimulation of the larynx and airways, histamine-induced bronchoconstriction, anaphylactic reactions in the lung, pulmonary arterial microembolism, mechanical stimulation by large inflations and deflations, pneumothorax, hyperpnea due to asphyxia or hypercapnea or to an increase in artificial ventilation, and pulmonary congestion due to left atrial obstruction.[15] Most of these diverse stimuli produce an increase in the distending force on the bronchial wall and, accordingly, probably activate pulmonary stretch receptors as well.

Although analysis is complicated when more than one receptor is involved,* the reflex responses from stimulating irritant receptors are bronchoconstriction, hyperpnea, constriction of the larynx during expiration, and possibly cough. It is noteworthy that the threshold for bronchoconstriction and laryngeal constriction appears to be considerably lower than that for cough.

The actual receptor sites are unknown. They may be the free unmyelinated nerve filaments that have been demonstrated in the superficial epithelium of the airways[23]; the endings in turn are attached to myelinated vagal nerve fibers (Figure 3–8). Axons that resemble free sensory endings located elsewhere in the body have been identified among and below ciliated cells, goblet cells, and basal cells in man and experimental animals (Figure 3–9). Judging from physiologic studies, irritant receptors are mainly concentrated in the larynx, trachea, and extrapulmonary bronchi, but intrapulmonary receptor activity has also been demonstrated in some animals.[15] There appears to be a variation among species because despite a careful search of the entire airways system in rats, superficial nerves with sensory morphology could be found only in extrapulmonary airways.[24]

3. *Type J pulmonary receptors* were thought originally to be chiefly involved in the reflexes to forced deflation of the lungs. Now, however, they are believed not to be sensitive to deflation of the lung but to cause rapid, shallow breathing when stimulated experimentally by pulmonary congestion and edema, microembolism, and inhalation of certain chemical substances.[15]

It was established that the receptor endings must be near the pulmonary capillaries, and hence they were called juxtapulmonary capillary receptors; now they are simply referred to as type J receptors.[16] Recently, small unmyelinated axons with the structural characteristics of sensory nerve endings have been described within the alveolar wall of rat lung (Figure 3–10); although scarce and difficult to demonstrate, these terminals are appropriately located to serve as J receptors.[25]

There is good reason to suppose

*Multiple receptors are nearly always involved because any primary response actuated by a single receptor system usually evokes secondary responses from other receptors.

Text continued on page 73

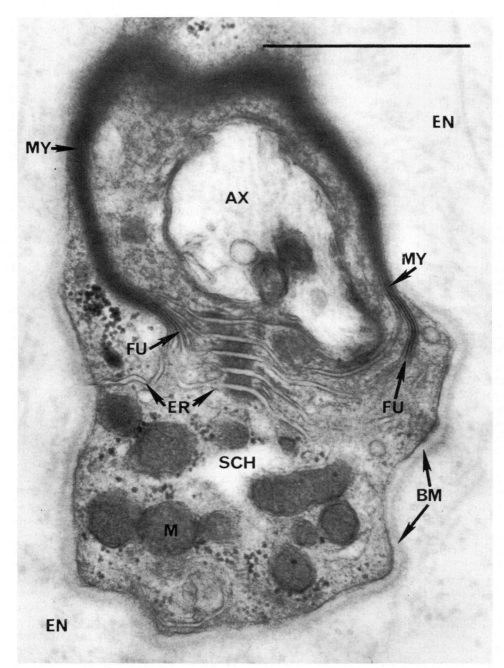

Figure 3–8   Electron photomicrograph of a myelinated nerve in the wall of a bronchus from an adult woman. The Schwann cell (SCH) containing mitochondria (M) rests on a basement membrane (BM) within the endoneurium (EN). The myelin sheath (MY), which is wrapped around an axon (AX), is formed by fusion (FU) of the endoplasmic reticulum (ER). Horizontal bar = 1 μm. ($\times$ 55,000. Courtesy of Dr. Donald McKay.)

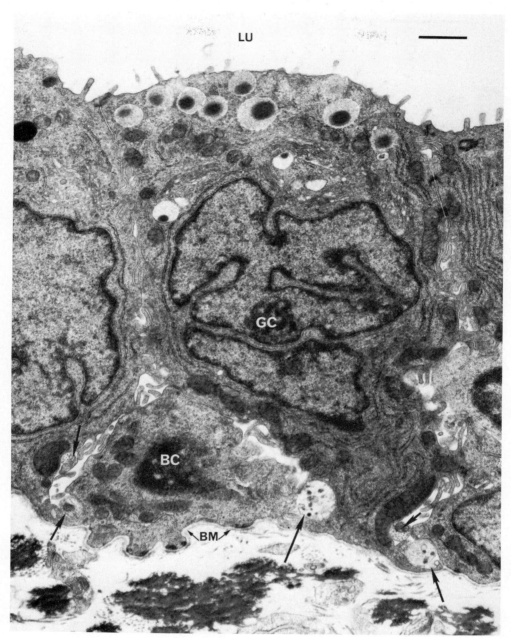

Figure 3–9 Electron photomicrograph showing a rat tracheal goblet cell (GC) facing the airway lumen (LU) and basal cell (BC) and five intraepithelial nerves (arrows) near the basement membrane (BM). Horizontal bar = 1 μm. (× 12,800. Courtesy of Dr. Peter K. Jeffery.)

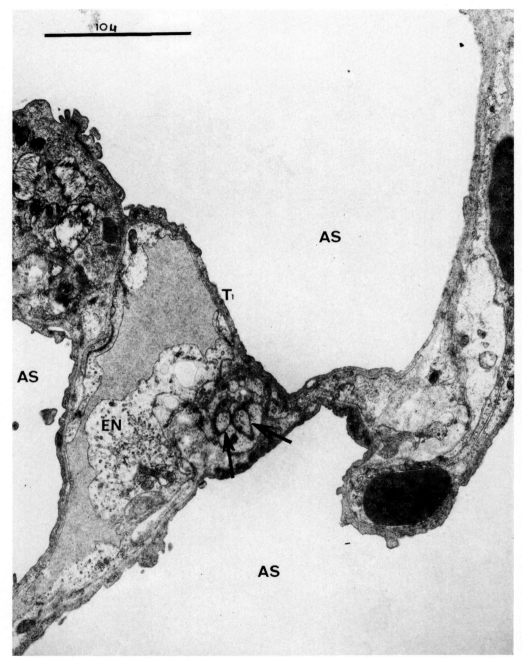

Figure 3–10   Electron photomicrograph of an intra-alveolar nerve. The two axons (arrows) lie between type I pneumocytes (TI) and capillary endothelium (EN) swollen because of adrenaline injection. AS = alveolar space. (× 3900. From Meyrick and Reid.[25] Reprinted by permission from the authors and publisher.)

that type J receptors contribute to the sensation of dyspnea that accompanies clinical conditions in which they are likely to be excited: pulmonary edema, pulmonary embolism, pneumonia, and inhalation of noxious chemicals. Paintal[26] has also proposed that type J receptors are involved in the breathlessness of severe muscular exercise and are activated by interstitial edema; this hypothesis has not been substantiated by studies of pulmonary extravascular water after one hour of strenuous exercise.[27]

Recently, it was demonstrated that stimulation of type J receptors causes marked expiratory narrowing of the larynx by reflex constriction that is sustained and often nearly complete.[28] This response may underlie the presence of expiratory grunting that characterizes the pattern of breathing in newborn infants with respiratory distress. Grunting expiration has been shown to be beneficial in this syndrome, and the stimulus for laryngeal constriction could originate in the extensive interstitial edema that is one of the pathologic hallmarks of the disorder. The absence of this response in adults with pulmonary edema may be explained by a weakening of the reflex similar to that of the pulmonary stretch reflex in normal babies within five days of birth.[22]

4. Pulmonary stretch receptors, irritant receptors, and type J receptors all can be stimulated by various suitable chemicals. In this sense, they are "chemosensitive." However, chemosensitivity to test substances does not confer chemoreceptor function to physiologic stimuli such as changes in the gaseous composition of blood or air.

The search for *pulmonary chemoreceptors* in the airways and blood

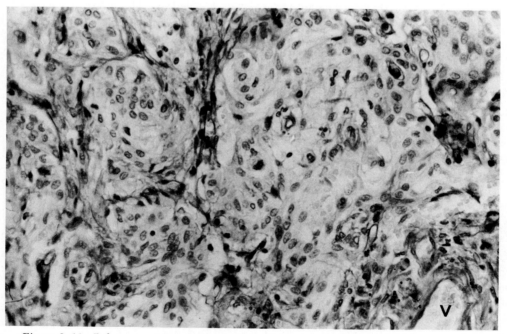

Figure 3–11 Pulmonary chemodectoma. Nests of chemoreceptor-like cells in the interstitium of the lung adjacent to a pulmonary vein (V). ($\times$ 420. Courtesy of Dr. Averill Liebow.)

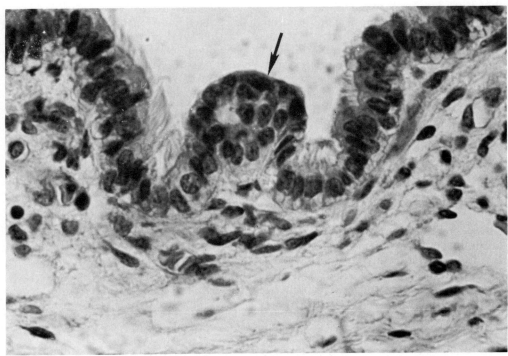

Figure 3–12 Neuroepithelial body (arrow) of a human infant showing the nonciliated lining on the luminal side and the protrusion slightly above the level of the surrounding ciliated epithelium. (× 1040. From Lauweryns and Peuskens.[30] Reprinted by permission from the authors and publisher.)

vessels has been long and exhaustive owing to the teleologic attractiveness of sensors that would "taste" the blood and "smell" the air. Although the reports of studies thus far have indicated far more negative than positive results, the quest nevertheless continues. The most promising clues are (1) the nests of cells that are found occasionally at autopsy and are believed to be tumors or hyperplasias of normal cellular constituents; because these cells resemble chemoreceptor cells elsewhere in the body, appear to be heavily innervated, and are invariably situated in close relationship to pulmonary veins (Figure 3–11), they are in a perfect location to monitor the composition of blood leaving the lung[29]; and (2) the neuroepithelial bodies found in airways (Figure 3–12) have an abundant nerve supply and are strategically located to sample and respond to changes in the gas com-

position entering and leaving regions of the lung.[30] However, much experimental work remains before the nervous pathways and physiologic roles for these structures are established.

The current state of knowledge about pulmonary vagal receptors and their responses can be summarized succinctly. Pulmonary stretch receptors are mainly important in controlling the pattern of breathing but are weakly active in man after the newborn period; irritant receptors and J receptors are mainly activated in lung disease and abnormal conditions and may interact with many reflex responses; pulmonary chemoreceptors that respond to changes in inspired air or blood gas composition have not been demonstrated convincingly, although some recently identified structures have been suggested as possible candidates for the role.

REFERENCES

1. Lauweryns, J. M., Claessens, S., and Boussauw, L.: The pulmonary lymphatics in neonatal hyaline membrane disease. Pediatrics, 41:917–930, 1968.
2. Nagaishi, C.: Functional Anatomy and Histology of the Lung. Baltimore, University Park Press, 1972, p. 148.
3. Lauweryns, J. M.: The juxta-alveolar lymphatics in the human adult lung. Histologic studies in 15 cases of drowning. Am. Rev. Resp. Dis., 102:877–885, 1970.
4. Lauweryns, J. M.: The blood and lymphatic microcirculation of the lung. In Sommers, S. C. (ed.): Pathology Annual 1971. New York, Appleton-Century-Crofts, 1971, pp. 365–415.
5. Trapnell, D. H.: The peripheral lymphatics of the lung. Brit. J. Radiol., 36:660–672, 1963.
6. Trapnell, D. H.: Radiological appearances of lymphangitis carcinomatosa of the lung. Thorax, 19:251–260, 1964.
7. Hall, J. G., Morris, B., and Woolley, G.: Intrinsic rhythmic propulsion of lymph in unanesthetized sheep. J. Physiol. (Lond.), 180:336–349, 1965.
8. Lauweryns, J. M., and Boussauw, L.: The ultrastructure of pulmonary lymphatic capillaries of newborn rabbits and of human infants. Lymphology, 2:108–129, 1969.
9. von Hayek, H.: The Human Lung. New York, Hafner Publishing Company, Inc., 1960, pp. 298–314.
10. Dyon, J. F.: Contribution à l'étude du drainage des lymphatiques du poumon. Ph.D. dissertation, Université Scientifique et Médicale de Grenoble, 1973, pp. 199.
11. Spencer, H., and Leof, D.: The innervation of the human lung. J. Anat., 98:599–609, 1964.
12. Cabezas, G. A., Graf, P. D., and Nadel, J. A.: Sympathetic versus parasympathetic nervous regulation of the airways in dogs. J. Appl. Physiol., 31:651–655, 1971.
13. Fillenz, M.: Innervation of blood vessels of lung and spleen. Bibl. Anat., 8:56–59, 1966.
14. Daly, I. deB.: Intrinsic mechanisms of the lung. Quart. J. Exp. Physiol., 43:2–26, 1958.
15. Widdicombe, J. G., and Sterling, G. M.: The autonomic nervous system and breathing. Arch. Intern. Med., 126:311–329, 1970.
16. Paintal, A. S.: Vagal sensory receptors and their reflex effects. Physiol. Rev., 53:159–227, 1973.
17. Clark, F. J., and von Euler, C.: On the regulation of depth and rate of breathing. J. Physiol. (Lond.), 222:267–295, 1972.
18. Fishman, N. H., Phillipson, E. A., and Nadel, J. A.: Effect of differential vagal cold blockade on breathing pattern in conscious dogs. J. Appl. Physiol., 34:754–758, 1973.
19. Margaria, C. E., Iscoe, S., Pengelly, L. D., Couture, J., Don, H., and Milic-Emili, J.: Immediate ventilatory response to elastic loads and positive pressure in man. Resp. Physiol., 18:347–369, 1973.
20. Mead, J.: Control of respiratory frequency. J. Appl. Physiol., 15:325–326, 1960.
21. Guz, A., Noble, M. I. M., Widdicombe, J. G., Trenchard, D., Mushin, W. W., and Makey, A. R.: The role of vagal and glossopharyngeal afferent nerves in respiratory sensation, control of breathing and arterial pressure regulation in conscious man. Clin. Sci., 30:161–170, 1969.
22. Cross, K. W., Klaus, M., Tooley, W. H., and Weisser, K.: The response of the newborn to inflation of the lungs. J. Physiol. (Lond.), 151:551–565, 1960.
23. Fillenz, M., and Woods, R. I.: Sensory innervation of the airways. In Porter, R. (ed.): Ciba Foundation Symposium: Breathing: Hering-Breuer Centenary Symposium. London, J. & A. Churchill, 1970, pp. 101–107.
24. Jeffery, P., and Reid, L.: Intra-epithelial nerves in normal rat airways: a quantitative electron microscopic study. J. Anat., 114:35–45, 1973.
25. Meyrick, B., and Reid, L.: Nerves in rat intra-acinar alveoli: an electron microscopic study. Resp. Physiol., 11:367–377, 1971.
26. Paintal, A. S.: The mechanism of excitation of type J receptors, and the J reflex. In Porter, R. (ed.): Ciba Foundation Symposium: Breathing: Hering-Breuer Centenary Symposium. London, J. & A. Churchill, 1970, pp. 59–71.
27. Vaughan, T. R., DeMarino, E. M., and Staub, N. C.: Extravascular lung water in prolonged heavy exercise. Circulation, 50 (Suppl. III):24, 1974.
28. Stransky, A., Szereda-Przestaszewska, M., and Widdicombe, J. G.: The effects of lung reflexes on laryngeal resistance and motoneurone discharge. J. Physiol. (Lond.); 231:417–438, 1973.
29. Liebow, A. A.: New concepts and entities in pulmonary disease. In Liebow, A. A. (ed.): The Lung. International Academy of Pathology Monograph No. 8. Baltimore, The William and Wilkins Company, 1967, pp. 332–365.
30. Lauweryns, J. M., and Peuskens, J. C.: Neuro-epithelial bodies (neuroreceptor or secretory organs?) in human infant bronchial and bronchiolar epithelium. Anat. Rec., 172:471–482, 1972.

Chapter Four

VENTILATION

INTRODUCTION

Respiration can be defined as "those processes that contribute to gas exchange—the uptake of O_2 and the elimination of CO_2—between an organism and its environment." The previous chapters demonstrated that the structure of the mammalian lung, which evolved over eons, is elegantly designed for the efficient transfer of gases between gas in the alveoli and blood in the pulmonary capillaries. Moreover, it should be apparent that

77

the lung is also elaborately furnished to carry out its nonrespiratory functions, such as filtering the bloodstream, transforming biochemical substances, and serving as a reservoir of blood.

Gas exchange in man can be subdivided into three principal, but interdependent, functional components: (1) those concerned with the volume and distribution of *ventilation* within the lungs (Chapter 4), (2) those concerned with the volume and distribution of blood flow through the pulmonary *circulation* (Chapter 5), and (3) those concerned with the *diffusion* of O_2 and CO_2 across the air-blood barrier (Chapter 6). The air-blood barrier in the terminal respiratory units is the site at which inspired fresh air (ventilation) is brought into apposition with the film of blood flowing through the pulmonary capillaries (circulation).

Ventilation consists of the bulk movement of air from outside the body through the upper air passages and the subdivisions of the conducting airways into the terminal respiratory units. The amount of inspired air that reaches the sites of gas exchange is determined by the distensibility of the lung parenchyma and the factors that govern the movement of air as it flows through the tracheobronchial tree. Muscular effort (or force from a mechanical ventilator) is required to enlarge the lungs and thorax and to cause air to flow through the system. In other words, ventilation depends upon the capabilities of the respiratory muscles and the mechanical properties of the conducting airways and distal respiratory units.

This chapter will consider certain basic aspects of ventilation and the mechanics of respiration to provide a background for analysis of most of the commonly used tests of ventilatory function and of the principles on which they are based. Excellent review articles are available, if additional details are desired.[1-4]

STATIC PROPERTIES

COMPLIANCE

Everyone who has witnessed an autopsy has had the opportunity to notice that when the thorax is incised it enlarges and the lungs collapse. This simple observation vividly displays two fundamental static properties of the respiratory system: (1) the lungs tend to recoil inward and (2) the chest wall tends to recoil outward. Movements in opposite directions by the lung and chest wall are possible when the force that ordinarily couples them into a functioning unit, the pleural pressure, is removed.

The recoil properties of both the lung and the chest wall, which includes not only the rib cage but also the diaphragm and abdominal contents, are displayed in the static volume-pressure diagrams of the two component structures. Volume-pressure curves may be determined experimentally by measuring the pressure change that results from adding or subtracting a given volume to the system or by determining the volume change that results from the application of a known amount of pressure to the system. The relationship between changes in volume and changes in pressure defines the compliance of a structure, and is expressed as follows:

$$\text{Compliance} = \frac{\text{change in volume}}{\text{change in pressure}}. \quad (1)$$

Under ordinary conditions, any change in volume of the lung must be equaled by a corresponding change in volume of the chest wall, assuming no change in intrapulmonary blood volume.* This means that changes in volume are equal throughout the respiratory system (lungs and chest wall combined). Because changes in vol-

---

*This is not true in pathologic disturbances such as pneumothorax or pleural effusion.

ume are similar, the compliances of the respiratory system and its lung and chest wall components vary according to the change in the pressure differences "across" (i.e., from the inside to the outside) the various structures. These pressures are referred to as the distending pressures and are shown schematically in Figure 4-1. Under static relaxed conditions, the distending pressures for the lung, chest wall, and respiratory system can be written as follows:

pressure difference across lung (transpulmonary pressure) = alveolar pressure minus pleural pressure,

$$P_l = P_{alv} - P_{pl};$$

pressure difference across chest wall = pleural pressure minus body surface pressure,

$$P_w = P_{pl} - P_{bs};$$

pressure difference across respiratory system (transthoracic pressure) = alveolar pressure minus body surface pressure,

$$P_{rs} = P_{alv} - P_{bs};$$

or transpulmonary pressure plus pressure difference across chest wall,

$$P_{rs} = P_l + P_w.$$

It follows that the compliances of the lung (C_l), chest wall (C_w), and respiratory system (C_{rs}) relate the change in volume (ΔVol), which is the same throughout, to the appropriate static distending pressures so that

$$C_l = \frac{\Delta Vol, L}{P_l, cm\ H_2O}, \tag{2}$$

$$C_w = \frac{\Delta Vol, L}{P_w, cm\ H_2O}, \tag{3}$$

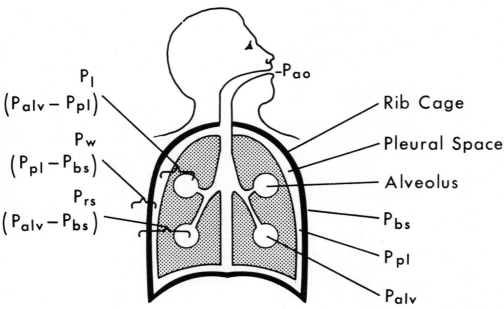

P_l

$(P_{alv} - P_{pl})$

P_w

$(P_{pl} - P_{bs})$

P_{rs}

$(P_{alv} - P_{bs})$

-P_{ao}

Rib Cage

Pleural Space

Alveolus

P_{bs}

P_{pl}

P_{alv}

Figure 4-1   Schematic representation of the pressures and pressure differences that determine ventilation. P_{ao} = pressure at the airway opening; P_{bs} = pressure at the body surface; P_{pl} = pressure within the pleural space; P_{alv} = pressure within the alveoli; P_l = pressure difference across the lung; P_w = pressure difference across the chest wall; and P_{rs} = pressure difference across the respiratory system.

$$C_{rs} = \frac{\Delta Vol, L}{P_{rs}, cm H_2O}, \text{ or}$$

$$= \frac{\Delta Vol, L}{(P_l + P_w), cm H_2O}.$$

(4)

A single value for compliance of the respiratory system or either of its components is of limited value for three reasons. (1) Volume-pressure curves for the separate structures and the structures combined are alinear. For example, the pressure-volume curve of the lung (Figure 4–2) is steepest at its origin and becomes flatter as inflation progresses; this means that compliance will have a higher value if derived from the lower part than from the upper part of the curve. (2) Conditions of measurement may affect the resulting values of compliance markedly. For example, volume-pressure curves of the lung obtained during inflation differ from those obtained during deflation due to hysteresis; similarly, the "volume-history" of the lungs (i.e., the pattern of ventilation) before the breathing sequence when volume and pressure are recorded will influence the measurements. (3) Total lung volume influences the absolute value of compliance. For example, a person with a large lung volume will have a higher lung compliance than a person with a small lung volume even though the lungs in both may be perfectly normal and have exactly the same distensibilities. The latter phenomenon has led to the use of the term *specific compliance*, or compliance divided by the lung volume at which it is measured, usually FRC.

In the discussion that follows, the volume-pressure curves through the entire range of vital capacity are shown, and it can be assumed that these are deflation curves (more reproducible than inflation curves) and that they were obtained after inflating the lung fully several times to ensure a constant volume history.

ELASTIC RECOIL OF THE LUNG

Because compliance is an expression of the distensibility of the elastic respiratory system, measured values of compliance depend upon the elastic recoil properties of the lung and chest wall. The lungs can be depicted for schematic purposes as two completely collapsible elastic balloons supported by a rigid Y-shaped tube (Figure 4–2A). As volume is added in increments through the tube to expand the collapsed lungs, pressure is generated within the system owing to the tendency for the elastic walls to recoil inward (Figure 4–2B). The magnitude and direction of the recoil forces are represented by the size and direction of the arrows in the figures. As more volume is added, the lungs continue to expand, but finally the volume-pressure curve begins to flatten as the elastic elements reach the limits of their distensibility (Figure 4–2C). At this pressure, the volume of the lung is maximal, and attempts to increase the volume further cause a huge rise in pressure due to the flatness of the volume-pressure curve, and the lungs are apt to rupture.

It can be seen from Figure 4–2 that under static conditions the pressure generated by the lung is determined solely by its elastic recoil pressure (P_{stl}). This means that when the airways are open and there is no airflow, static elastic recoil pressure is equal to transpulmonary pressure ($P_{sl} = P_l = P_{alv} - P_{pl}$). It follows that under static conditions, when $P_{alv} = 0$, both P_{sl} and P_l are equal and opposite to P_{pl}. This is easy to understand by considering the situation of a subject holding his breath at any lung volume with his glottis open (so that $P_{alv} = 0$). Because the tendency of the lungs to recoil inward establishes the transpulmonary pressure, to keep the lungs inflated to that volume, pleural pressure must be equal and opposite to recoil pressure ($-P_{pl} = P_l = P_{stl}$).

The relationship between elastic

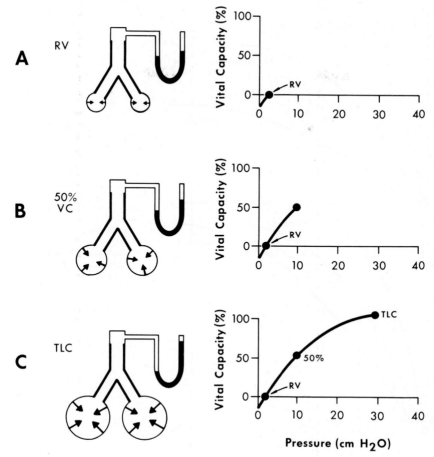

Figure 4–2 Schematic representation of the volume-pressure relationships of isolated lungs. *A*, Because excised lungs collapse to less than residual volume (RV), at RV a small recoil pressure (indicated by small arrows facing inward) is evident; this pressure is reflected in the slight deflection of the column in the manometer and the value on the horizontal (pressure) axis. *B*, At 50 per cent vital capacity (VC), the recoil pressure is increased (more and larger arrows than in *A*); thus more pressure is reflected in the manometer and on the horizontal axis. *C*, At total lung capacity (TLC), recoil pressure is maximal (normally about 30 cm H_2O).

recoil and compliance is also depicted in Figure 4–2. Because compliance is defined as a change in volume resulting from a change in pressure, it is derived from the volume-pressure curve as the *slope* of the line ($\Delta Vol/\Delta P$) at any point along the line. The *position* of the line depends upon the elastic recoil of the lungs.

The lungs of patients with emphysema are more distensible and the lungs of patients with diffuse intersti-

tial fibrosis or other infiltrative diseases are less distensible, or stiffer, than normal lungs. Representative volume-pressure curves from adults with normal lungs, with emphysema, and with pulmonary fibrosis are shown in Figure 4–3; the curves were compiled assuming that the three persons are similar in age and body build so that they should have lungs with similar vital capacities and volume-pressure relationships. The curve from the pa-

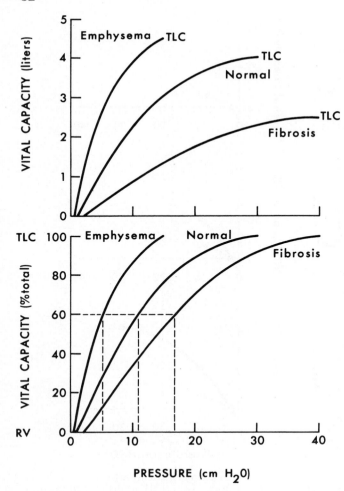

Figure 4–3 Representative volume-pressure curves from adult subjects of the same age, sex, and body size showing changes caused by emphysema and pulmonary fibrosis compared with normal lungs. *Upper panel* depicts volume-pressure relations in terms of measured (i.e., observed) vital capacity and demonstrates that emphysematous lungs are larger and fibrotic lungs smaller than normal. When expressed in terms of percentage of measured vital capacity (*lower panel*), at any given vital capacity (e.g., 60 per cent, shown by dashed lines), elastic recoil pressure is less than normal in emphysema and greater than normal in fibrosis. TLC = total lung capacity; RV = residual volume.

tient with emphysema is steeper and shifts above the normal curve, whereas the curve from the patient with fibrosis is flatter and shifts below. When expressed at any given lung volume or per cent of vital capacity (e.g., 60 per cent, as shown in Figure 4–3), elastic recoil is lower than normal in the patient with emphysema and higher than normal in the patient with fibrosis. Thus, values of elastic recoil can be used to describe the static properties of normal and abnormal lungs; but, as will be described subsequently, elastic recoil also is an important determinant of the dynamic behavior of the lungs.

MEASUREMENT OF PLEURAL PRESSURE

A measurement of pleural pressure is obviously necessary for the assessment of the pulmonary elastic recoil properties of both normal subjects and patients with pulmonary diseases. Although it is difficult and dangerous to measure pressure directly from the pleural space in human beings, the problem has been largely overcome through the use of pressure recordings from a balloon positioned in the subject's esophagus. Because the esophagus is located between the two pleural spaces, esophageal pressure measurements, when carried out correctly, provide a close approximation of pleural pressure at the level of the balloon in the thorax.[5] Static volume-pressure (elastic recoil) curves of the lung can be obtained by measuring esophageal pressure at different lung volumes while the subject holds his breath with his glottis open to eliminate the effect of changes in alveolar pressure. Values are usually recorded after the subject has maximally inflated his lungs a few times to ensure a constant volume history. Measurements are made first at full inspiration and then at successively decreasing lung volumes to FRC to provide a deflation volume-pressure curve; studies between FRC and residual volume are less reliable owing to inaccuracies in the measurement of esophageal pressure at low lung volumes.

ORIGIN OF LUNG ELASTIC RECOIL

The total force causing the inflated human lung to recoil inward has two

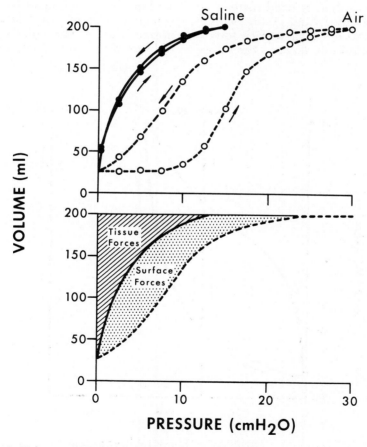

Figure 4–4 Volume-pressure curves of lungs filled with saline and with air (*upper panel*). The use of saline eliminates the effect of surface forces at the air-liquid interface and allows subdivision of the total pressure required to inflate the lung into the amounts necessary to overcome tissue forces and surface forces (*lower panel*). The arrows indicate whether the lung is being inflated or deflated; note that when using saline, hysteresis (i.e., the difference between inflation and deflation limbs of the curve) is virtually eliminated. (Adapted from Clements and Tierney.[7] Reprinted by permission from the authors and publisher.)

different origins: part arises from the elastic properties of the lung tissue itself and part arises from the film of surface-active material that lines the terminal respiratory units. The two components of elastic recoil were first deduced by von Neergaard[6] over 40 years ago, and their separate influences can be demonstrated by repeating his classic experiment of comparing the volume-pressure relationships of the air-filled lung with those of the saline-filled lung. It can be seen in Figure 4–4 that less pressure is required to inflate the lung to a given volume and that hysteresis is nearly absent when saline is used instead of air. Filling the lung with saline eliminates the effect of surface forces at the air-liquid interfaces in the lungs

and demonstrates the effect of surface forces on pulmonary compliance and hysteresis.

Surface Forces. The surface forces at the air-liquid interfaces are determined by the surface tension of the thin film of surfactant that covers the surface of terminal respiratory units and probably also lines the luminal surface of terminal bronchioles. (The cellular origin, metabolism, and anatomic location of the surface-active material are described in Chapters 1 and 2.) The important property of pulmonary surfactant is that its surface tension decreases remarkably as the area of the surface layer is reduced, as shown in Figure 4–5. Surfactant from normal lung is particularly unique in its behavior and demonstrates the

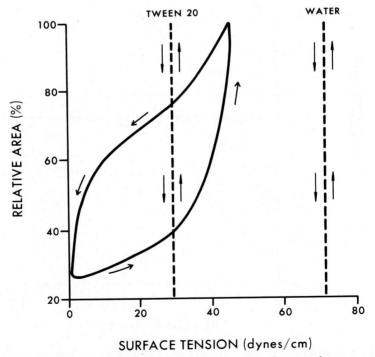

Figure 4–5 Surface area–surface tension relationships for lung washings containing normal surfactant (solid lines) and for Tween 20 (a detergent) and H_2O (dashed lines). Note that when the surface film containing surfactant is reduced in area, its surface tension decreases nearly to 0 dynes/cm. The arrows indicate expansion (upward) or compression (downward) of the material. Note the similarity between the hysteresis loops in lung washings and normal lungs (Fig. 4–4). (Adapted from Clements and Tierney.[7] Reprinted by permission from the authors and publisher.)

lowest surface tension of any biologic substance ever measured. Furthermore, when studied *in vitro*, lung surfactant displays a striking hysteresis loop (Figure 4–5) that is qualitatively similar to and presumably accounts for the hysteresis encountered when filling and emptying the normal lung with air (Figure 4–4).

To summarize, the presence of surface forces at the air-liquid interface adds to the pressure required to distend the lung (i.e., compliance is decreased); however, the special properties of surfactant minimize this effect: surface tension is low to begin with and decreases even further when surface area (i.e., lung volume) decreases. Furthermore, if surface tension did not decrease with decreasing lung volumes, peripheral airspaces and airways would become unstable and tend to collapse; thus, the presence of the surface-active substance in normal amounts and location serves to stabilize the lung and prevent atelectasis.[7] In diseases in which surfactant is either inactivated or decreased in amount (e.g., neonatal respiratory distress syndrome), pulmonary compliance is characteristically low and multiple areas of atelectasis develop.

Tissue Forces. It is not known precisely in which structural elements the lung tissue elasticity resides. In contrast to previous concepts, recent evidence (from experiments in rats in which different connective tissue elements were digested with specific enzymes) suggests that elastin rather than collagen is the chief connective tissue determinant of the lung's tissue forces.[8]

The respective contributions of tissue and surface forces to total compliance differ at low and high lung volumes; it can be seen in Figure 4–4 that at low lung volumes, surface forces are the chief determinant of the lung's distensibility, but at high lung volumes, tissue forces predominate. This difference is attributable to the changing pressure-volume relations of the elastic structures and to the aug-

mented effects of surface tensions (T) on pressure (P) when the radius of curvature (r) is small. These relationships are expressed in the Laplace equation for a spherical structure:

$$P = \frac{2T}{r}. \qquad (5)$$

Therefore, even though the surface tension of the surface layer decreases strikingly as lung volume is reduced, the effects are more than offset by the effects of deflation on alveolar geometry and on the radius of curvature. Moreover, at low lung volumes the elastic elements are operating on the steepest segments (i.e., most distensible) of their pressure-volume curve. Conversely, the mechanical advantage gained by the effects of increasing lung volume on the radius of curvature during inflation more than offsets the effects of increasing surface tension from surface area expansion; at high lung volumes, the elastic elements are reaching the limits of their distensibility and are operating on the flat portion of the pressure-volume curve.

ELASTIC RECOIL OF THE CHEST WALL

The chest wall can be depicted for schematic purposes as a compressible and distensible structure that contains an appreciable volume in its resting state (Figure 4–6A). If the volume of the thorax-diaphragm is reduced by contraction of the muscles of expiration, the chest wall tends to resist compression and by recoiling outward to its resting volume creates a negative pressure within the system (Figure 4–6B). The pressure exerted by the expiratory muscles to empty the thorax a given volume must, therefore, overcome the outward recoil pressure generated by the chest wall at that volume. Conversely, if the thorax is made to

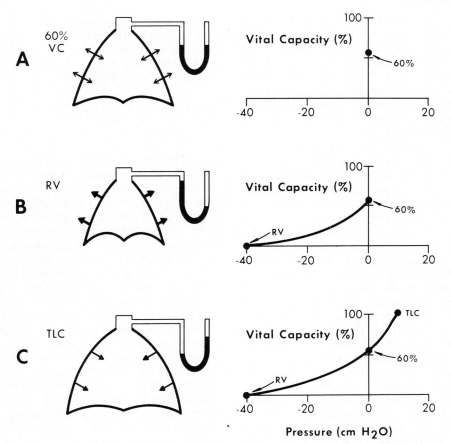

Figure 4-6 Schematic representation of the volume-pressure relationships of the isolated chest wall. *A*, The chest wall in the relaxed position (zero pressure) has a volume approximately 60 per cent of vital capacity (VC). *B*, When the chest wall is compressed to residual volume (RV), it tends to recoil outward to its resting position and thus generates the negative pressure shown on the manometer and horizontal axis. *C*, When the chest wall is expanded to total lung capacity (TLC), the chest wall tends to recoil inward and thereby generates the positive pressure shown on the manometer and horizontal axis.

accommodate a larger volume by contraction of the inspiratory muscles (Figure 4–6*C*), the muscular effort must overcome the positive pressure generated by the tendency of the chest wall to recoil inward back to its resting position.

ELASTIC RECOIL OF THE RESPIRATORY SYSTEM

It is useful for introductory purposes to describe the recoil characteristics of the lung and chest wall separately, but obviously they have to be considered in concert, because their physiologic functions are interdependent. The two structures can be viewed as being in series with each other, and therefore, the pressure of the (total) respiratory system is the algebraic sum of the pressure generated by both the lung and the chest wall: $P_{rs} = P_l + P_w$. Because any given volume change is equal throughout the respiratory system, the lungs and the chest wall, the separate volume-pressure curves shown in Figures 4–2 and 4–6 can be combined into one for the total respiratory system by simply adding the pressures at a chosen volume (Figure 4–7). The resulting curve indicates the pressure that must be applied by contraction of the respiratory muscles, or by a mechanical respirator, to achieve a volume change throughout the respiratory system; under static conditions, the total pressure must equal the sum of the pressures required to offset the elastic recoil pressures of the lung and chest wall at that volume.

LUNG VOLUMES

The volume-pressure diagram of the respiratory system and its components also provides an easily understood explanation about the determi-

nants of normal lung volumes. Moreover, abnormalities in these relationships account for the characteristic lung volume changes in various diseases such as pulmonary emphysema and interstitial fibrosis. It can be seen in Figure 4–7 that FRC occurs normally at the volume of the total system at which the inward recoil force of the lung is equal and opposite to the outward recoil force of the chest wall; in other words, the resting volume (FRC) is that volume at which the net force in the respiratory system is zero.

During a continuous inspiration, the net force developed by the contracting muscles of respiration (agonist and antagonist groups) meets progressively increasing recoil forces from the combined expansion of the lung and chest wall. Furthermore, as

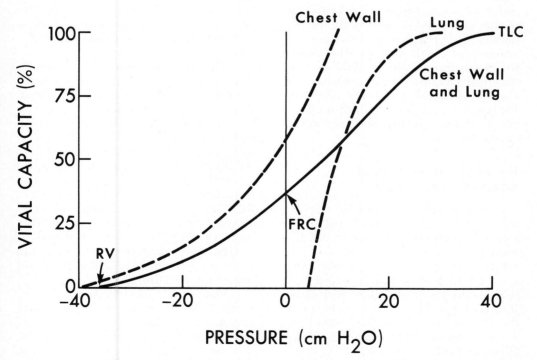

Figure 4–7   Schematic representation of the volume-pressure relationships of the chest wall and lung combined (solid line). The combined curve is obtained by summation of the recoil pressures of the isolated chest wall (dashed line and Figure 4–6) and the isolated lung (dashed line and Figure 4–2). TLC = total lung capacity; FRC = functional residual capacity; RV = residual volume. (Adapted from Rahn, Otis, Chadwick, and Fenn.[9] Reprinted by permission from the authors and publisher.)

the contracting muscle fibers shorten, they generate progressively less force. Finally, *total lung capacity* (TLC) is the volume at which inspiration ceases because the opposing forces are balanced (i.e., the weakening forces of inspiration can no longer overcome the increasing force required to distend the lungs and chest wall).

Similarly, during a continuous expiration the net force developed by the contracting muscles encounters increasing opposition from the recoil force in the system, which originates chiefly from the chest wall (Figure 4–7). In children and young adults, expiration ceases at the volume at which the opposing forces are equal (i.e., expiratory muscle force is insufficient to cause a further reduction in chest wall volume); *residual volume* (RV), therefore, in young subjects is determined by the balance of forces operating in the chest wall. In older persons, however, RV appears to be governed increasingly by the factors that regulate the caliber and patency of small airways; this means that even though the respiratory muscles are capable of compressing the chest wall and emptying the lung further, they are prevented from doing so by airway closure and trapping of gas in the lung.[10]

FACTORS HOLDING LUNG AGAINST CHEST WALL

As just described, at FRC the lung and chest wall tend to recoil in opposite directions, creating forces that tend to separate the visceral from the parietal pleura; if the layers were allowed to part, a space would form that would need to be filled with either liquid or gas. The lung and chest wall do *not* separate from each other but remain apposed throughout their ventilatory excursions owing to the mechanisms that prevent gas and liquid from collecting in the pleural space. Moreover, the same mechanisms operate to cause the removal of gas from a pneumothorax or liquid from a pleural

effusion, if either is formed as part of a pathologic process.

The pleural space, though an anatomically delimited cavity, is otherwise analogous to a tissue space and is therefore governed by the same mechanisms that regulate the pressure of gases everywhere in the body. This subject is treated more fully in the section on Gas Exchange (Chapter 6) because it depends upon the respective shapes of the oxyhemoglobin and the CO_2 dissociation curves. The net result of the exchange of respiratory gases between blood and cells determines that the sum of the partial pressures of all the individual gases in capillaries and venous blood (O_2, CO_2, N_2, H_2O) will be about 700 mm Hg and that interstitial tissues will be exposed to a gas pressure that is nearly 60 mm Hg subatmospheric (760 − 700 mm Hg). The high negative pressure serves to keep the pleural space free of gas and to cause the absorption of gases once they are introduced into any part of the body.

The pleural cavity is not totally devoid of liquid, and under normal conditions a small amount is present. The volume has never been determined accurately in healthy man but is presumed to be only a few milliliters at most; in the normal dog, weighing about 10 kg, pleural liquid collections averaged 2.4 ml.[11] The liquid forms a very thin film of uniform thickness that couples the parietal and visceral pleural surfaces, enabling them to slide over each other and allowing the instantaneous transmission of forces between the chest wall and the contiguous lung.

The exact site of formation of pleural liquid under normal circumstances is not known but is believed to be through the parietal pleura. Thus, the rate of transudation is governed primarily by the permeability characteristics of the parietal pleural membrane and the opposing hydrostatic and osmotic forces across the endothelium of capillaries in the chest wall (see Chapter 5 for a discussion of the factors that affect liquid movement).

Once formed, pleural liquid is removed either by the bloodstream or by lymphatics. The evidence favors absorption of most of the liquid by lymphatic capillaries located within the visceral pleura; lymphatic uptake may be facilitated during inflation by the formation of intermittent dehiscences between adjacent mesothelial cells of the visceral surface of the lung that provide access to underlying lymphatic vessels.[11] In contrast, cells and particles appear to be removed through preformed stomata within the parietal pleura that connect the pleural and lymphatic spaces. Although the precise mechanisms of pleural liquid formation and removal are incompletely understood, it is clear that the balance of forces serves to keep the pleural space virtually free of liquid. This balance appears to be finely regulated and easily disrupted, judging from the frequency with which pleural effusions are encountered in different diseases.

The pressure in the pleural liquid is slightly more negative than that on the pleural surface, which is determined by the elastic recoil of the lung. The difference between the two pressures is due to the added effect in the liquid of the pressure from the forces of deformation in the walls of the pleural cavity (those forces which resist a closer apposition of the pleural surfaces). Pleural liquid pressure is an important determinant of the movement of liquid into and out of the pleural cavity in normal subjects and in patients with pleural effusions. But when considering the transmission of mechanical forces between the lung and chest wall, the pleural (surface) pressure is the one that counts.[11]

PLEURAL PRESSURE GRADIENT

In the discussion thus far, pleural pressure has been considered to have a single uniform value at any given lung volume. Not only is this useful

for descriptive purposes, but also the customary method of measuring pleural pressure in man by the esophageal balloon technique yields a single value for a given lung volume. However, it is now well established from evidence obtained by several different experimental approaches that there is a gradient in pleural pressure between top and bottom of the lung; the result is that pleural pressure is lowest, or most negative, at the top and is highest or least negative, at the bottom of the lung. The magnitude of the gradient is about 0.20 to 0.25 cm H_2O per cm vertical distance in the normal human lung. This means that in the upright position, transpulmonary pressure ($P_{alv} - P_{pl}$) is greatest, or most positive, at the apices of the lung and is lowest, or least positive, at the bases. At lung volumes above and below FRC, the data on the vertical distribution of pleural pressure are controversial, but a gradient is observed to a varying degree in all body positions. From the studies available, it can be inferred in man that at FRC, pleural pressure and transpulmonary pressure vary, as shown in Table 4-1.[11]

The factors that contribute to the gradient of pleural pressure are complex and appear to include the effects of lung weight, the effect of gravity on the chest wall, and the support of the lung afforded by the hilum and abdominal contents. Although the causes of the

Table 4-1   Representative Pleural Pressures (P_{pl}) and Transpulmonary Pressures (P_l) in cm H_2O at the Top and Bottom of the Lung in a Normal Man at FRC*

	TOP		BOTTOM	
POSITION	P_{pl}	P_l	P_{pl}	P_l
Sitting	−8	8	−2	2
Lateral	−6	6	0	0
Supine	−4	4	0	0
Prone	−3.5	3.5	0	0

*Data from Agostoni.[11]

vertical gradient of pleural pressure are not fully understood, its consequences and those of the resulting gradient in transpulmonary pressure have been examined extensively in recent years. The functional implications of the higher transpulmonary pressure at the top compared with that at the bottom of the lung are the following.

1. Regional differences in lung volumes are created, such that alveoli at the top of the lung are more fully expanded at FRC than those at the bottom; these differences have been thoroughly documented in studies of both man[12] and experimental animals.[13] Functional evidence for the presence of regional differences in lung volumes in man is reproduced in Figure 4–8, and morphometric evidence from experimental animals is presented in Figure 4–9. Regional discrepancies in volume become less marked as the lung is progressively inflated, and at TLC, alveoli at the top and bottom are virtually equal in size.

2. Because the volume-pressure curve is believed to be the same for different regions regardless of their location within the normal lung, the higher distending pressure at the top compared with that at the bottom means that alveoli in the two regions are operating on different portions of the same curve. This causes them to expand differently when a given *change* in distending pressure, which is uniformly distributed throughout the lung, is added to the different initial values (Figure 4–10). For this reason, at lung volumes above FRC, alveoli at

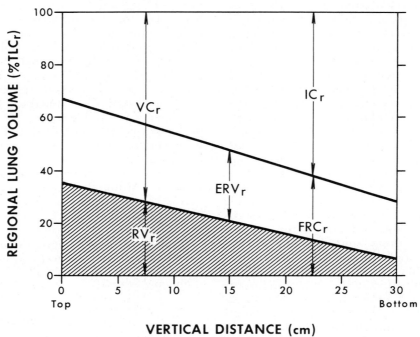

Figure 4–8   Schematic representation of the changes in regional lung volumes, expressed as a percentage of regional total lung capacity (%TLC$_r$), at varying distances from the top to the bottom of the vertical lungs of healthy men. Measurements were made at full expiration (lower heavy line) and at resting end-expiratory lung volume (upper heavy line). VC$_r$ = regional vital capacity; RV$_r$ = regional residual volume; ERV$_r$ = regional expiratory reserve volume; IC$_r$ = regional inspiratory capacity; FRC$_r$ = regional functional residual capacity. (Adapted from Milic-Emili, Henderson, Dolovich, Trop, and Kaneko.[12] Reprinted by permission from the authors and publisher.)

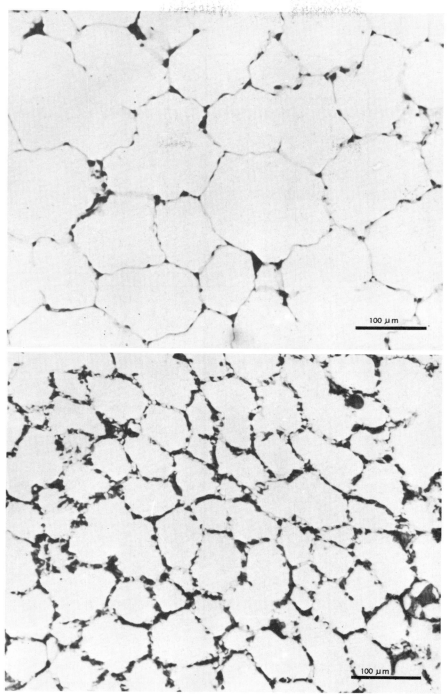

Figure 4–9 Sections of lung from the apex (*upper panel*) and 20 cm below the apex (*lower panel*) obtained from a greyhound dog frozen in the vertical position. At functional residual capacity it is obvious that the alveolar spaces are larger at the apex than near the base. Horizontal bar = 100 μm. ($\times$ 188. Courtesy of Dr. Jon B. Glazier.)

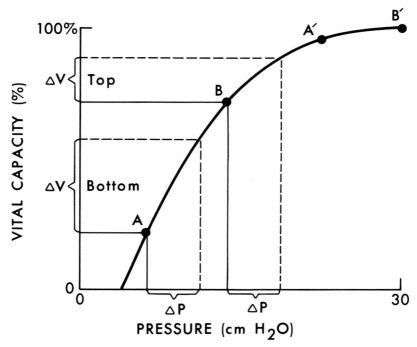

Figure 4–10 Volume-pressure curve of a normal lung (heavy solid line). At functional residual capacity, distending pressure is less at the bottom than at the top; accordingly, alveoli at the bottom (A) are smaller (i.e., lower per cent vital capacity) than those at the top (B). When a given amount of distending pressure (ΔP) is applied to the lung, alveoli at the bottom increase their volume (ΔV) more than alveoli at the top, owing to the varying steepness of the volume-pressure curve. When fully expanded to total lung capacity (100% VC), alveoli at the bottom (A′) are nearly the same size as alveoli at the top (B′) because both points lie on the flat portion of the curve.

the bottom expand considerably more than those at the top. Accordingly, during normal breathing at rest, the lowermost regions ordinarily ventilate more than the uppermost regions; this difference increases the efficiency of gas exchange because, under these same conditions, there is also more blood flow to the bottom of the lungs than to the top (Chapter 6).

3. When pleural pressure in the lowermost lung regions becomes positive, or, in other words, transpulmonary pressure becomes negative, there is a compressing force that tends to close airways. If blood flow continues to the terminal respiratory units distal to the site of airway closure, gas exchange is impaired. Airway closure may occur in the dependent lung regions of normal elderly persons breath-

ing at FRC, and premature closure is characteristic of certain diseases such as obesity, emphysema, and bronchitis. This phenomenon is a subject of considerable interest because it can now be studied by relatively simple tests, described below, for "closing volume."[14–16]

CLOSING VOLUME

The closing volume test measures the lung volume at which lower lung zones cease to ventilate, presumably as a result of airway closure. The closing volume has been measured using a variety of techniques that fall into two general categories: those that use a bolus of foreign gas such as Xe, Ar, or He (the bolus method) and those that use the N_2 normally present in alveolar gas (the resident gas or N_2 method). Both techniques depend on the creation, at full inspiration, of a pre-expiratory concentration difference of a marker gas between the top and bottom of the lung with the upper zones relatively rich in marker gas and the lower zones relatively poor.

The principle of the bolus method for measuring closing volume depends upon the fact that the distribution in the lungs of a test gas when inhaled is determined by the lung volume at which the gas is introduced into the air stream. As stated earlier, when a subject breathes normally at FRC, the inspired air is distributed predominantly to the dependent lung regions. However, when inspiration begins at or near RV, the usual pattern of distribution is reversed. Most of the initial inspirate goes to the upper regions because airways leading to the lower (dependent) regions are nonventilated.

The bolus method of measuring closing volume is performed by having a subject exhale to RV and hold his breath momentarily. The initial part of the next inspirate is labeled with a small bolus of a test gas (e.g., ^{133}Xe, He, Ar) as the subject inhales slowly to TLC. A record of the subsequent expiration (Figure 4–11) reflects the appearance of the test gas, and its concentration in the expirate measured at the mouth varies according to the sequence of regional emptying. During slow expiration, emptying normally takes place in an orderly and sequential fashion from bottom to top of the lungs. Because most of the bolus is inhaled to the uppermost regions of the lung, after airway closure begins to occur at the bases late in expiration, the expirate progressively reflects the high concentration of the preferentially labeled upper regions.

The record, as shown, can be sub-

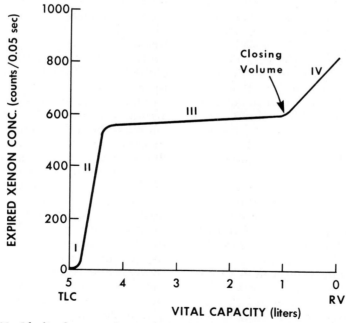

Figure 4–11 Idealized tracing of expired xenon concentration during a slow exhalation from total lung capacity (TLC) to residual volume (RV) after the previous breath has been labeled with a bolus of xenon. Explanation for the breathing maneuver and the four phases (I to IV) of washout is given in the text. Closing volume (arrow) is the vital capacity remaining at the junction between phase III and phase IV.

divided into four phases: phase I, gas from conducting airways (anatomic dead space gas); phase II, mixed dead space and alveolar gas; phase III, the "alveolar plateau" consisting of mixed alveolar gas—the upward slope of the plateau is explained by the combination of gravity-dependent regional inequality of gas distribution (i.e., between lobes) and stratified inhomogeneity of gas mixing within lung units (i.e., within lobes; see subsequent section for additional details); and phase IV, closure of airways in the dependent lung regions and extension of this phenomenon into more and more of the neighboring lung regions. The steep slope of phase IV is caused by airways progressively closing in the bases so that the expirate contains more and more gas of high concentration from alveoli at the top of the lung.

Closing volume is defined as the volume of gas remaining in the vital capacity at the intersection of phases III and IV and is usually expressed as per cent of vital capacity (CV/VC, %). The term "closing capacity" is used to express the combination of closing volume and RV (CC = CV + RV) and is usually expressed as per cent of TLC (CC/TLC, %). Because the CC/TLC ratio has less variability than the CV/VC ratio and because closing capacity includes RV, which itself changes early in diseases causing airway obstruction, the CC/TLC ratio is perhaps the better measurement of the two.

The principle of the resident gas method also depends on establishing a regional gradient of a gas, in this case N_2, during a single breath of 100 per cent O_2 from RV to TLC. Figure 4–8 shows that the RV of alveoli at the base of the lung is less than that of alveoli at the top. Because both inflate to nearly the same volume at TLC, alveoli at the base receive more O_2 and have a lower N_2 concentration than alveoli at the top. Thus, a gradient of N_2 concentrations, highest at the top

and lowest at the bottom, is created. When a subject whose lungs are "labeled" with these N_2 differences exhales, a recording of expired N_2 concentration plotted against expired volume yields a tracing similar to the one shown in Figure 4–11.

Closure is believed to occur in small (< 1 mm) airways whose patency is determined normally by the transpulmonary pressure across them and by the compliance of their walls; in addition, the stability of small airways at low lung volumes may depend, in part, upon the presence of surfactant that is believed to line the luminal surface. Thickening of the airway wall or excessive secretions will narrow the lumen and cause premature closure. Physiologic[17] and morphologic[18] evidence in favor of airway closure has been obtained from animal experiments, but no convincing data are available in man. It is possible that dynamic compression of airways (see subsequent section on flow-volume relations) and slowing of emptying, rather than complete closure and cessation of flow, accounts for phase IV.[19] Regardless of whether flow stops entirely or just slows markedly, the size of the lumen of small airways depends in part upon the distending pressure and tethering effect of elastic elements acting upon them. Because these are known to be low in young children, to increase during maturation, and to diminish with advancing age, the airways of a child and an old person will not be "held open" as well as those of a young adult. Therefore, closing volume, as a percent of vital capacity, decreases during growth and increases during senescence.[14, 20] Although closing volume remains relatively constant despite variations in body position, FRC decreases upon changing from the upright to the supine position and under these conditions may be less than closing volume. When closing volume exceeds FRC (as in young and old persons, and especially in the recumbent position), dependent regions of the lung are poorly ventilated and abnormalities of gas exchange may result (see Chapter 7 for discussion of mechanisms).

The value of the closing volume test in the early detection of lung disease remains to be established. However, the implications of variations in airway closure caused by age, changes in body position, and lung disease on gas exchange in normal subjects and in patients are extremely important and are considered further in Chapters 6 and 12.

DYNAMIC PROPERTIES

To cause air to move from outside the body into the terminal respiratory units, a force must be applied to the respiratory system that is sufficient to overcome three opposing forces: (1) the elastic recoil of the lungs and chest wall, (2) the frictional resistance afforded by the airways and by the tissues of the lungs and thorax, and (3) the inertance (impedance of acceleration) of the entire system. The elastic forces of the lung and chest wall, as discussed in the previous section, depend upon the volume introduced into the system and are not affected by motion (i.e., rate of deformation) within the system. In contrast, frictional resistance is determined by the *rate* of change of volume (i.e., flow) and not by the magnitude of the change in volume *per se*. Inertance depends upon the rate of change of flow (i.e., acceleration) of the gas and of the tissues that compose the system.

Analysis of the mechanical properties of the respiratory system can be simplified because inertance has been found to be a negligible quantity during normal breathing and because the contributions of elastic forces and flow-resistance forces can be separated by studying the system under static and dynamic conditions, respectively.

FRICTIONAL RESISTANCE

Resistance to airflow in the respiratory system is computed from simultaneous measurements of the airflow and the pressure difference causing the airflow. Resistance is calculated according to the general equation:

$$\text{Resistance} = \frac{\text{pressure difference}}{\text{rate of flow}}. \quad (6)$$

Airflow is easy to measure, but the pressure differences that cause air to flow require specialized recording equipment. However, by measuring the appropriate individual pressure differences that are described subsequently, the flow-resistance properties of individual components of the respiratory system can be analyzed separately, i.e., the airways, the tissues of lung parenchyma, and the tissues of the thorax and abdomen that surround the respiratory tract and are deformed by its movements. The various resistances that can be calculated by measurement of different "driving pressures" are as follows.

1. *Airway resistance* (R_{aw}) is defined as the frictional resistance afforded by the entire system of air passages to airflow from outside the body to within the alveoli. Airway resistance is determined from the simultaneous measurements of the flow and the pressure difference between the airway opening (P_{ao}) and the alveoli. These variables can all be measured accurately in the body plethysmograph[21]; accordingly,

$$R_{aw} = \frac{P_{ao} - P_{alv}, \text{cm H}_2\text{O}}{\text{flow, L/sec}}. \quad (7)$$

2. *Pulmonary resistance* (R_1) is defined as the frictional resistance afforded by the lungs and air passages combined. Hence, pulmonary resistance is the sum of lung-tissue resistance and airway resistance and is

determined from the simultaneous measurements of the flow and the pressure difference between the airway opening and the pleural space. The total pleural pressure must be corrected by subtracting, either graphically or electronically, the lung elastic pressure to obtain the lung resistive pressure ($P_{pl[cor]}$). Given these variables,

$$R_l = \frac{P_{ao} - P_{pl(cor)}, \text{cm H}_2\text{O}}{\text{flow, L/sec}}. \quad (8)$$

Because pulmonary resistance consists of both the frictional resistance of the airways (R_{aw}) and the *frictional (viscous) resistance of lung tissue* (R_{lt}), the latter, which cannot be measured separately, may be derived by subtraction:

$$R_{lt} = R_l - R_{aw}, \text{cm H}_2\text{O per L/sec}. \quad (9)$$

3. *Chest wall tissue resistance* (R_w) is defined as the frictional resistance of the chest wall and abdominal structures. Chest wall tissue resistance is determined from the simultaneous measurements of the flow and the pressure difference from the pleura to the body surface, after subtracting from the total pressure difference the amount required to overcome the elastic recoil of the chest, leaving a corrected value ($P_{bs[cor]}$):

$$R_w = \frac{P_{pl} - P_{bs(cor)}, \text{cm H}_2\dot{\text{O}}}{\text{flow, L/sec}}. \quad (10)$$

Chest wall resistance can be measured by using a respirator[1] or the oscillation technique[22] and an esophageal balloon to record the appropriate pressure difference across the chest wall; by either method, however, it is difficult to avoid the spurious effects from respiratory muscle contractions.

PARTITIONING OF FRICTIONAL RESISTANCE

Only a limited number of complete studies have been performed on normal subjects to assess the total frictional resistance of the entire respiratory system and to subdivide the total into the parts contributed by the various components of the system.[3] A graphic representation of how frictional resistance is partitioned is shown in Figure 4–12. The flow resistance contributions of the various components vary depending upon the flow rate. For reference purposes, it should be pointed out that the peak flow rates achieved during quiet breathing are about 0.4 L/sec and between 1.25 and 1.50 L/sec during mild exercise (minute volume 25 to 30 L/min). Figure 4–12 also shows that the resistance offered by the nose is the largest single component, comprising one-half to two-thirds of the airway resistance during nasal breathing at low flow rates. The resistance of the nose, which is markedly nonlinear, increases proportionately much more than flow as flow increases and must become prohibitively large during heavy exercise. The transition from nose to mouth breathing presumably occurs for this reason when flow through the nasal passages requires pressures of 6 to 8 cm H_2O.[23]

The resistance offered by the oropharynx and larynx is also nonlinear and accounts for about 40 per cent of the resistance offered by all the air passages during quiet mouth breathing. As flow rate increases, the partition of frictional resistance becomes weighted toward an increased contribution of either the nose or the oropharynx owing to their nonlinear flow-resistance characteristics. The contribution of the larynx is minimized by the widening that occurs from reflex activity during deep breathing.

By the technique of measuring pressures in the trachea and small

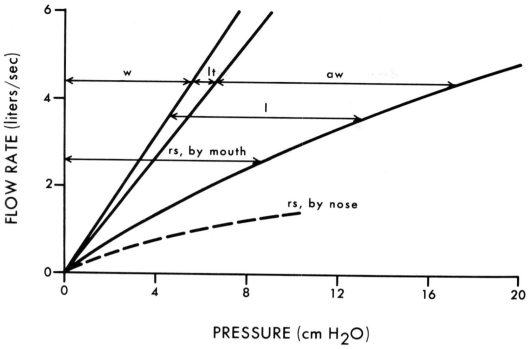

Figure 4–12 Schematic representation of the flow-pressure relationships of the respiratory system (rs) of normal man breathing through the nose or mouth. The distance from the vertical axis to the curves or between one curve and another indicates the pressure necessary to overcome the frictional resistance imposed by the various components of the respiratory system at a given flow (e.g., the horizontal lines). w = chest wall; lt = lung tissue; aw = airway; l = pulmonary (lung tissue + airway). (Adapted from Fenn and Rahn[3] [Chapter 14 by Mead and Agostoni]. Reprinted by permission from the authors and publisher.)

airways, resistance of the tracheobronchial tree can be partitioned into contributions from the large or central airways (trachea and all branches out to about 2 mm diameter) and from the small or peripheral airways (< about 2 mm diameter).[24] Studies of excised human lungs and of both living and excised animal lungs (Figure 4–13) revealed that peripheral airways resistance is only a small proportion of the total resistance afforded by the entire tracheobronchial tree.[24, 25] This conclusion is in agreement with recent morphometric data and calculations that reveal a progressively increasing total cross-sectional area of all airways of a given generation as airway size decreases[26] (see also Figure 2–2). However, the distribution of resist-

ance probably varies in normal subjects, and undoubtedly does in patients, depending upon vagal activity and the extent and location of bronchomotor tone.

The observations about the partitioning of tracheobronchial resistance are important in clinical disorders that affect the caliber of small bronchi and bronchioles. Because these airways contribute very little to total flow resistance, significant disease may occur in them that will not be detected by simple routine pulmonary function tests. For this reason, Mead[27] has called peripheral airways the "quiet zone" of the lung, and much effort has been directed toward developing new tests and methods for identifying obstruction in small airways.[28] It is im-

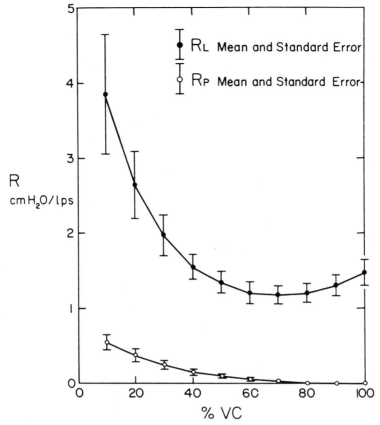

Figure 4–13 Mean values of measurements of pulmonary flow resistance (RL) and peripheral resistance (RP) at different percentages of vital capacity (%VC) in eight living dogs. The vertical lines indicate ± one standard error of the mean. (From Macklem and Mead.[24] Reprinted by permission from the authors and publisher.)

portant to recognize that the methods currently used to document diseases of small airways are essentially tests of the distributive capabilities of all airways; therefore, indistinguishable functional abnormalities can result from localized (or nonuniform) disease of large airways.

Resistance in the tracheobronchial tree is nearly linear up to flow rates of 2 L/sec, and during quiet mouth breathing it accounts for about 60 per cent of total airway resistance. Lung tissue resistance is small compared with airway resistance; of the total pulmonary resistance (tissue plus airway), lung tissue resistance accounts

for about one-sixth (or less) and airway resistance about five-sixths of the total.[29] Chest wall resistance is also approximately linear up to flow rates of 2 L/sec and contributes about 40 per cent and 19 per cent of the total respiratory resistance during mouth and nose breathing, respectively, at flow rates of 1 L/sec.[23]

FACTORS AFFECTING AIRWAY RESISTANCE

Airway resistance depends upon the number, length, and cross-sectional area of the conducting airways. The number of airways in the normal lung is determined by the pattern of branching that is established by the sixteenth week of fetal life. Airways do not form thereafter, and in fact, the total number of small airways becomes reduced during the first few years of life by the transformation of conducting bronchioles into respiratory bronchioles. At times, the number of airways may be reduced further by surgical resection and pulmonary diseases. The length of airways varies considerably from person to person, depending upon age and body size; airway length also varies in an individual, depending upon the phase of ventilation, lengthening during inspiration as lung volume increases, and shortening during expiration. Because resistance to airflow in a given airway changes according to the fourth power of the radius of the airway, the cross-sectional area within the tracheobronchial tree is by far the most important, as well as potentially the most variable, determinant of airway resistance.

The cross-sectional area of any given intrathoracic airway must be determined by the balance between those forces tending to contract the walls, primarily tension of airway smooth muscle and elastic elements, and those forces providing outward traction on the walls, either from the attached lung parenchyma in the case of intrapulmonary airways (bronchioles) or from pleural pressure in the case of intrapulmonary bronchi and all extrapulmonary airways. Airway resistance is significantly influenced by the following variables.

Lung Volume. Airway resistance can be shown to vary with changes in lung volume according to the relationship shown in Figure 4–13; changes in lung volume above FRC have little effect on airway resistance, but between FRC and RV airway resistance increases rapidly and may be infinite at RV. The curvilinear relationship between changes in airway resistance and lung volume can be transformed into a nearly linear diagram by plotting the reciprocal of airway resistance, *airway conductance* ($G_{aw} = 1/R_{aw}$), against lung volume. Furthermore, the marked variations in individual values of airway resistance and conductance among children and adults of both sexes, primarily the result of differences in body size, can be reduced if conductance is related to lung volume.[30] This relationship has led to the use of the term *specific airway conductance*, or airway conductance divided by the lung volume at which it was measured. Although it is useful to relate measurements of airway conductance to those of lung volume, the determinant of the relationship between lung volume and airway resistance is the elastic recoil at the given lung volume. When elastic recoil and lung volume are made to vary independently (e.g., by chest strapping), it can be shown that elastic recoil and not lung volume is the variable that determines airway resistance.[31]

Elastic Recoil. The elastic recoil properties of the lung affect the caliber of both bronchioles and bronchi but by different mechanisms: first, by providing direct traction on small intrapulmonary airways, and second, by being one of the two determinants (alveolar pressure being the other) of intrapleural pressure, which provides the pressure surrounding bronchi and extrapulmonary airways and distends them.* Therefore, elastic recoil establishes airway size and becomes the chief determinant of intrathoracic airway resistance in normal subjects breathing under conditions in which flow is not limited by airway compression (see subsequent section on Flow-Volume Relationships).

Geometry of Airways. Changes in the geometry of normal bronchi de-

---

*Peribronchial pressure is at least as negative as and probably slightly more negative than pleural pressure.[32]

pend not only on the transmural pressure across their walls but also on the distensibility of the elements composing the walls. These phenomena are reflected in the diameter-pressure and length-pressure relationships of the airways. However, only limited information is available on this topic and mainly from studies in excised dogs' lungs.[33, 34] A bronchus increases its diameter about 60 per cent and its length about 40 per cent during inflation from the airless state to TLC.[33] In the absence of smooth muscle tone, virtually all the increase in bronchial diameter is achieved by the time distending pressures of 6 to 10 cm H_2O are reached, and very little change occurs at higher pressures; in contrast, bronchial length continues to change throughout inflation. Both small (<3 mm diameter) and large bronchi demonstrate similar behavior.[34] This means that there is a considerable difference between the volume-pressure relationships of the lung and the diameter-pressure relationships of the airways. The consequences of this difference are that airways enlarge early during the course of lung inflation and are nearly completely distended at about FRC; thereafter, airways change mainly in length while the lung expands to TLC.

There is a small amount of resting smooth muscle tone in the walls of normal airways that serves to narrow their lumen and decrease their distensibility. Administration of bronchodilator drugs to normal subjects causes bronchial smooth muscle to relax and produces a corresponding decrease in airway resistance. An increase in smooth muscle tone (i.e., bronchospasm) not only narrows the lumen of the airway but also decreases the distensibility of the walls. In addition to bronchospasm, a variety of other pathologic processes can affect the geometry of airways by causing thickening of the walls, secretions in the lumen, or narrowing from external compression.

FLOW-VOLUME RELATIONSHIPS

It has long been recognized that there is a maximum limit to the flow rate that can be attained during expiration and that once this limit is achieved, greater muscular effort does not further augment flow. The concept that flow is limited despite additional effort emerged from a series of experiments carried out in the late 1950s and early 1960s concerning isovolumic pressure-flow relationships.[35, 36] The best explanation of an isovolumic pressure-flow curve lies in understanding how one is constructed. Flow, volume, and esophageal (i.e., pleural) pressure are measured simultaneously during the performance of repeated expiratory vital capacity maneuvers by a subject seated in a volume plethysmograph, which corrects for gas compression. The subject is instructed to exhale with varying amounts of effort that are reflected by changes in pleural pressure. From these data, it is possible to plot flow rate against pleural pressure at any given lung volume, for example, 60 per cent of vital capacity, as shown in Figure 4-14. It is apparent from the figure that flow rate reaches a plateau at a relatively low positive pleural pressure and that once maximum flow for that lung volume is reached, it remains constant despite increasing pleural pressure to substantially higher values.

Figure 4-15 depicts a family of isovolumic pressure-flow curves at different lung volumes; they show that at high lung volumes (i.e., near TLC) expiratory flow is not limited by a flow maximum but that below about 70 per cent vital capacity, plateaus develop and maximum flow is limited.[37] From the left-hand panel in Figure 4-15, it is possible to construct a maximum expiratory flow-volume curve (right-hand panel). It can be seen that peak flow is achieved shortly after beginning a forced exhalation from full inspiration; thereafter, as lung volume is reduced flow declines but is *the maximum*

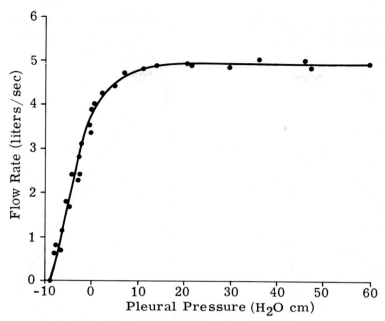

Figure 4-14   An example of an isovolume flow-pressure curve at 60 per cent vital capacity from an idealized series of measurements. The points depict the relationship between flow rate and pleural pressure at 60 per cent vital capacity during a series of vital capacity maneuvers with varying amounts of expiratory effort. It is evident that after a certain flow is reached, increasing effort, reflected by increasing pleural pressure, does *not* cause flow rate to increase.

flow for that particular lung volume. Peak flow varies with effort, and thus is regarded as *effort-dependent*; in contrast, flow on the downslope of the curve is maximal for that particular lung volume and hence is considered *effort-independent.*

Carrying out the measurements necessary to construct isovolumic pressure-flow curves is cumbersome and requires specialized equipment. However, important and clinically useful information is available from maximum flow-volume curves recorded using the equipment available in many respiratory function laboratories. (These curves usually differ only slightly from those recorded using a plethysmograph.) Also, because interpretation of flow-volume curves is based primarily on the downslope of the curve — in other words, on the effort-independent portion — a high degree of patient cooperation is not necessary to obtain a satisfactory tracing. Patient

effort is paramount in determining the values for the conventional tests of forced expiratory volume in 1 sec and maximum expiratory flow rate; these tests depend upon performance in the early, or effort-dependent, part of the expiratory maneuver and are therefore liable to variability. Maximum flow-volume measurements may prove superior to values of forced expiratory volume in 1 sec and maximum expiratory flow rate in studies of the mechanical properties of the respiratory system because additional information is provided and less patient cooperation is required.

DYNAMIC COMPRESSION

Limitation of flow results from dynamic compression of the airways, which in turn depends upon changes in intrathoracic pressures during forced expiration. Alveolar pressure provides the "pressure head" that ex-

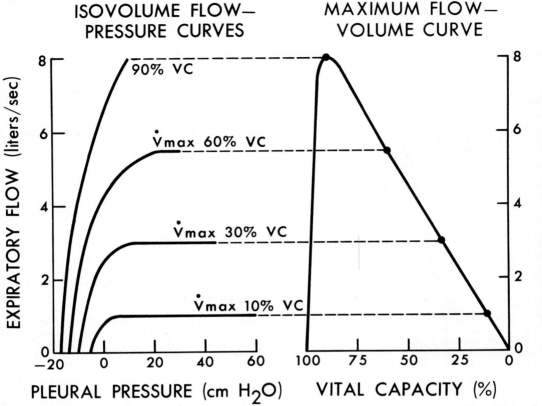

Figure 4-15 From a series of isovolume flow-pressure curves at varying vital capacities (VC) (*left diagram*), it is possible to construct a maximum flow-volume curve (*right diagram*). V̇max = maximum expiratory flow. A similar flow-volume curve can also be obtained by simply plotting expired flow rate against volume using an X-Y recorder during a single forced expiratory vital capacity maneuver.

pels air from the terminal gas exchange units to outside the body during expiration. The determinants of transpulmonary pressure (Figure 4–1) can be revised to show that alveolar pressure is the sum of transpulmonary pressure and pleural pressure ($P_{alv} = P_l + P_{pl}$). Transpulmonary pressure is always positive in sign and, as indicated, equals the static elastic recoil pressure of the lung. Pleural pressure is usually negative in sign during normal breathing but becomes positive during vigorous expiratory efforts. During forced expiration, therefore, alveolar pressure is the algebraic sum of two positive values and provides the total pressure that must be dissipated—overcoming flow-resistance—along the airway from alveolus to mouth where the pressure is zero. It

follows, as shown in Figure 4–16, that there must be a point somewhere along the intrathoracic airway at which the pressure within the lumen of the airway equals the pressure surrounding the wall. The site at which the intraluminal and pleural pressures are equal, and hence pressure difference across the wall is zero, is called the equal pressure point. "Downstream" (i.e., toward the mouth) from the equal pressure point, lateral pressure within the lumen is less than the compressive pressure on the walls, and compression of the airway develops.

It can be seen from the model in Figure 4–16 that as effort and pleural pressure increase, the equal pressure point moves "upstream" (i.e., toward the alveolus) but becomes fixed when

QUIET EXPIRATION

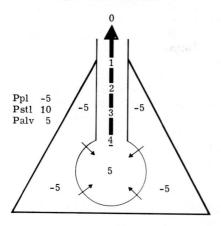

FORCED EXPIRATION

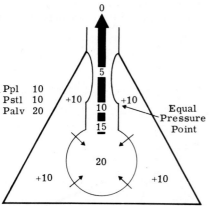

Figure 4–16 A schematic representation of the equal pressure point concept in which pleural pressure (P_{pl}), static elastic recoil pressure (P_{stl}), and alveolar pressure (P_{alv}) are in cm H_2O. *Upper diagram,* During expiration with little muscular effort from a given lung volume at which static elastic recoil pressure (P_{stl}) is 10, pleural pressure (P_{pl}) at the beginning of expiration may be −5; therefore, alveolar pressure at that instant is +5, and this pressure must be dissipated, moving gas to the airway opening where the pressure is 0 (hence $5·4 \cdots → 0$). *Lower diagram,* During vigorous expiration from the same lung volume, P_{pl} becomes positive. When this value is added to the same P_{stl}, P_{alv} equals 20. In this case, as pressure is dissipated during airflow ($20·15 \cdots → 0$) there must be a point at which the pressures inside and outside the airway wall are equal — the equal pressure point. Compression occurs downstream from this point, because lateral pressure in the lumen is less than the pressure surrounding the wall.

maximum flow rate occurs. Further increases of pleural pressure only augment the degree of compression of the downstream segment.

Because the transmural pressure at the equal pressure point is zero, the pressure inside and outside the wall at that point must be equal to pleural pressure. Under these conditions, the driving pressure of the upstream segment from the alveolus (where $P_{alv} = P_{pl} + P_1$) to the equal pressure point (where the pressure = P_{pl}) is the elastic recoil pressure of the lung ($P_1 = P_{stl}$), and the resistance to flow is that offered by the airways from alveolus to the constricted orifice at the junction of the upstream and downstream segments. Therefore, both driving pressure (i.e., elastic recoil) and resistance (i.e., caliber of airways of the upstream segment) are fixed.[37] Flow limitation occurs owing to the fortuitous relationships between progressive effort-induced increases in pleural pressure and the resulting changes in the geometry of the airways downstream from the equal pressure point; for any given increase in effort, the compression of the downstream airways is such that resistance increases proportional to the pressure change and flow is limited.

The obvious value of dynamic compression of the airways is to improve the effectiveness of cough even though maximum flow rates are not increased. Cough is most effective downstream from the equal pressure point at which compression occurs, and a greater shearing force develops owing to the increased linear velocity of airflow that serves to dislodge secretions and particles along the walls of the airways. At mid-lung volume, the equal pressure point is near the origins of the segmental bronchi so that dynamic compression involves only the lobar and mainstem bronchi and intrathoracic trachea. Although the equal pressure point probably moves farther toward the alveoli at low lung volumes,[38] it probably remains within segmental bronchi; this means that coughing is effective in clearing only relatively large airways.

Inspiratory flow is not normally limited by effort because compression does not occur. As greater inspiratory efforts are made, intrathoracic airways become progressively distended and flow is enhanced.

Figure 4–17 shows a combined maximum flow-volume diagram for inspiration and expiration, as well as the usual values for flow rates and tidal volumes in a normal subject during heavy exercise. The figure indicates that values for maximum flow are not reached ordinarily even during maximum exercise.[38] Although normal subjects seldom attain maximum flow rates during ordinary breathing ma-

neuvers, except when coughing, substantial impairment in maximum expiratory flow-volume relationships occurs in patients with pulmonary diseases such as asthma, bronchitis, and emphysema. This mechanism seriously affects ventilatory capacity and may be the chief cause of disability in these conditions. Moreover, tests of maximum expiratory flow-volume relationships may prove useful in the early diagnosis of diseases with airway obstruction.[40]

FREQUENCY DEPENDENCE OF COMPLIANCE

The recent interest in frequency dependence of compliance, like the interest in maximum expiratory flow-

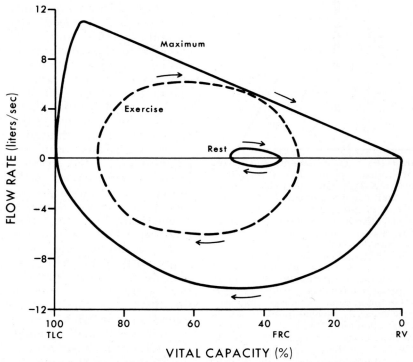

Figure 4–17 Schematic representation of a maximal inspiratory and expiratory flow-volume curve from a normal subject, showing for comparison the flow rates attained during heavy exercise and while at rest. TLC = total lung capacity; FRC = functional residual capacity; RV = residual volume.

volume relationships, derives from the potential usefulness of both these tests of ventilatory function in the early recognition of certain lung diseases.[41] In contrast to the testing procedure for recording maximum expiratory flow-volume relationships, measurement of frequency dependence of compliance is complicated and extremely difficult to perform accurately. However, knowledge of the physiologic principles that result in normal or abnormal tests of frequency dependence of compliance provides insight into the pathogenesis of the disturbances in the mechanics of ventilation and the distribution of inspired gas.[42] Static compliance of the lung, as described previously, is used to define the static volume-pressure relationships of the lung and is determined while the subject holds his breath. Lung compliance can also be determined during a normal breathing cycle without breath holding from measurements of lung volumes and esophageal pressures at the end of inspiration and expiration; in other words, at the instants when flow at the mouth has ceased. These values may be obtained at varying breathing frequencies and under these conditions yield a measurement of *dynamic compliance.*

In normal subjects, dynamic compliance is approximately equal to static compliance, even at high breathing frequencies; but in patients with various bronchopulmonary disorders, dynamic compliance falls as respiratory rate increases.[41] These two patterns of response are depicted in Figure 4–18. Dynamic compliance in normal subjects can be seen to be relatively independent of respiratory frequency; in contrast, the patients with bronchial asthma demonstrated a fall of compliance to less than 80 per cent of the extrapolated value at zero frequency; this reduction signifies abnormal frequency dependence of compliance.

The origin of frequency depend-

ence of compliance can be displayed in the three lung models shown in Figure 4–19. In the normal subjects, model A, most of the flow resistance in the tracheobronchial tree resides in the central airways (shown by the thick wall), and only a small amount originates in the peripheral airways (shown by their thin walls); furthermore, both alveoli are equally distensible (shown by similar springs). In this system, the major source of flow resistance is common to both peripheral pathways and the peripheral pathways have similar resistances and distensibility characteristics. Another way of expressing the equality of the mechanical properties of the peripheral units is to say that their "time constants"* are the same. If the "subject" breathes at a given tidal volume and a slow respiratory rate, both alveoli will expand and contract the same amount and at the same time (i.e., there is no phase lag between them). If the subject now breathes at the same tidal volume but increases his respiratory rate, both alveoli will continue to respond identically.

Model B simulates the condition of partial obstruction of a peripheral bronchus. When the same tidal volume as in model A is applied to this system at low breathing frequencies so that the flow rate of air within the peripheral airways is very low, both alveoli will expand and contract identically. When respiratory frequency and flow rate begin to increase, there will be a progressively increasing pressure drop across the resistance in the partially obstructed airway, which causes a corresponding decrease in the pressure "available" to fill the

---

*The term "time constant" derives from the use of an electrical analogue of the condition in which a resistance (resistor) and a compliance (capacitor) are in series with each other. Time constants can be used to calculate the phase shift in current that will occur when a phasic voltage is applied to the circuit.[42]

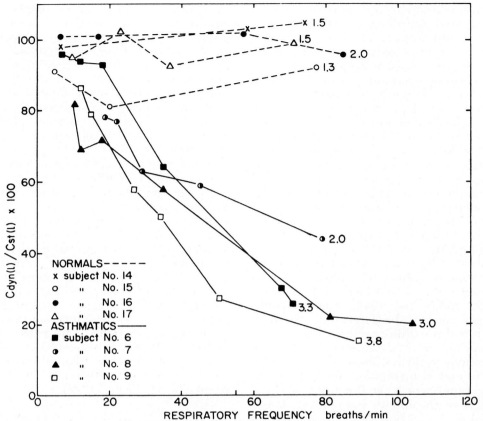

Figure 4–18 Dynamic compliance [Cdyn(l)] as a percentage of static compliance [Cst(l)] at different breathing frequencies in four normal subjects (-----) and four patients of similar age with asthma (———). The number to the right of each person's graph is the value of pulmonary resistance obtained at the time of the study. (From Woolcock, Vincent, and Macklem.[41] Reprinted by permission from the authors and publisher.)

alveolus distal to the obstruction. Because tidal volume is constant, the unobstructed alveolus will fill more than it does in model A, and the partially obstructed alveolus will fill less than it did at slower frequencies of breathing; this means that the system is showing frequency dependence of compliance.

Exactly the same argument pertains to model C, in which the peripheral airway to one alveolus is completely obstructed but the unit does not become atelectatic owing to the presence of a collateral ventilatory pathway from the unobstructed alve-

olus. At low respiratory rates, both units will fill and empty equally and synchronously. When respiratory frequency increases, there will be frequency dependence of compliance because, owing to the resistance offered by the collateral channel, the distal alveolus will fill less and less and the proximal "normal" alveolus will fill more and more.

Because most of the flow resistance occurs in the central airways, as illustrated in the three models in Figure 4–19, the resistance of the parallel peripheral airways is small, and hence their time constants are also

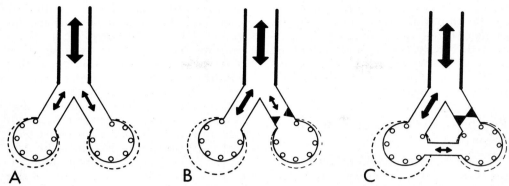

Figure 4–19 Three models of the lung showing the origin of frequency dependence of compliance. In A, because resistance in the two peripheral airways and compliance of the two distensible alveoli are equal, the amount of gas distributed to the two units at constant tidal volumes (shown by the size of the arrows) is equal at all breathing frequencies. In B and C, there is a high resistance pathway to one of the units. At low breathing frequencies, the effects of increased resistance are trivial, and the distribution of inspired air is equal; however, at increasing frequencies, the effects of resistance become progressively important, and the distribution of inspired air shifts from the partially obstructed alveolus to the nonobstructed unit. Thus a phase lag and frequency dependence of compliance occur. (For details, see text.)

small. This distribution of resistances is advantageous because it allows for considerable variation in time constants (up to fourfold) among the peripheral pathways before their compliances become frequency-dependent.[38] If more resistance resided peripherally than is encountered normally, less discrepancy in time constants would be possible before frequency dependence would occur.

It can be inferred from the models that when frequency dependence of compliance occurs, unevenness in the distribution of inspired gas must also occur. Moreover, as in model B, whenever the time constants of parallel pathways differ sufficiently to produce a phase shift in the time course of gas flow, the slowly ventilating unit will receive part of its inspired volume from the rapidly ventilating unit ("pendelluft") because the former is still inspiring while the latter is exhaling. A unit dependent upon collateral ventilation, as in model C, is in series with its proximal alveolus and is totally parasitic upon it for inspired air.

Although the use of models considerably oversimplifies the complexity of pathophysiologic abnormalities, they realistically depict the disturbances in distribution of ventilation that may be produced by numerous common lung diseases.[43] The consequences of these events are important because any change in the distribution of ventilation is likely to lead to an abnormality of gas exchange.

DISTRIBUTION OF VENTILATION

The regional distribution of ventilation during inspiration depends upon the distensibility of peripheral gas exchange units and the resistance of the airways leading to them. On the one hand are the mechanical consequences of the vertical gradient of pleural pressure that lead to nonuniformity in the distribution of inspired air. On the other hand are three additional mechanisms that operate to cause terminal units to inflate and deflate synchronously and thus serve to make the distribution of ventilation uniform: (1) the magnitude of the dif ferences in compliance and resistance in the uppermost and lowermost regions of the lung, (2) the interdependence that exists between adjacent lung units and between the lung and chest wall, and (3) the presence of collateral pathways for ventilation.

REGIONAL COMPLIANCE AND RESISTANCE

The vertical gradient of pleural pressure means that airways and alveoli at the top of the lung are more distended than those at the bottom; this in turn implies that there must be time constant differences among units throughout the lung. At first glance, this observation appears to conflict with the absence of frequency dependence of compliance in normal lungs. The apparent discrepancy is explained by the previously mentioned calculation that a fourfold variation in peripheral time constants could occur before asynchronous behavior is detectable.[38] Furthermore, because regional gravity-dependent unevenness of ventilation can be demonstrated by using various inert gases, it can be concluded that these tests are more sensitive methods of detecting asynchronous behavior than are tests of frequency dependence.[43]

INTERDEPENDENCE

The lung parenchyma, as pointed out in Chapters 1 and 2, has a connective tissue framework containing elastic elements. Because contiguous units are attached to each other, they are not free to move independently; instead, the behavior of one unit should influence the behavior of its neighbors. This summarizes the concept of interdependence among peripheral units introduced by Mead and co-workers[32] and now generally accepted as an important mechanism promoting uniformity of ventilation. The magnitude of interdependence depends upon the number of elastic

elements and the forces transmitted by each and the area of the surface involved. The effect, however, is always unifying because it serves to offset (in part) any coexisting tendency that would otherwise make units larger or smaller than they should be.

A somewhat similar analogy has been applied to movement between the lung and the adjacent chest wall and is illustrated in Figure 4-20. Any lag in inflation of the lower lobe induces a distortion in the shape of the chest wall. The pleural pressure surrounding the lower lobe is amplified according to the extent that the chest wall resists distortion (i.e., attempts to assume its static configuration). Amplification of the pleural pressure tends to expand the lower lobe and thus counterbalance its tendency to resist inflation.[44] Experimental evidence supports the presence of interdependence between the lung and chest wall,[45] and it is likely that this mechanism is of physiologic significance and serves to minimize lag during normal breathing maneuvers.

COLLATERAL VENTILATION

Pathways for collateral ventilation occur between adjacent alveoli (pores of Kohn), contiguous lobules (Lambert's canals), and possibly even larger units (Chapter 2); despite the presence of numerous communications, the contribution of collateral ventilation to uniformity of ventilation in normal human lungs is unknown. However, there is abundant evidence from studies in both man and experimental animals that collateral ventilation is of considerable importance in determining the mechanical behavior and distribution of ventilation of lungs with airway obstruction.[43]

REGIONAL INHOMOGENEITY

Regional inhomogeneity derives from the anatomy of the tracheobronchial tree and the vertical gradient

Figure 4-20 Illustration of the mechanism by which dynamic pleural pressure changes may be amplified to a region of the lung that lags behind other parts of the lung. The *left diagram* depicts the normal relationship between the lung and chest wall under static conditions at a given lung volume. The *right diagram* depicts the relationships at the same lung volume under dynamic conditions during which the lower lobe may lag behind the upper. If this occurs, it introduces a distortion in the chest wall; the extent to which the chest wall resists distortion and attempts to assume its static configuration (arrow and dashed lines) determines the magnitude of pleural pressure amplification over the lower lobe. (From Macklem.[44] Reprinted by permission from the author and publisher.)

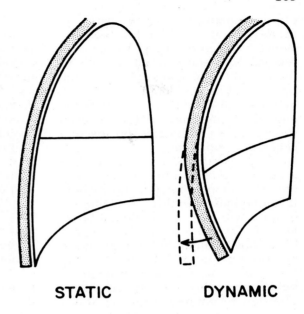

STATIC   **DYNAMIC**

of pleural pressure. It has already been pointed out that the length of various pathways within the tracheobronchial tree varies considerably, depending upon whether the pathways lead to a central or a peripheral gas exchange unit. Because the bronchial tree is asymmetric, so is the volume of gas occupying different pathways, the so-called *anatomic dead space*; this means that the amount of dead space gas that precedes inspired fresh air into central and peripheral gas exchange units during inhalation must also vary. Consequently, unequal alveolar gas concentrations must result from the mixing of the incoming boluses of fresh air with varying volumes of dead space gas.

The vertical gradient of pleural pressure (see section on Pleural Pressure Gradient) causes regional changes in alveolar geometry and airway caliber. Accordingly, topographic variations in the distribution of inspired gas result; these vary with the lung volume at which inspiration begins. Furthermore, because body position influences the magnitude of the

difference in pleural and transmural pressures between the top and bottom of the lung (Table 4-1), the subject's position during breathing also affects the regional distribution of the inspired fresh air.

Studies using radioactive gases have provided convincing documentation of the effects of the vertical gradients of pleural pressure on the distribution of inspired air. During breathing at slow respiratory frequencies from FRC, it has been demonstrated that each breath is distributed according to regional compliances.[46] In other words, the lowermost regions receive more of the inspirate because they are functioning on a steeper, more compliant part of the lungs' volume-pressure curve than the uppermost regions (see Figure 4-10). However, of considerable importance is the additional observation that when breathing frequency increases, the distribution of the inspirate becomes more uniform.[46] At inspiratory flows beginning at 0.2 L/sec and up to 1.5 L/sec, there is a progressive redistribution of ventilation until the apex and base receive approximately equal shares. At these inspiratory flow rates, it can be shown from an electrical analogue of regional time constant differences that there ought to be a phase lag between upper and lower lobes.[44] However, under these conditions, interdependence between lung and chest wall should serve to minimize any discrepancies in ventilation.

The "wisdom of the body" is again apparent. Ventilation is distributed to those regions of the lung where it can be most useful in maintaining a balance with the distribution of blood flow. Thus, while the body is at rest, blood flows chiefly to the lung bases, but during exercise, blood flow becomes more uniformly distributed as pulmonary artery pressure increases. The slow respiratory frequency at rest and the increased breathing rate during exercise cause the distribution of ventilation to correspond to that of blood flow.

STRATIFIED INHOMOGENEITY

Because the total cross-sectional area of conducting airways becomes progressively larger from the trachea to the terminal bronchioles and because the cross-sectional area of respiratory bronchioles increases proportionately more (because several orders of branching occur with virtually no change in the diameter of the component bronchioles), the forward velocity of the inspired airstream moving peripherally through the airways slows markedly. Finally, in the neighborhood of the alveolar ducts, forward velocity is probably so slow that it becomes superseded by movement of gas molecules owing to thermal agitation. Thus, inspired gas reaches alveolar ducts by mass flow (sometimes called bulk flow) through the airways, but alveoli are "ventilated" owing to movement of molecules by gaseous diffusion. The completeness of mixing determines whether or not stratified inhomogeneity will occur.[47]

Diffusion of molecules within a mixture of gases depends upon the physical properties of the gases involved, the volume through which they have to move, and the time available for carrying out the process. The distance for gas-phase diffusion between alveolar ducts and their adjacent alveoli is sufficiently small that in normal subjects breathing at slow (resting) rates, stratified inhomogeneity is barely discernible. During the determination of closing volume, for example, the procedure is such that the slope of the alveolar plateau (phase III, Figure 4–11) is mainly influenced by sequential emptying of regions owing to the vertical gradient of pleural pressure; stratified inhomogeneity contributes very little to the changing alveolar gas concentration, primarily because the breathing maneuver is a slow one, and gas-phase mixing is complete. However, the presence of stratified inhomogeneity can be demonstrated in normal subjects by varying the pattern of breathing, especially by using high inspiratory flow rates and beginning inspiration above FRC.[48] Furthermore, incompleteness of gas mixing has been shown to be an important factor in determining the distribution, and hence the adequacy of gas exchange, in patients with various forms of lung diseases.[47]

REFERENCES

1. Otis, A. B., Fenn, W. O., and Rahn, H.: Mechanics of breathing in man. J. Appl. Physiol., 2:592–607, 1950.
2. Mead, J.: Mechanical properties of lungs. Physiol. Rev., 41:281–330, 1961.
3. Fenn, W. O., and Rahn, H.: Handbook of Physiology, Section 3. Respiration. Vol. I. Washington, D.C., American Physiological Society, 1964, pp. 357–476.
4. Campbell, E. J. M., Agostoni, E., and Davis, J. N.: The Respiratory Muscle: Mechanics and Neural Control. 2nd Ed. London, Lloyd-Luke (Medical Books) Ltd., 1970.
5. Milic-Emili, J., Mead, J., Turner, J. M., and Glauser, E. M.: Improved technique for

estimating pleural pressure from esophageal balloons. J. Appl. Physiol., *19*:207–211, 1964.

6. von Neergaard, K.: Neue Auffassungen über einen Grundbegriff der Atemmechanik. Die Retraktions-Kraft der Lunge, abhängig von der Oberflächenspannung in den Alveolen. Z. Ges. Exp. Med., *66*:373–394, 1929.

7. Clements, J. A., and Tierney, D. F.: Alveolar instability associated with altered surface tension. *In* Fenn, W. O., and Rahn, H. (eds.): Handbook of Physiology, Section 3. Respiration. Vol. II. Washington, D.C., American Physiological Society, 1964, pp. 1565–1583.

8. Johanson, W. G., Jr., and Pierce, A. K.: Effects of elastase, collagenase, and papain on structure and function of rat lungs in vitro. J. Clin. Invest., *51*:288–293, 1972.

9. Rahn, H., Otis, A. B., Chadwick, L. E., and Fenn, W. O.: The pressure-volume diagram of the thorax and lung. Am. J. Physiol., *146*:161–178, 1946.

10. Leith, D. E., and Mead, J.: Mechanisms determining residual volume of the lungs in normal subjects. J. Appl. Physiol., *23*:221–227, 1967.

11. Agostoni, E.: Mechanics of the pleural space. Physiol. Rev., *52*:57–128, 1972.

12. Milic-Emili, J., Henderson, J. A. M., Dolovich, M. B., Trop, D., and Kaneko, K.: Regional distribution of inspired gas in the lung. J. Appl. Physiol., *21*:749–759, 1966.

13. Glazier, J. B., Hughes, J. M. B., Maloney, J. E., and West, J. B.: Vertical gradient of alveolar size in lungs of dogs frozen intact. J. Appl. Physiol., *23*:694–705, 1967.

14. Leblanc, P., Ruff, F., and Milic-Emili, J.: Effects of age and body position on "airway closure" in man. J. Appl. Physiol., *28*:448–451, 1970.

15. McCarthy, D. S., Spencer, R., Greene, R., and Milic-Emili, J.: Measurement of "closing volume" as a simple and sensitive test for early detection of small airway disease. Am. J. Med., *52*:747–753, 1972.

16. Buist, A. S., and Ross, B. B.: Predicted values for closing volumes using a modified single breath nitrogen test. Am. Rev. Resp. Dis., *107*:744–752, 1973.

17. Burger, E. J., Jr., and Macklem, P.: Airway closure: demonstration by breathing 100% O_2 at low lung volumes and by N_2 washout. J. Appl. Physiol., *25*:139–148, 1968.

18. Hughes, J. M. B., Rosenzweig, D. Y., and Kivitz, P. B.: Site of airway closure in excised dog lungs: histologic demonstration. J. Appl. Physiol., *29*:340–344, 1970.

19. Hyatt, R. E., Okeson, G. C., and Rodarte, J. R.: Influence of expiratory flow limitation on the pattern of lung emptying in normal man. J. Appl. Physiol., *35*:411–419, 1973.

20. Mansell, A., Bryan, A., and Levison, H.: Airway closure in children. J. Appl. Physiol., *33*:711–714, 1972.

21. DuBois, A. B., Botelho, S. Y., and Comroe, J. H., Jr.: A new method for measuring airway resistance in man using a body plethysmograph: values in normal subjects and in patients with respiratory disease. J. Clin. Invest., *35*:327–335, 1956.

22. DuBois, A. B., Brody, A. W., Lewis, D. H., and Burgess, B. F., Jr.: Oscillation mechanics of lungs and chest in man. J. Appl. Physiol., *8*:587–594, 1956.

23. Ferris, B. G., Jr., Mead, J., and Opie, L. H.: Partitioning of respiratory flow resistance in man. J. Appl. Physiol., *19*:653–658, 1964.

24. Macklem, P. T., and Mead, J.: Resistance of central and peripheral airways measured by a retrograde catheter. J. Appl. Physiol., *22*:395–401, 1967.

25. Hogg, J. C., Macklem, P. T., and Thurlbeck, W. M.: Site and nature of airway obstruction in chronic obstructive lung disease. New Eng. J. Med., *278*:1355–1360, 1968.

26. Pedley, T. J., Schroter, R. C., and Sudlow, M. F.: The prediction of pressure drop and variation of resistance within the human bronchial airways. Resp. Physiol., *9*:387–405, 1970.

27. Mead, J.: The lung's "quiet zone." New Eng. J. Med., *282*:1318–1319, 1970.

28. Macklem, P. T.: Obstruction in small airways—a challenge to medicine. Am. J. Med., *52*:721–724, 1972.

29. Marshall, R., and DuBois, A. B.: The measurement of the viscous resistance of the lung tissues in normal man. Clin. Sci., *15*:161–170, 1956.

30. Briscoe, W. A., and DuBois, A. B.: The relationship between airway resistance, airway conductance and lung volume in subjects of different age and body size. J. Clin. Invest., *37*:1279–1285, 1958.

31. Stubbs, S. E., and Hyatt, R. E.: Effect of increased lung recoil pressure on maximal expiratory flow in normal subjects. J. Appl. Physiol., *32*:325–331, 1972.

32. Mead, J., Takishima, T., and Leith, D.: Stress distribution in lungs: a model of pulmonary elasticity. J. Appl. Physiol., *28*:596–608, 1970.

33. Marshall, R.: Effect of lung inflation on bronchial dimensions in the dog. J. Appl. Physiol., *17*:596–600, 1962.

34. Hyatt, R. E., and Flath, R. E.: Influence of lung parenchyma on pressure-diameter behavior of dog bronchi. J. Appl. Physiol., *21*:1448–1452, 1966.

35. Hyatt, R. E., Schilder, D. P., and Fry, D. L.:

Relationship between maximum expiratory flow and degree of lung inflation. J. Appl. Physiol., 13:331–336, 1958.

36. Fry, D. L., and Hyatt, R. E.: Pulmonary mechanics. A unified analysis of the relationship between pressure, volume and gasflow in the lungs of normal and diseased human subjects. Am. J. Med., 29: 672–689, 1960.

37. Mead, J., Turner, J. M., Macklem, P. T., and Little, J. B.: Significance of the relationship between lung recoil and maximum expiratory flow. J. Appl. Physiol., 22:95–108, 1967.

38. Macklem, P. T., and Mead, J.: Factors determining maximum expiratory flow in dogs. J. Appl. Physiol., 25:159–169, 1968.

39. Olafsson, S., and Hyatt, R. E.: Ventilatory mechanics and expiratory flow limitation during exercise in normal subjects. J. Clin. Invest., 48:564–573, 1969.

40. Gelb, A. F., Gold, W. M., Wright, R. R., Bruch, H. R., and Nadel, J. A.: Physiologic diagnosis of subclinical emphysema. Am. Rev. Resp. Dis., 107:50–63, 1973.

41. Woolcock, A. J., Vincent, N. J., and Macklem, P. T.: Frequency dependence of compliance as a test for obstruction in the small airways. J. Clin. Invest., 48:1097–1106, 1969.

42. Otis, A. B., McKerrow, C. B., Bartlett, R. A., Mead, J., McIlroy, M. B., Selverstone, N. J., and Radford, E. P.: Mechanical factors in distribution of pulmonary ventilation. J. Appl. Physiol., 8:427–443, 1956.

43. Macklem, P. T.: Airway obstruction and collateral ventilation. Physiol. Rev., 51:368–436, 1971.

44. Macklem, P. T.: Relationship between lung mechanics and ventilation distribution. Physiologist, 16:580–588, 1973.

45. Zidulka, A., Demedts, M., and Anthonisen, N. R.: Lobar obstruction in dog lungs. Fed. Proc., 31:321, 1972.

46. Robertson, P. C., Anthonisen, N. R., and Ross, D.: Effect of inspiratory flow rate on regional distribution of inspired gas. J. Appl. Physiol., 26:438–443, 1969.

47. Cumming, G.: Gas mixing efficiency in the human lung. Resp. Physiol., 2:213–224, 1967.

48. Anthonisen, N. R., Robertson, P. C., and Ross, W. R. D.: Gravity-dependent sequential emptying of lung regions. J. Appl. Physiol., 28:589–595, 1970.

Chapter Five

CIRCULATION

INTRODUCTION

The chief function of the pulmonary circulation is to deliver blood in a thin film to the terminal respiratory units so that gas exchange can take place. The anatomy of the pulmonary circulation is well suited for this purpose because it consists of inflow and outflow vessels that supply and drain an extensive capillary bed that occupies 85 to 95 per cent of the total alveolar surface. Although the lung is designed as an efficient gas exchanger, numerous factors operate continuously to influence gas transfer between air and blood by affecting whether or not incoming blood and inspired air are brought into apposition in proportionate amounts. The previous chapter considered the mechanisms that regulate the volume and distribution of inspired air to the terminal respiratory units; this chapter deals similarly with the volume and distribution of pulmonary blood flow.

The pulmonary circulation has additional functions besides gas exchange.[1] Some of these have been alluded to briefly elsewhere but are summarized as follows: (1) it acts as a filter of the venous drainage from virtually the entire body; (2) it provides O_2 and substrates for the nutrition and metabolic needs of the lung parenchyma, including the synthesis of surfactant; (3) it serves as a reservoir of blood for the left ventricle; (4) it modifies the pharmacologic properties of a variety of circulating substances by biochemical transformation; and (5) it provides a large surface for the absorption of lung liquid that must occur immediately after birth or may take place in unusual circumstances (instillation of liquids therapeutically, drowning).

This chapter also considers the important aspects of liquid and solute movement across pulmonary blood vessels and certain metabolic functions, apart from the provision of substrates, of the pulmonary circulation.

PULMONARY BLOOD FLOW

After fetal shunt pathways have closed, the pulmonary circulation of a normal infant accommodates the entire output of the right ventricle, regardless of the amount ejected. Total pulmonary blood flow, as described earlier, is considerably different during fetal life from what it is after the newborn period; it may also differ from normal in persons with cardiovascular diseases, especially congenital heart abnormalities with shunts of blood from left to right or right to left. The output of the right ventricle is normally a little less than that of the left ventricle—the difference being due to drainage through bronchial veins and thebesian veins that bypass the right ventricle. Cardiac output averages about 5 to 8 L/min in an adult at rest and may rise to 20 to 30 L/min during heavy exercise.

INTRAVASCULAR PRESSURES

Although blood flow to the lung is higher than that to any other organ of the body, the pressure within pulmonary arteries is low, being about one-fifth of that within systemic arteries. A comparison of intravascular pressures in the pulmonary and systemic circulations is presented in Table 5–1. Not only is the pulmonary circulation a high flow–low pressure system in a subject at rest, but also it can accommodate increases in cardiac output of up to three or four times resting values with only a small rise in inflow pressure. This means that pulmonary vascular resistance is low in a resting subject and is capable of substantial further reductions when pulmonary blood flow increases. The physiologic and clinical importance of changes in pulmonary vascular resistance have been recognized for many years and are considered in greater detail in subsequent sections of this chapter.

Pulmonary venous pressure must

Table 5–1   Comparison of Pulmonary and Systemic Hemodynamic Variables During
Rest and Exercise of Moderate Severity in Normal Adult Man

CONDITION	REST (SITTING)	EXERCISE
Oxygen consumption	300	2000 ml/min
Blood flow		
Cardiac output	6.3	16.2 L/min
Heart rate	70	135 beats/min
Stroke volume	90	120 ml/beat
Intravascular pressures		
Pulmonary arterial pressure	20/10	30/11 mm Hg
Mean	14	20 mm Hg
Left atrial pressure, mean	8	10 mm Hg
Brachial arterial pressure	120/70	155/78 mm Hg
Mean	88	112 mm Hg
Right atrial pressure, mean	5	1 mm Hg
Resistances		
Pulmonary vascular resistance	0.95	0.62 unit°
Systemic vascular resistance	13.2	6.9 units°

°Units = mm Hg/L/min.

be slightly higher than, but for practical purposes can be regarded as equal to, left atrial pressure. Left atrial pressure is normally higher than right atrial pressure, a condition that accompanies the increase in pulmonary blood flow at birth and serves to close the foramen ovale. Knowledge of pulmonary venous and/or left atrial pressure values is essential to an assessment of the pulmonary circulation, but it is technically more difficult to measure pressures within the left atrium than pressures within the right heart chambers and pulmonary arterial circulation during cardiac catheterization. This presented a serious practical limitation to studies of the pulmonary circulation until it was learned that "wedge" pressures from an accessible pulmonary artery were almost identical with simultaneously measured pressures from the left atrium.[2]

A wedge pressure is obtained by occluding blood flow through a branch of the pulmonary artery by either wedging the end of a cardiac catheter or inflating a balloon surrounding the catheter in the vessel. Pressures recorded from the tip of the catheter under conditions of "no flow" reflect the pressure downstream within the vascular network at the site of the next freely communicating channels, i.e., pulmonary capillaries or small pulmonary veins.

The fact that wedge pressures from the pulmonary artery and left atrial pressures are nearly the same means that the decrease in pressure along the entire pulmonary venous system is very small. It has also been pointed out recently that pulmonary arterial end-diastolic pressure in normal subjects and patients without lung diseases provides a close approximation of their wedge pressure. This correspondence occurs because the total pressure difference across the lungs is small to begin with and because the pressure difference will be least at the end of diastole when blood flow through the pulmonary circulation is lower than at any other instant during the cardiac cycle. This relationship, however, is not maintained in the presence of disorders of the pulmonary circulation, and, therefore, the method should *not* be used as a substitute for more accurate techniques of left atrial pressure recording in patients with any form of lung disease.[3]

Pulmonary arterial and wedge pressures can now be measured outside the cardiac catheterization laboratory through the use of specially designed flexible catheters that can be "floated" through the venous system and right heart into the pulmonary circulation.[4] This technique is being widely applied to studies of the pulmonary circulation in both healthy subjects and seriously ill patients.

DISTRIBUTION OF PULMONARY BLOOD FLOW

Soon after the technique of cardiac catheterization was introduced and direct measurements of pulmonary arterial pressures became available, Dock[5] suggested that the distribution of blood flow within the lung must be uneven because the pulmonary circulation is a low pressure system that is operating in a gravitational field. He also speculated that the presence of uneven blood flow would create important differences between regions of the lung in their local defense capabilities and adequacy of gas exchange. Fifteen years later, the discovery of radioactive gas techniques for assessing the distribution of pulmonary blood flow provided convincing confirmation of Dock's theory.

Regional pulmonary blood flow can be measured using radioactive tracers whose uptake, release, or retention is a reflection of blood flow and whose presence can be detected by external counting. (1) Radiolabeled CO_2 ($C^{15}O_2$) was the first material to be used to study the pulmonary circulation.[6] Its suitability depends upon monitoring the disappearance of an inhaled gas whose uptake from alveoli is determined by the blood flow to them; because the indicator gas is breathed into the lung, a region must be ventilated before perfusion to the region can be detected by diffusion of $C^{15}O_2$ into the bloodstream. (2) A radioactive, insoluble gas (such as ^{133}Xe) can be used to identify gas-filled alveoli that are perfused by pulmonary capillary blood.[7] A small amount of tracer gas dissolved in saline is injected intravenously, and as the blood containing the injectate flows through the lung, the gas diffuses from the blood, owing to its low solubility, into air-containing spaces; hence, the presence of radioactivity signifies perfusion of gas-filled alveoli in a given region. (3) Radiolabeled particles (such as ^{125}I-labeled macroaggregated albumin) of sufficient size to be trapped within small pulmonary blood vessels during an attempted passage through the lungs will be retained in and can be detected over perfused regions of the lung.[8]

Each of the procedures described has its advantages and disadvantages, but all have yielded similar evidence concerning the presence of a vertical gradient of blood flow from the top to the bottom of the lung. The topographic gradient of blood flow is determined by hydrostatic pressure differences in the pulmonary circulation caused by gravity and not, as is the case with the regional distribution of ventilation, by the vertical gradient of intrapleural pressure.* The difference between the factors affecting the distribution of ventilation on the one hand and the distribution of blood flow on the other can easily be demonstrated by studies performed with isolated lungs or open-chest animals; in these preparations, the vertical gradient of intrapleural pressure is abolished, but that due to hydrostatic pressure remains.

The importance of hydrostatic pressure differences is shown schematically in Figure 5–1. In the diagram, alveolar pressure is set realistically and for convenience at 0 cm H_2O;

---

*Gravity, in fact, contributes in part to the vertical gradient of pleural pressure because the weight of the lung is involved. However, the pleural pressure gradient is determined in addition by the support of the lung and the configuration of the chest wall (Chapter 4), factors that do not affect the vertical gradient of blood flow.

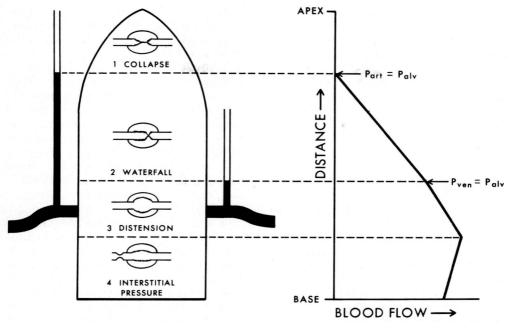

Figure 5–1 Schematic representation of the four zones of the lung in which different hemodynamic conditions govern blood flow. Alveolar pressure (Palv) is assumed to be 0; the heights of the
black columns on the left and right of the lung represent the magnitude of pulmonary arterial (Part)
and pulmonary venous (Pven) pressures, respectively. For discussion, see text. (Adapted from Hughes,
Glazier, Maloney, and West.[9] Reprinted by permission from the authors and publisher.)

the importance of changes in alveolar
pressure is considered below. It can
be seen in Figure 5–1 that pulmonary
arterial pressure, reflected by the
height of the column in the manometer,
is insufficient to cause blood to rise all
the way to the apex of the lung in
the upright position. The column
of blood will rise in the lung as
well as in the manometer to the level
at which the pressure at the top
of the column equals alveolar pressure. At 5 cm below the top of the
column the perfusion pressure is 5 cm
H_2O, and at 15 cm below the top of
the column, the perfusion pressure is
15 cm H_2O. Because the hydrostatic
pressure varies, more blood will perfuse a region 15 cm below the "top" of
pulmonary arterial pressure than a region 5 cm below the top. Therefore, inflow pressure to any region of the lung
is determined by the maximum pres-

sure within the pulmonary artery (i.e.,
the top of the column in the manometer) and by how far the given region is
below this level.

On the basis of these considerations, Dock[5] predicted and West and
co-workers[6, 10] demonstrated that the
topographic distribution of perfusion
must be affected by the level of pulmonary artery pressure in relation to the
total vertical dimensions of the lung.
This explains why the apex of the
lung receives less blood flow than the
base in the upright position and why
at a constant pulmonary arterial pressure the lung is more evenly perfused
in the recumbent than in the upright
position.

Figure 5–1 also demonstrates an
important relationship between the
pulmonary venous (or outflow) pressure and the distribution ·of blood
within the lung. Pulmonary venous

pressure is customarily low (Table 5–1), and its hydrostatic effect, therefore, is to support a column of venous blood that reaches only partway up the total vertical height of the lung. This column, like the column on the inflow side, will also rise to the level within the lung and manometer, at which the pressure at the top of the column equals alveolar pressure. Below this level, the hydrostatic effect of venous pressure becomes increasingly great and will cause those vessels exposed to its influence either to open or to dilate, or both. Conversely, the amount of blood flow to the lung above the level at which venous pressure equals alveolar pressure is not influenced by (i.e., is out of "reach" of) venous pressure.

Alveolar pressure was deliberately assigned a value of zero in Figure 5–1, but it can be visualized that if alveolar pressure were changed, it would displace the column of blood a corresponding amount in the lung, but *not* in the manometer. For example, if alveolar pressure were plus 5 cm H_2O and inflow and outflow pressures were unchanged, the profile of blood flow shown in the right-hand panel of Figure 5–1 would be displaced downward 5 cm, and the lungs accordingly would be perfused less completely.

These descriptions should suffice to show that all three pressures, pulmonary arterial, pulmonary venous, and alveolar, govern the distribution of blood in the lungs. The relationships among these pressures have been employed to subdivide the lung, as shown in Figure 5–1, into four zones with differing conditions of blood flow.

1. In Zone 1, alveolar pressure (P_{alv}) exceeds both pulmonary arterial (P_{PA}) and venous (P_{PV}) pressures $(P_{alv} > P_{PA} > P_{PV})$. There is no blood flow to this region because inflow pressure is everywhere lower than alveolar pressure.

2. In Zone 2, pulmonary arterial pressure exceeds alveolar pressure, but alveolar pressure exceeds pulmo-

nary venous pressure $(P_{PA} > P_{alv} > P_{PV})$. In this region, blood flow increases progressively down the lung from the level of no flow $(P_{PA} = P_{alv})$ to the level at which alveolar and pulmonary venous pressures are equal $(P_{alv} = P_{PV})$. Because the effect of venous pressure is not transmitted to Zone 2, the resistance to blood flow through the zone is determined by the pressure difference from pulmonary artery to alveolus. This condition has been likened to a "sluice" or "waterfall" and can be simulated by a Starling resistor.[11, 12]

3. In Zone 3, pulmonary arterial pressure exceeds pulmonary venous pressure and pulmonary venous pressure exceeds alveolar pressure $(P_{PA} > P_{PV} > P_{alv})$. Resistance to blood flow in this region is determined by the pressure difference from pulmonary artery to pulmonary vein. Because this difference remains constant throughout Zone 3, at first glance there seems to be no reason for blood flow to increase below the level at which pulmonary venous and alveolar pressures are equal $(P_{PV} = P_{alv})$. However, the transmural distending pressure across the vessel wall increases with distance down the zone because pulmonary arterial and venous pressures both increase while alveolar pressure remains constant. The progressively increasing distending force alters the geometry of the intervening vascular pathways and lowers the resistance to blood flow through them.

In Figure 5–1, the junction between Zones 2 and 3 is recognizable by an increase in the slope of the line depicting blood flow at a given level of the lung. This is not always the case, and in some experiments the incremental change in blood flow may be the same within the two zones so that the slope remains constant.

4. In Zone 4, the relationships between intravascular and alveolar pressures are the same as in Zone 3, but other factors are present that cause vascular narrowing.[9] Resistance to

blood flow in the dependent lung regions may increase, and hence blood flow will decrease if vascular caliber is reduced owing to the possible effects of increasing interstitial pressure (see next section) and local alveolar hypoxia (if airways leading to the region are closed or narrowed, as described in Chapter 4).

"ALVEOLAR" AND "EXTRA-ALVEOLAR" VESSELS

The model shown in Figure 5-1 certainly provides the best explanation that is currently available for the varying patterns of pulmonary blood flow observed in man and experimental animals under physiologic and pathologic conditions. However, the applicability of the model depends upon two special requirements inherent in the behavior and location of vessels designated as collapsible: (1) that the vessels offer virtually no resistance to the collapsing pressure, in other words, the pressure difference across the vessel wall is negligible, and (2) that the vessels are exposed to alveolar pressure, in contrast to vessels elsewhere in the lung that are exposed to a pressure that is more closely approximated by pleural pressure.[13]

Proponents of the model, however, have been careful not to delineate the anatomic boundaries of the collapsible segments. The pulmonary capillaries seem like logical sites because they lie unsupported in the interalveolar septum; but because it has been shown that one of the effects of the film of surfactant which lines alveolar walls is to hold capillaries open, it is possible that vessels further downstream (e.g., pulmonary venules) might be more susceptible than capillaries to a collapsing force.

Despite the absence of precise information about which vessels are involved, it is clear that some pulmonary blood vessels are exposed to alveolar pressure and others are exposed to a different pressure. The two "types" of vessels, called *alveolar* and *extra-alveolar*,[14] are depicted schematically in Figure 5-2. Although, as mentioned, the *site* of collapse of alveolar vessels under Zone 2 conditions is not known, and recent theoretic considerations suggest that collapse need not develop to account for the pattern of blood flow,[15] histologic examination of the lung in Zone 1 revealed that few vessels with a diameter less than 30 μm contained red blood cells.[16] This morphometric observation, coupled with

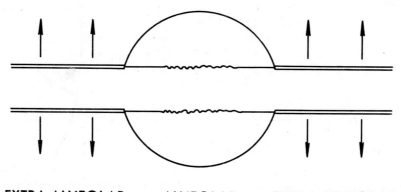

EXTRA-ALVEOLAR   ALVEOLAR   EXTRA-ALVEOLAR

Figure 5-2 Schematic representation of extra-alveolar and alveolar vessels. The pressure surrounding extra-alveolar vessels (arrows) is approximately the same as pleural pressure. In contrast, the pressure surrounding alveolar vessels is approximately the same as alveolar pressure. In addition, extra-alveolar vessels are thick walled and resist collapse, whereas alveolar vessels are thin walled and readily collapsible. (Adapted from Hughes, Glazier, Maloney, and West.[9] Reprinted by permission from the authors and publisher.)

the fact that vessels less than 100 μm in diameter have virtually no elastic tissue and smooth muscle to support their walls, strengthens the concepts that vessels at least as large as 30 μm in diameter are exposed to alveolar pressure and that vessels greater than 100 μm in diameter are exposed to a different perivascular pressure that is much nearer to pleural than to alveolar pressure.

TOTAL INTERSTITIAL PRESSURES

Both alveolar and extra-alveolar vessels are surrounded by a perivascular space, but, as indicated, the pressures in the two interstitial compartments are different. The customary practice of referring to "tissue pressure" or "interstitial pressure" is no

longer tenable. Guyton and associates[17] emphasized recently that the total pressure applied to a tissue surface is the sum of the liquid pressure (from the force of kinetic bombardment of the surface by molecules of the liquid) and the solid pressure (from the force attributable to actual points of contact between the surface and neighboring solid structures), so that

Total interstitial pressure =
interstitial liquid pressure +
interstitial solid pressure.   (1)

These concepts have been applied to the local factors that contribute to total interstitial pressures surrounding alveolar and extra-alveolar vessels and are shown schematically in Figures 5–3 and 5–4.[18] In both examples, a

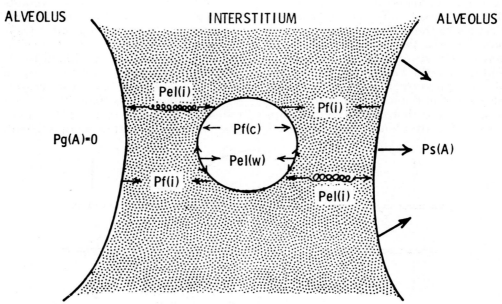

Figure 5–3 Schematic diagram of the forces determining the pressure surrounding *alveolar* vessels (i.e., total pericapillary pressure in the interstitium of the interalveolar septum). The arrows indicate the direction of action but not the magnitude of the pressures acting on the alveolar and capillary membranes. Pg(A) = alveolar gas pressure; Ps(A) = pressure arising from tension in the alveolar membrane (mainly surface tension); Pel(i) = solid elastic pressure arising from packing together of the solid elements in the interstitium; Pf(i) = fluid pressure in interstitial liquid; Pf(c) = fluid pressure in pulmonary capillaries; Pel(w) = pressure arising from elastic tension due to stretching of the capillary wall (assumes no active tension). The net balance of these forces is believed to result in a pericapillary pressure slightly less than alveolar pressure. For discussion, see text. (From Hughes.[18] Reprinted by permission from the author and publisher.)

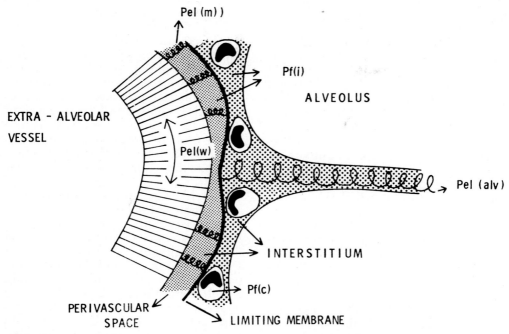

Pel (m))

Pf(i)

ALVEOLUS

EXTRA - ALVEOLAR
VESSEL

Pel(w)

Pel (alv)

INTERSTITIUM

Pf(c)

PERIVASCULAR
SPACE

LIMITING MEMBRANE

Figure 5–4 Schematic diagram of the forces determining the pressure surrounding *extra-alveolar* vessels (i.e., perivascular interstitial pressure). Abbreviations as in Figure 5–3. Absorption of interstitial liquid from the perivascular space proceeds until deformation of the solid elements creates an elastic recoil pressure of the limiting membrane (i.e., the perivascular connective tissue sheath) itself [Pel(m)]. The limiting membrane is also exposed to the elastic recoil pressure of the alveolar parenchyma [Pel(alv)] generated by expansion of the lung. The net balance of these forces is believed to result in a pressure in the perivascular space slightly less than pleural pressure. (See Chapter 4 for discussion of the relationship between pleural pressure and elastic recoil pressure of the lung parenchyma.) (From Hughes.[18] Reprinted by permission from the author and publisher.)

force exists that favors liquid absorption from within the perivascular space into the bloodstream; the absorptive force is due to the fact that colloid osmotic (oncotic) pressure exceeds the hydrostatic pressure within the blood vessel. Accordingly, liquid is absorbed from the interstitial space until the pressure generated by packing the solid tissue elements is sufficient to resist further absorption, and equilibrium is attained.

The difference between total interstitial pressure around alveolar and extra-alveolar vessels is accounted for by the different lung structures that determine the point of equilibrium. For alveolar vessels (Figure 5–3), the balance occurs across the alveolar mem-

brane (including surfactant layer) and the capillary membrane. It is believed that pericapillary total interstitial pressure is less than alveolar pressure by an amount determined by alveolar surface forces. Both calculations from presumed values of geometry and surface tension and data from animal experiments suggest that pericapillary total interstitial pressure is approximately minus 3 to 5 cm H_2O.[18, 19]

For extra-alveolar vessels (Figure 5–4), the balance of forces that affect perivascular total interstitial pressure operates across the perivascular sheath that is attached to the lung parenchyma; consequently, the pressure on the alveolar side of the membrane (i.e., opposite the blood vessel lumen) is determined by the elastic recoil of the lung. Because elastic recoil pressure is equal and opposite to pleural pressure, it can be appreciated why extra-alveolar perivascular total interstitial pressure is nearly the same as pleural pressure. Moreover, as mentioned in the case of conducting airways, the pressure surrounding extra-alveolar vessels is believed to be at least as negative as and probably slightly more negative than pleural pressure; the increment of additional negativity is related to the extent to which the vessels do not follow the expansion of the remainder of the lung.[20] This phenomenon can also be visualized from Figure 5–4. During lung inflation, elastic recoil and the outward "pull" on the perivascular sheath increase; if the blood vessel wall resists this pull, the total interstitial pressure becomes more negative than if the vessel enlarged in proportion to the increase in lung volume.

Because the interstitial spaces throughout the lung are continuous, it follows that there must be a hydrostatic gradient of interstitial liquid pressure of 1 cm H_2O for every 1 cm of vertical distance in the lung. However, it is generally assumed that total interstitial pressure at any level within the lung is not affected by gravity because any change in interstitial liquid pressure is offset by an equal and opposite change in interstitial solid pressure. However, in pathologic disorders associated with pulmonary edema, the separation of tissue elements by the excess liquid accumulation nullifies the effect of solid pressures; under these conditions, a vertical hydrostatic gradient of total interstitial pressure can be demonstrated.[18]

EFFECTS OF LUNG INFLATION

Figure 5–5 shows the results of mean regional blood flow measurements at different lung volumes in seated normal subjects. It can be seen that the vertical gradient of blood flow

is most evident when measured at TLC and that the gradient is reversed when measurements are made at RV. These variations cannot be explained by changes in the relationships among pulmonary arterial, pulmonary venous, and left atrial pressures, which presumably remained relatively constant during the study, but are believed to result from the influence of lung expansion on total interstitial pressure and on the caliber of extra-alveolar vessels.[9]

At RV, the entire parenchyma is collapsed and total interstitial pressure is increased sufficiently to influence the topographic distribution of blood flow throughout the entire lung. At FRC, the upper half of the lung is expanded more than the lower half, which therefore still demonstrates the effect of raised total interstitial pressure. When the lung is fully expanded to TLC, the only region where total interstitial pressure is still high enough to affect the caliber of extra-alveolar vessels and reduce blood flow is a small area at the bottom of the lung.

STRATIFICATION OF BLOOD FLOW

Although the distribution of pulmonary blood flow is governed chiefly by the transmural distending pressure and the distensibility of the vessel wall, other mechanisms can be detected as well. Morphometric studies of the pulmonary circulation leave no doubt that there is considerable variation in the length of available pathways from the main pulmonary artery to the terminal respiratory units; this must lead to different transit times for red blood cells traveling between the pulmonary valve and gas exchange units in various locations throughout the lung. In one carefully studied human lung specimen, it was found that the length of the pulmonary arteries from pulmonary valve to branches of the order of 50 μm in diameter averaged about 14 cm, with a range of 7 to 23 cm.[21] Thus, variation occurs

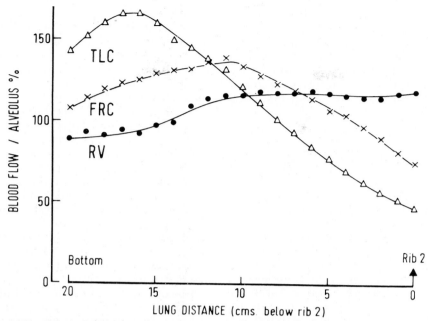

Figure 5–5   Blood flow per alveolus as a percentage of that expected if all alveoli were perfused equally, plotted against vertical distance from the bottom of the lung to the second rib. Points represent the mean values of both right and left lungs of subjects studied at total lung capacity (TLC), functional residual capacity (FRC), and residual volume (RV). Note the reduction in blood flow to the bottom of the lung that is more marked at FRC and RV than TLC. (From Hughes, Glazier, Maloney, and West.[9] Reprinted by permission from the authors and publisher.)

between one distal unit and another. There is, moreover, variation within a single terminal respiratory unit; incoming blood reaches the first order respiratory bronchioles and their alveoli sooner than it reaches more distal alveolar ducts and alveolar sacs.

The branching system of pulmonary arteries is analogous to that in the airways in which the presence of pathways of different lengths causes varying transit times of inhaled gas moving between the mouth and the alveoli. And the physiologic consequences of the anatomic similarities are the same: unevenness of the distribution of blood flow from stratification of perfusion and unevenness of the distribution of inspired air from stratification of ventilation. It might be anticipated that since the variations in transit times affect the distribution of both ventilation and perfusion, gas exchange might

be facilitated because matching of the two is maintained. This is a difficult problem to study, but experimental data suggest that, contrary to expectation, gas exchange is worse when both ventilation and perfusion are stratified than when only blood flow is unevenly distributed.[22]

PULMONARY VASCULAR RESISTANCE

GENERAL CONSIDERATIONS

Resistance to blood flow through the pulmonary circulation is calculated using the same general equation for frictional resistance described on p. 95; as before, the flow resistance offered by a system is computed from the pressure difference "across" the system and the flow through it. *Pul-*

monary vascular resistance (PVR) is determined by the inflow pressure in the pulmonary artery, the outflow pressure in the pulmonary veins or left atrium (P_{LA}), and the blood flow through the lungs (pulmonary blood flow) according to the equation.

$$PVR, \text{ units} = \frac{P_{PA} - P_{LA}, \text{ mm Hg}}{\text{pulmonary blood flow, L/min}} . \quad (2)$$

Pulmonary blood flow is normally equal to the cardiac output, but at times may be larger or smaller if intracardiac or other shunts exist. Values for normal pulmonary vascular resistance at rest and during moderately severe exercise are given in Table 5–1 and compared with values of systemic vascular resistance. The striking feature of the pulmonary circulation is its ability to accommodate huge increases in cardiac output with only a slight increase in pulmonary arterial pressure. This means that pulmonary vascular resistance decreases markedly.

SITES OF PULMONARY VASCULAR RESISTANCE

A decrease of pulmonary vascular resistance, in the presence of a constant or slightly increased pulmonary arteriovenous pressure difference, indicates that the cross-sectional area of those vessels that are the principal sites of resistance to blood flow must increase. Unfortunately, despite extensive investigation, there is still considerable doubt about how total pulmonary vascular resistance is partitioned among the various blood vessels that compose the human pulmonary circulation. Even in dogs, the subjects of many different experimental approaches, the issue has not been completely resolved. However, in contrast to the systemic circulation, in which resistance to blood flow through capillaries is a small fraction of the total

systemic vascular resistance, it appears that a substantial portion of the total pulmonary vascular resistance in dogs resides in capillaries—34 per cent in one study[23] and 53 per cent in another.[24] Whether or not this holds true for man remains to be determined.

Regardless of uncertainties about the site(s) of resistance, it can be inferred that an increase in cross-sectional area of the vascular bed can be produced either by distension (an increase in volume of those vessels already containing circulating blood) or by recruitment (blood flow through previously empty vessels). It is difficult to differentiate between recruitment and distension in the human vascular bed, but presumably both occur when pulmonary blood flow increases as, for example, during exercise. Reference to Figure 5–1 again shows that even a slight increase in pulmonary arterial pressure raises the column of blood on the inflow side somewhat. An increase in perfusion pressure "reaches" and recruits additional blood vessels toward the top of the lung, and the new (higher) pressure at all levels throughout the lung tends to distend vessels previously open and to open vessels previously closed because their opening pressures had not been exceeded.

Studies in dogs showed that the increase in blood flow from the top to the bottom of the upright lung was associated with morphologic evidence of increased capillary filling; this was attributed chiefly to recruitment of capillaries in upper Zone 2 and to distension of capillaries in lower Zones 2 and 3.[16] However, these conclusions were challenged by the results of other studies that indicated that the predominant mechanism was recruitment throughout the lung.[25]

The pattern of filling in the pulmonary capillary bed has been examined because it was reasoned that if recruitment were determined by the opening of a previously closed small artery, all capillaries in the region supplied by that artery would be filled with blood. This would lead to a "patchwork" pattern of filling in Zone 2 because all arteries would not open simultaneously, but owing to variations in their critical opening pressures, some would be open and some would remain closed at a given level of pressure in the lung.[26] It was discovered, however, that capillary recruitment did not vary from one arteriolar "domain" to another, but changes occurred within the network supplied by a single arteriole; this was revealed by finding red blood cells in some capillaries of an interalveolar septum while adjacent capillaries were empty. Under Zone 3 conditions, all capillaries in a given septum were filled. The random filling of capillaries in a network suggests that the pressure drop across a single channel of the network must be small and that hemodynamic changes occurring in one part of the segment probably affect those in neighboring segments. Thus, unstable flow conditions are created, which helps to account for the intermittency of pulmonary capillary flow that has been observed directly in many experimental preparations.

Efforts to study the pulmonary circulation by means of a descriptive model have led to a dispute over the most valid representation of the vascular bed. The pattern of filling, the histologic appearance of septal walls, and the area of the alveolar septum occupied by capillaries when the pulmonary circulation was intensely congested in dogs have led to a model of a network of branching vessels[26]; in contrast, morphometric studies of the interalveolar capillary bed of the cat were believed to be consistent with a model of sheet-flow in which the microcirculation was depicted as a sheet-like endothelium-lined space bridged by avascular endothelium-lined posts.[15] Differences between the species of animals examined may account for differences in the models used to display the pattern of blood

flow within capillaries. Further morphologic studies of the human pulmonary circulation are needed to determine which of the two models more closely represents the capillary bed in man.

PULMONARY BLOOD VOLUME

An expected corollary of any change that occurs in the cross-sectional area of the pulmonary vascular bed, which as indicated must underlie increases or decreases in pulmonary vascular resistance, is that corresponding changes should occur in the volume of blood contained within the pulmonary circulation. Accordingly, if vascular resistance decreases, owing to an increase in the cross-sectional area of the vascular bed, pulmonary blood volume should also increase, and vice versa. This straightforward analysis, though accurately describing the changes that take place in the resistance vessels, is an oversimplification of the events in the entire vascular bed. The relationship between volume and resistance is a complicated one, because the change in volume at the principal site(s) of vascular resistance may not be in the same direction as the changes in volume elsewhere in the circulation. This means that pulmonary vascular resistance is determined chiefly by variations in the caliber of the *major* resistance vessels; however, these changes may not be reflected by changes in total pulmonary blood volume because total volume is affected by increases and decreases of the *entire* pulmonary vascular bed. Differences in the behavior of resistance vessels and the rest of the vascular bed are evident during inflation of the lung from FRC. Pulmonary vascular resistance increases, implying a decrease in caliber of the resistance vessels; however, the blood volume of large vessels increases.

The total volume of blood in the lungs can be estimated in man by means of the indicator dilution technique. Normal values are about 295 ml/m² body surface, or roughly 10 per cent of the total circulating blood volume.[27] Although reliable data are limited, it is now generally recognized that during exercise, pulmonary blood volume tends to remain constant, and increases of more than 20 per cent seldom occur despite marked increases in cardiac output.[28] Furthermore, during experiments in man in which total circulating blood volume was rapidly expanded, pulmonary blood volume did not change, although cardiac output and pulmonary arterial pressure both increased significantly.[27] These studies also demonstrate that serial measurements of pulmonary blood volume do not necessarily reflect changes in pulmonary vascular resistance.

PULMONARY VASCULAR DISTENSIBILITY

The observations just cited, which emphasize the constancy of pulmonary volume, may seem at first glance to conflict with reports that emphasize the distensibility of the pulmonary vascular bed. It is known, for example, that nearly 70 per cent of the right ventricular stroke volume is retained in pulmonary arteries during systole for distribution to the pulmonary capillaries during the ensuing diastole.[29] Although the "storage capacity" is affected by changes in heart rate and pulmonary arterial pressure, its presence appears to belie statements about the constancy of pulmonary blood volume.

This apparent paradox can be explained by the fact that measurements of pulmonary blood volume by the conventional method utilizing the indicator dilution technique (multiplying mean transit time and blood flow through the pulmonary circulation) eliminate variations in volume during a single heartbeat. Thus, in any given segment of the pulmonary circulation

the volume varies from moment to moment during the cardiac cycle, but when averaged during several beats, the volume in the entire pulmonary vascular bed tends to remain constant despite changing cardiac output.

Accommodation of blood during systole and its release during the subsequent diastole means that the pulmonary arterial system is pulsatile, a feature that has been recognized for decades through the use of fluoroscopy. It is now known from studies performed with the body plethysmograph that blood flow through the pulmonary capillaries is also pulsatile.[30] Recent experimental data demonstrated that venous blood flow is pulsatile as well, reflecting the transmission of pulsations through "open" arteries and capillaries into the veins.[31] Figure 5–6 shows examples of the pulse wave characteristics of pulmonary arteries, pulmonary capillaries, and pulmonary veins. The transmission of pulse waves through the pulmonary circulation depends on the characteristics of the blood vessel walls and on the frequency of the impulses (determined by heart rate).[32] Pulmonary vasoconstriction induced by drugs (e.g., serotonin) or hypoxia in experimental animals has been shown to produce a decrease in arterial distensibility and, as expected, an increase in pulse wave velocity.[29]

In man, pulmonary blood volume did not change proportionately the same amount as total circulating blood volume when total volume was increased or decreased[27]; this constancy indicates that changes in pulmonary vasomotor tone must have occurred. In addition, similar experiments in which autonomic blocking drugs were used provide convincing evidence that the distensibility of the pulmonary circulation is regulated by neurogenic influences that operate to keep blood volume in the lungs constant within fairly narrow limits.[33] Thus, factors seem to be acting to prevent "over-

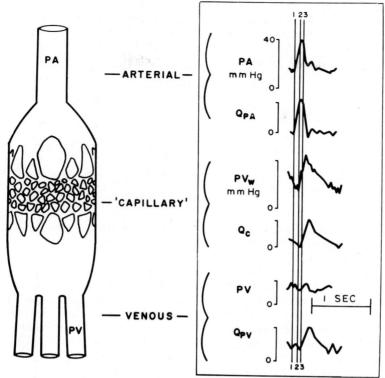

Figure 5-6 Schematic diagram showing the transformation of the pressure and flow pulses from the pulmonary artery to the pulmonary vein. PA = pulmonary arterial pressure; Q_{PA} = pulmonary arterial flow; PV_W = pulmonary venous wedge pressure; Q_c = pulmonary capillary flow; PV = pulmonary venous pressure; Q_{PV} = pulmonary venous flow. The interval 1–2 is the transmission time (0.09 sec) for the pulse from the pulmonary artery to capillaries; the interval 2–3 is the transmission time (0.03 sec) from the capillaries to pulmonary veins. (From Morkin, Collins, Goldman, and Fishman.[31] Reprinted by permission from the authors and publisher.)

loading" of the pulmonary circulation; if this assumption is true, these mechanisms can be considered "protective" and if they are deficient or overwhelmed, pulmonary vascular congestion may develop.

FACTORS AFFECTING VASCULAR RESISTANCE

A logical extension of the considerations analyzed in previous sections is that total pulmonary vascular resistance is determined by the interaction of several different mechanisms. These can be conveniently divided into *passive* (Table 5–2) and *active* (Table 5–3) influences. Altera-

tions in resistance from a "passive" process indicate that changes in the caliber of pulmonary blood vessels are secondary responses to changing mechanical conditions within the lung or to hemodynamic events in the systemic circulation. In contrast, alterations in pulmonary vascular resistance from an "active" process imply that contraction or relaxation of the smooth muscles of blood vessel walls has occurred in response to neural, humoral, or chemical stimuli.

Two points should be stressed about interpretation of studies that have attempted to discover the mechanisms underlying any induced changes in pulmonary vascular resist-

Table 5–2 A List of Factors That When Varied Cause "Passive" Changes in Pulmonary Vascular Resistance (PVR) and the Direction of the Responses

FACTOR	RESPONSE
Pulmonary arterial pressure (P_{PA})	Increased P_{PA} causes decreased PVR
Left atrial pressure (P_{LA})	Increased P_{LA} causes decreased PVR
Transpulmonary pressure (P_l)	Increase and decrease of P_l from value at FRC cause increased PVR
Total interstitial pressure (P_{is})	Increased P_{is} causes increased PVR
Pulmonary blood volume	Shift of blood from systemic vessels into lung vessels causes decreased PVR
Whole blood viscosity	Increase in viscosity causes increased PVR

ance. First, the investigation must include measurements of left atrial pressure, or a suitable substitute such as wedge pressure, before any meaningful conclusions about resistance changes can be reached; this is an important constraint because the pulmonary arteriovenous pressure difference is small to begin with, and thus even small changes in left atrial pressure have a considerable influence on the calculated value for pulmonary vascular resistance. Second, it is impossible to demonstrate conclusively active pulmonary vasoconstriction or vasodilatation in the presence of changing conditions that also cause passive alterations in the caliber of the vessels.[34] (An exception to this occurs if the vasomotor responses are opposite to and prevail over those from associated passive variations.)

PASSIVE CHANGES IN VASCULAR RESISTANCE

Included in Table 5–2 are six factors that, when changed, cause secondary changes in pulmonary vascular resistance by imposing a passive increase or decrease in the caliber of blood vessels. Changing one mechanical variable in the respiratory system frequently causes changes in another variable; for example, increasing left atrial pressure or alveolar pressure causes an increase in pulmonary arterial pressure and pleural pressure, respectively. For this reason, in order to study the effects of variations of a single factor, it is necessary (although difficult experimentally) to hold all other factors constant. It is obvious that these rigorous requirements cannot be met in a study of the

Table 5–3 A List of Important Causes of "Active" Changes in Pulmonary Vascular Resistance (PVR) and the Direction of the Responses

Neurogenic stimuli
    Sympathetic stimulation increases PVR in experimental animals; no effect in man
    Parasympathetic stimulation causes no detectable response
Humoral substances
    Vasoconstrictors: catecholamines, serotonin (no effect in man), histamine,
        angiotensin, fibrinopeptides, prostaglandin F
    Vasodilators: acetylcholine, bradykinin, prostaglandin E
Chemical stimuli
    Alveolar hypoxia increases PVR
    Alveolar hypercarbia increases PVR in experimental animals; no effect in man
    Acidemia (decreased pH) increases PVR

human pulmonary circulation, so most of the available evidence was derived from studies of isolated lungs from experimental animals. Despite this limitation, there is good reason to believe that the general conclusions from these studies describe the behavior of pulmonary blood vessels in man.

Pulmonary Arterial Pressure. As pulmonary arterial pressure is raised (either by raising the height of a perfusion reservoir or by increasing flow), with lung volume and left atrial pressure held constant, pulmonary vascular resistance decreases.[35] The increase in inflow pressure causes an increase in transmural distending pressure, which, by increasing the cross-sectional area of the pulmonary arterial system and capillary network through dilatation and recruitment, decreases

resistance to blood flow. As shown in Figure 5–7, the effect of changing pulmonary arterial pressure on pulmonary vascular resistance is lessened when left atrial pressure is high to begin with, because this maneuver separately dilates and recruits pulmonary blood vessels.[36]

Left Atrial Pressure. When left atrial pressure is raised, and pulmonary arterial pressure and lung volume are kept constant, pulmonary vascular resistance decreases, as shown in Figure 5–8.[35] As might be expected from the relationships between pulmonary arterial and left atrial pressures, the effect of changing left atrial pressure on pulmonary vascular resistance diminishes if pulmonary arterial pressure is high at the outset. Similarly, the effect on vascular resistance is augmented if pulmonary

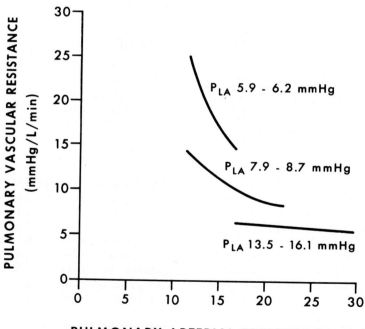

Figure 5–7 Diagrammatic representation of the results of perfusion experiments showing the effects of changes in pulmonary arterial pressure on pulmonary vascular resistance at three different ranges of left atrial pressure (P_{LA}). As pulmonary arterial pressure is increased, pulmonary vascular resistance decreases; but the effect progressively lessens as left atrial pressure is raised. (Adapted from Borst, McGregor, Whittenberger, and Berglund.[36] Reprinted by permission from the authors and the American Heart Association, Inc.)

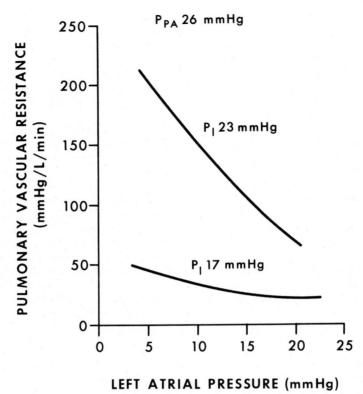

Figure 5–8 Diagrammatic representation of the results of perfusion experiments showing the effects of changes in left atrial pressure on pulmonary vascular resistance at two different values of transpulmonary pressure (P_1); pulmonary arterial pressure (P_{PA}) was held constant at 26 mm Hg throughout. As left atrial pressure is increased, pulmonary vascular resistance decreases. The influence of transpulmonary pressure is explained by the effects of lung inflation on pulmonary vascular resistance (see text and Figure 5–9). (Adapted from Roos, Thomas, Nagel, and Prommas.[35] Reprinted by permission from the authors and publisher.)

arterial pressure is allowed to increase as left atrial pressure is raised, a circumstance more closely resembling normal relationships than a change in left atrial pressure alone.

Transpulmonary Pressure. A distinction has already been made between alveolar vessels and extra-alveolar vessels on the basis of the different pressures surrounding the two "types" of vascular channels (see earlier section on Interstitial Pressure). Because these pressures are one component of the transmural pressures that exist across vessel walls and hold them open and because the pressures vary differently during lung inflation,

alveolar and extra-alveolar vessels are exposed to different distending forces as the lung expands. This, in turn, affects the cross-sectional area of the vessels, which, in addition to mechanical changes in length, governs the resistance to blood flow through them. As shown schematically in Figure 5–9, the resistance offered by alveolar and extra-alveolar vessels changes in opposite directions during inflation of the lung from RV to TLC.[13, 14]

At low lung volumes, the relatively high total interstitial pressure and the kinking that occurs as extra-alveolar vessels shorten increase resistance to flow through them; these two effects diminish as lung volume increases. At high lung volumes, although extra-alveolar vessels are maximally dilated but lengthened, alveolar vessels are stretched and flattened and thus offer increased resistance to blood flow. The curves shown in Figure 5–9 must be regarded as speculative owing to uncertainties about the partitioning of vascular resistance among different vessels; the diagram accurately reflects, however, the belief that total pulmonary vascular resistance is minimal at FRC, and both increases and decreases in lung volume from the resting position are associated with increased resistance to blood flow. The magnitude of the changes depicted is arguable.

In theory, the lung should be ex-panded equally well by applying either positive pressure to the airways or negative pressure around the lungs. If the transpulmonary pressure is equal in the two conditions, the amount of lung inflation and thus the effects on pulmonary vascular resistance must be the same. Despite this certainty, there is still a lively debate on the origin of the hemodynamic differences between positive and negative pressure breathing. Suffice it to say that the chief differences between the methods cannot be accounted for by differences in the mechanical effects of static lung inflation on vascular resistance and must be due to other hemodynamic phenomena, especially the influences on venous return to the thorax.

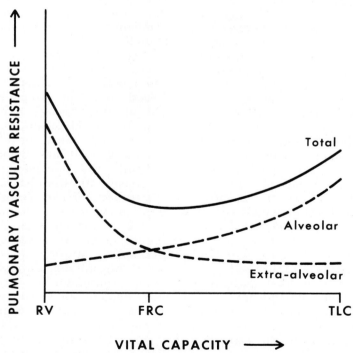

Figure 5–9 Schematic representation of the effects of changes in vital capacity on total pulmonary vascular resistance and the contributions to the total afforded by alveolar and extra-alveolar vessels. During inflation from residual volume (RV) to total lung capacity (TLC), resistance to blood flow through alveolar vessels increases, whereas resistance through extra-alveolar vessels decreases. Thus changes in total pulmonary vascular resistance form a U-shaped curve during lung inflation, with the nadir at functional residual capacity (FRC).

Perivascular Pressure. All vessels have pressure applied to their outside walls, and as indicated earlier, the perivascular (total interstitial) pressure differs between the two "types" of pulmonary blood vessels. Perivascular pressure surrounding alveolar vessels is normally slightly lower than alveolar pressure, owing to the retractive force created by the film of surfactant that lines alveolar walls. If surface tension rises, so does the inward "pull" of the film, and the pericapillary pressure will become more negative. This phenomenon lowers resistance to blood flow through alveolar vessels, but it also has important implications for the movement of liquid and solute (see next section). The total interstitial pressure surrounding extra-alveolar vessels is normally equal to or less than pleural pressure, and thus is affected by changing lung volumes. Total interstitial pressure around extra-alveolar vessels is increased at low lung volumes and also by the accumulation of fluid, blood, or air in the interstitial space; under these conditions, resistance to blood flow through extra-alveolar vessels increases.

Pulmonary Intravascular Volume. Although pulmonary intravascular volume tends to remain relatively constant, it may increase or decrease under certain normal circumstances and in a variety of pathologic conditions. Regardless of the mechanism, if blood volume increases, it must distend previously perfused blood vessels or recruit new ones, and pulmonary vascular resistance will tend to decrease. As emphasized previously, the fall in total pulmonary vascular resistance depends upon how much (local) resistance decreases in those vessels whose size increases in order to accommodate the extra volume.

Blood Viscosity. Blood viscosity depends upon the intravascular hematocrit ratio, the characteristics of red blood cells (especially their deformability), and the composition of plasma. Although measurement of these components presents difficulty and the contribution of blood viscosity to total pulmonary vascular resistance is hard to assess, convincing experimental evidence is now available (Figure 5–10) that demonstrates that an increase in pulmonary vascular resistance accompanies an increase in blood viscosity induced by changing hematocrit ratio.[37]

ACTIVE CHANGES IN VASCULAR RESISTANCE

Table 5–3 lists the chief neurogenic, humoral, and chemical causes of active pulmonary vasomotor reactions. But in view of the difficulties inherent in designing suitable experiments, it is not surprising that considerable doubt still exists about the mechanism of action of numerous common physiologic or pharmacologic stimuli.

Neurogenic Stimuli. Pulmonary arteries and veins are richly innervated with nerve fibers that are believed to be of sympathetic origin. Despite the presence of an extensive vascular nervous plexus, which (as a first assumption) must have functional significance, it has been extremely difficult to document vasomotor responses to stimulation of either sympathetic or parasympathetic pathways in experimental animals. Studies in dogs have demonstrated that sympathetic nerve stimulation increased pulmonary arterial tone and pulse wave transmission through the circulation[38]; although no vasoconstriction was evident in these experiments, recent investigations, using different methods, revealed a vasoconstrictor response.[39] Intrathoracic nerve stimulation experiments are obviously impossible to carry out in man; however, studies with neurogenic blocking drugs have been performed and have led to the conclusion that the auto-

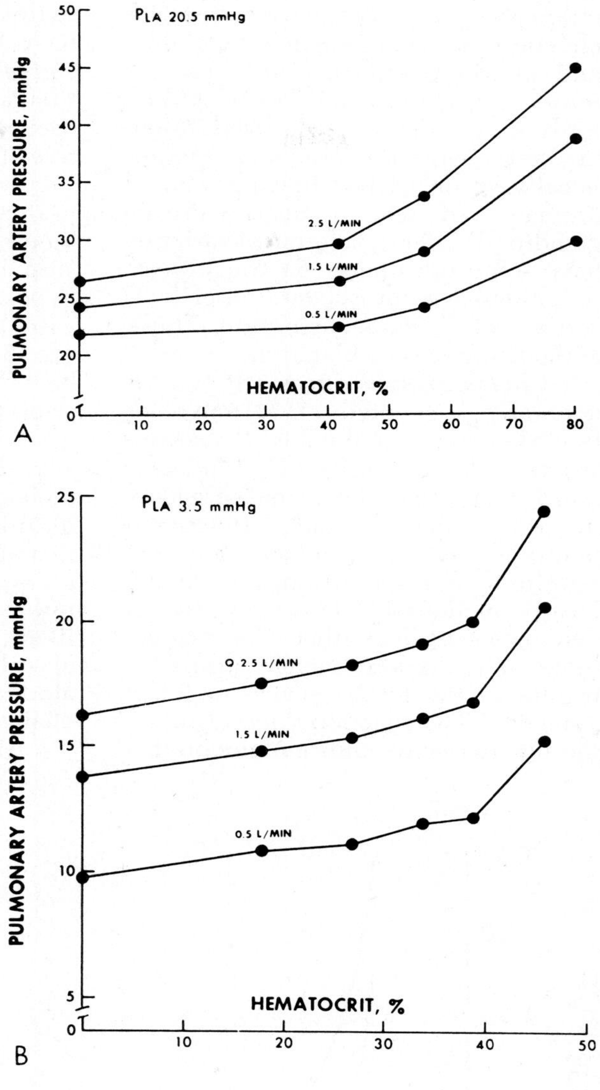

Figure 5-10 Experimental results showing the effect of changes in hematocrit on the pulmonary arterial pressure required to produce a given blood flow. Left atrial pressure (P_{LA}) was constant at 20.5 mm Hg in *A* and 3.5 mm Hg in *B*. As hematocrit increases, progressively more pressure is required to overcome the contribution of increasing blood viscosity to resistance to blood flow. (From Murray, Karp, and Nadel.[37] Reprinted by permission from the publisher.)

nomic nervous system exerts little or no control over the pulmonary circulation in the normal human adult.[40]

Humoral Agents. Several naturally occurring humoral agents are thought to initiate either vasoconstrictor or vasodilator responses from different segments of the pulmonary vascular bed. Most of this information was derived from studies of animals that were given large doses of the test substance. Because it is well known that drugs have different effects in different species, and the action may be dose-dependent, some reservation is always necessary about translating the results from animal studies into inferences about the regulation of the human pulmonary circulation. Within these limitations, it is believed that several humoral substances exert vasomotor control of the pulmonary circulation[34]: *vasoconstrictors* — catecholamines, angiotensin, histamine, and fibrinopeptides; and *vasodilators* — bradykinin and acetylcholine (only in an already constricted vascular bed). Serotonin produces unequivocal vasoconstriction in experimental animals but not in man.[34] Prostaglandins of different chemical varieties have opposing effects on the pulmonary circulation: prostaglandins of the F series cause vasoconstriction, those of the E series vasodilatation.

Chemical Substances. It is now generally accepted that alveolar hypoxia causes pulmonary vasoconstriction, presumably of pulmonary arteries. Because the response occurs in the isolated lung, functional neurohumoral mechanisms are not required, and the response may be locally mediated.[41] However, recent evidence suggests that the sympathetic nervous system may also contribute to the total reponse in intact animals.[42] The reaction depends upon the P_{O_2} in the alveolus and not on that

in the bloodstream. These observations have led to the hypothesis that some sort of receptor is present on the adventitial surface of pulmonary arteries that "senses" alveolar P_{O_2} (or some derivative of it) and initiates vasoconstriction.

Several studies in man[43] and experimental animals[44] have documented the synergistic interrelationship between the effects of alveolar hypoxia and acidosis on pulmonary vascular resistance. As shown in Figure 5–11, the influence of hypoxia becomes progressively greater as arterial pH is lowered. At the present time it is impossible to say what, if any, direct effect CO_2 has on the pulmonary circulation. In studies in man, its influence was trivial.[45] Because an increase and decrease in $[H^+]$ causes a respective increase or decrease in pulmonary vascular resistance, it is likely that any effects of changes in alveolar or blood P_{CO_2} will be mediated in large part by the corresponding changes in pH.

Many endogenous vasoactive hor-

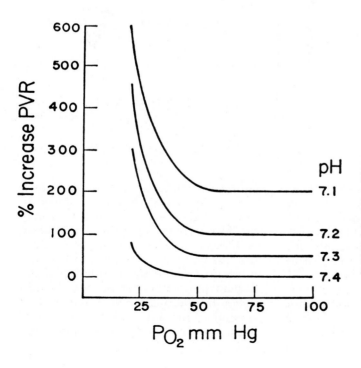

Figure 5–11 Diagram of the average results from experiments in newborn calves showing the effect of changes in inspired P_{O_2} on pulmonary vascular resistance (PVR) under conditions of different arterial blood pH. As inspired P_{O_2} is decreased, pulmonary vascular resistance increases; this effect becomes exaggerated and occurs at progressively higher P_{O_2} values as pH is decreased. (From Rudolph and Yuan.[44] Reprinted by permission from the authors and publisher.)

mones have been synthesized and are available as drugs. Most of the naturally occurring agents just listed have been given to man and have elicited the responses indicated. Other pulmonary vasoconstrictors are metaraminol, phenylephrine, and bretylium tosylate; other vasodilators are isoproterenol and aminophylline.[34] Virtually all the conclusions about the actions of drugs, both in man and experimental animals, were derived from acute studies; the chronic effects of drugs on the human pulmonary circulation remain a complete mystery.

LIQUID AND SOLUTE MOVEMENT

Among the significant developments of the past few years are the results of investigations concerning both the anatomy and physiology of liquid and solute movement in the lungs. These data allow inferences to be made about the basic mechanisms involved in the formation and removal of extravascular extracellular liquid in the lungs and how disturbances in these processes cause pulmonary edema (defined as an abnormal accumulation of extravascular liquid). The new formulation has resulted in a drastic revision of older concepts that the lung is a "dry" organ. Although many knowledge gaps remain, the handling of liquid and solutes by the lungs provides one of the best examples of the interdependence of pulmonary structure and function.

Normally, some liquid (the exact amount is not known) continuously escapes from small pulmonary blood vessels, and an equal amount is removed from the lungs, chiefly by pulmonary lymphatics. Liquid leaks principally through the walls of pulmonary capillaries, but arterioles and venules may be involved to some extent as well. The site at which the earliest *excess* of liquid can be de-

tected in the lungs by electron microscopy under certain experimental conditions is the interstitial space of the interalveolar septum.[46] Presumably, a leak of liquid from the pulmonary capillaries accounts for the recognizable accumulation, and this observation has led to the belief that the capillary endothelium is the source of the extravascular liquid that is continuously being produced under normal circumstances. Furthermore, and as a corollary to the above, it is now widely accepted that a considerable amount of liquid must be accommodated within the distensible interstitial spaces of the lung before any liquid appears in alveolar spaces.[47] Thus, the familiar clinical hallmarks of pulmonary edema, rales and frothy sputum, are relatively late manifestations of the sequence of liquid accumulation. Awareness that interstitial edema must precede alveolar edema has resulted in extensive efforts to develop techniques that will allow the early stages to be identified before the late life-threatening manifestations appear.

ANATOMIC CONSIDERATIONS

The interalveolar septum, it will be recalled (Chapter 2), is composed of several pulmonary capillaries that are supported within the septal wall lined by alveolar epithelium on both sides (Figure 5–12). Each capillary consists of a tube of endothelial cells supported by a basement membrane. The endothelium is primarily a thin cytoplasmic layer because nuclei comprise only a small portion of the surface area covered by each cell. It can be seen in Figure 5–12 that the basement membranes of the endothelium and epithelium appear to be fused over about half of the capillary perimeter, but that elsewhere the two basement membranes are separated by an interstitial space that contains chiefly connective tissue elements and occasionally macrophages and fibroblasts. The region where the base-

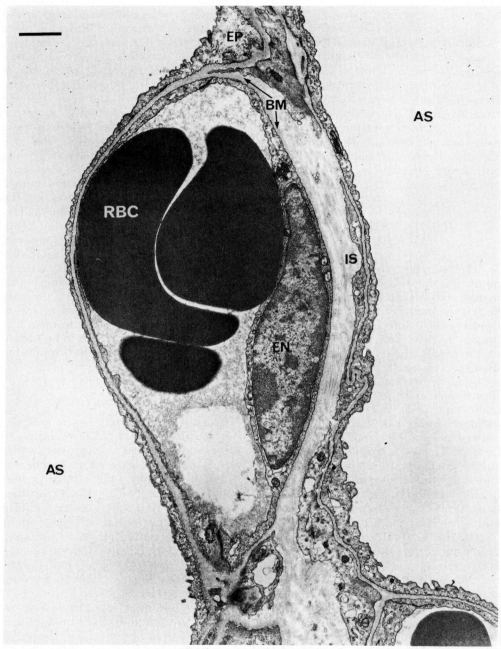

Figure 5–12 Electron photomicrograph of a human lung. Two capillaries containing red blood cells (RBC) are suspended in the interalveolar septum between two alveolar spaces (AS). The basement membranes (BM) of the epithelium (EP) and endothelium (EN) appear to be fused over the thin portion of the septum (or air-blood barrier) and are separated over the thick portion of the septum containing the interstitial space (IS). Horizontal bar = 1 μm. (× 11,000. Courtesy of Dr. Ewald R. Weibel.)

ment membranes are fused is called the thin portion of the alveolar-capillary septum, or air-blood barrier, and because of its narrowness must be the preferential location for the diffusion of gases; conversely, the region that contains the interstitial space is called the thick portion of the septum and presumably is the site of initial fluid accumulation. This is a beneficial arrangement because, as can be visualized in Figure 5–12, the spatial separation of functions means that the interstitial space of the alveolar septum may accommodate increased amounts of fluid without necessarily impairing gas exchange. Moreover, as will be discussed in greater detail later, physical forces exist that drain liquid from the interstitial space of the thick portion of the septum into the interstitial space surrounding conducting airways and blood vessels; this mechanism also serves to limit liquid accumulation in the terminal respiratory units and its possible interference with gas transfer.

Adjacent cells in both endothelium and epithelium either abut bluntly or overlap each other and produce in both instances a narrow cleft between cells (Figure 5–13). However, the junctions between endothelial cells are only partially fused in their narrowest portions (maculae occludentes), and tiny slits about 40 Å in width remain that allow communication between the intravascular and extravascular (interstitial) spaces. In contrast, the clefts between adjacent type I and type II alveolar epithelial cells are virtually completely fused toward the alveolar spaces. The alveolar epithelium is thereby "tighter" than the capillary endothelium and provides a more impenetrable barrier against liquid movement. This arrangement means that liquid and solute molecules that are continuously moving across the endothelium into the interstitial space in response to normally occurring forces do not enter the alveolar gas spaces. Furthermore, differences in the calculated sizes of pores in the alveolar and capillary membranes are consistent with demonstrated differences in their electron microscopic characteristics.[48]

It can be inferred from the previous statement that the size of pores is important because it determines whether or not a given molecule can pass through a membrane. Liquid movement can occur through cellular junctions, through cell membranes, or by way of endocytosis; each of these processes can be represented as a "pore" of certain dimensions. Thus, pores are not necessarily open interstices but are a means of describing physiologic phenomena that must have anatomic counterparts. To account for water and solute movement across the pulmonary capillary endothelium,* the pore theory assumes that there are sets of channels with different dimensions, and thus differing permeability characteristics. Most recent models of lung permeability use four sets of pores to account for the different rates of movement of all the various intravascular constituents that are known to cross the endothelial barrier. Some believe that large molecules exchange via pinocytosis in endothelial and epithelial cell vesicles (Figure 5–14), which thereby can be viewed as the anatomic pathways of the large pore system.[49] There is, however, general uncertainty about the structural equivalents of the pore system. Prevailing evidence indicates that the junctions between adjacent endothelial cells serve as sieves that govern exchange of water and solutes. Moreover, by changing hemodynamic

---

*Ultrastructural examination and physiologic studies of permeability reveal that pulmonary capillaries resemble skeletal and heart muscle capillaries but differ from capillaries in visceral organs.[48]

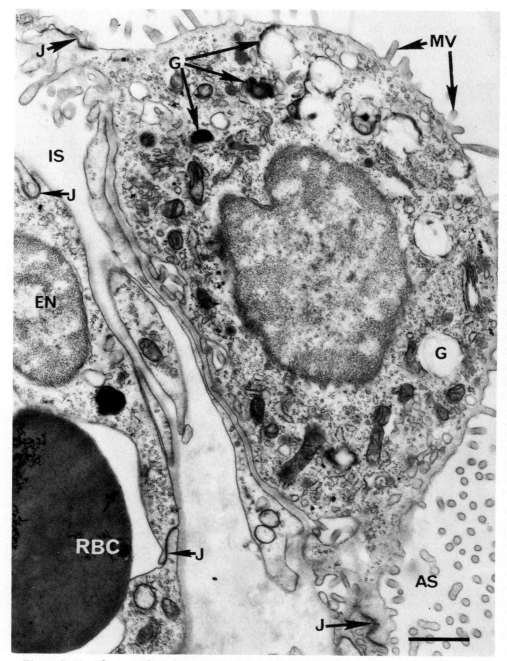

Figure 5–13 Electron photomicrograph of the alveolar-capillary membrane from an adult man showing: alveolar epithelium composed of a type II cell, recognized by its characteristic inclusions (G) and microvilli (MV), that abuts type I cells at intercellular junctions (J). Two junctions (J) between adjacent endothelial cells (EN) are also demonstrated. RBC = red blood cell; IS = interstitial space; AS = alveolar space. Horizontal bar = 1 μm. ($\times$ 16,000. Courtesy of Dr. Donald McKay.)

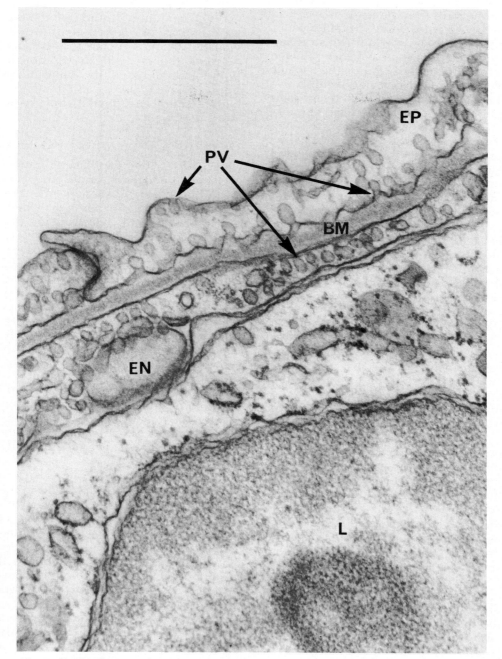

Figure 5–14 Electron photomicrograph of the air-blood barrier from an adult man showing pinocytotic vesicles (PV) in the epithelium (EP) and endothelium (EN). The basement membranes (BM) of the two layers appear to be fused. L = lymphocyte in pulmonary capillary. The horizontal bar = 1 μm. (× 56,400. Courtesy of Dr. Donald McKay.)

conditions experimentally, endothelial permeability can be made to vary as if the pores were being stretched wider; although there was no ultrastructural evidence to support a change in size of intercellular junctions, the results clearly showed that permeability is a dynamic rather than a fixed characteristic of the endothelial membrane.[46]

The lung has an extensive network of lymphatic channels, which do not extend into the alveolar septum but terminate in the interstitial space surrounding terminal bronchioles and small blood vessels (Chapter 3). However, the "juxta-alveolar" lymphatics (see Figure 3–3) are strategically located to drain liquid that has passed along the interstitial space of the interalveolar septum[50]; it is likely that the pulmonary capillaries, the chief sites of transvascular liquid formation, are all within a few hundred, or at most 1000 μm (1 mm) of a lymph channel. The ultrastructural appearance of pores and gaps in the endothelium and basement membrane of lymph capillaries suggests strongly that liquid in the interstitial spaces of the lung has ready access to lymphatic drainage pathways.[51]

Pulmonary vascular congestion, probably through its interstitial component, is known to stimulate J (juxtacapillary) receptors, one of the three well-established vagal afferent systems arising in the lungs (Chapter 3). Five unmyelinated axons have been identified in the rat lung (Figure 3–10), but the function of these structures, whether or not they are J receptors, and the presence of their counterparts (if any) in man remain to be demonstrated. However, despite the morphologic uncertainties, stimulation of J receptors and possibly other receptors probably plays a role in the genesis of the sensation of breathlessness in patients with a variety of cardiopulmonary disorders (see Table 3–1) in which interstitial liquid accumulation is known to occur.

PHYSIOLOGIC FACTORS

The amount of liquid in the interstitial space at a given moment obviously depends upon the balance between the rate of extravasation of liquid and the rate of its removal. Net liquid flow ($\dot{Q}_f$) across an endothelial barrier can be described by the classic Starling equation,[52]

$$\dot{Q}_f = K_f \left[(P_{cap} - P_{is}) - \sigma(\pi_{pl} - \pi_{is}) \right], \quad (3)$$

where K_f is the capillary filtration coefficient, which describes the permeability characteristics of the endothelial membrane through which exchange occurs; P_{cap} and P_{is} are the hydrostatic pressures in the capillary and pericapillary interstitial spaces, respectively; π_{pl} and π_{is} are the colloid osmotic (oncotic) pressures in the plasma and interstitial liquids; and σ is the reflection coefficient, a term that defines the effectiveness of the membrane in preventing the flow of solute compared with the flow of H_2O. Although only one of these (π_{pl}) can be measured with precision, recent experimental data allow reasonable estimates to be made about the remaining factors that contribute to liquid exchange and the direction in which they operate; these are shown schematically in Figure 5–15.*

Permeability. Permeability is not affected directly by changes in the surface area of the membrane involved; although K_f (Equation 3) does not include the dimensions of the membrane, if the area is doubled and other conditions are constant, filtration will also double. Quantification of the permeability characteristics of the barriers to liquid movement in the lung has proved extremely difficult. It is known that pulmonary capillaries are highly permeable to H_2O and also, but to a

---

*Because the reflection coefficient is nearly 1.0, it is ignored in the simplified model.

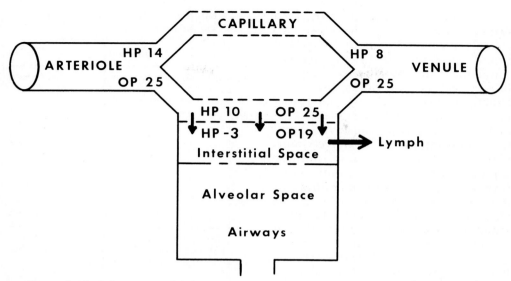

Figure 5–15 Schematic model showing the hydrostatic pressure (HP) and colloid osmotic pressure (OP) relationships under normal resting conditions in the pulmonary arteriole, capillary, venule, and pericapillary interstitial space. The arrows indicate the direction of liquid movement.

lesser degree, to small solutes (Na^+, K^+, Cl^-) and certain uncharged metabolites (urea, glucose, sucrose).[53] The greater opposition to the movement of most substances, including H_2O and low molecular weight solutes, afforded by the alveolar epithelium compared with the capillary endothelium has already been emphasized.

Filtration varies in healthy subjects during normal activities such as lying down, which shifts blood into the pulmonary circulation, and exercise, which increases capillary hydrostatic pressure. An abnormal increase in membrane leakiness appears to underlie many forms of noncardiogenic pulmonary edema; in these conditions, edema may be generalized or regional, as in pulmonary infections or chemical injuries (circulating, aspirated, or inhaled).

Capillary Hydrostatic and Osmotic Pressures. Pulmonary capillary hydrostatic pressure, a force which serves to drive liquid out of the vessel, is normally about 10 mm Hg, a value considerably below the inward or retaining force afforded by the colloid osmotic pressure of plasma proteins (25 mm Hg). Although capillary pressure is not uniform throughout the lung, owing to the effects of gravity, the difference between capillary hydrostatic and osmotic pressures is clearly in favor of intravascular retention of liquid. This imbalance led to the early hypothesis that the lung is a "dry" organ, but it is now known that alveolar surfaces are persistently moist and, more important, that there is constant drainage of liquid from the lungs through the pulmonary lymphatic vessels.

Continuous drainage of liquid means it must continually be formed. However, because intravascular pressures by themselves do not provide the required outward "driving" force, it means that values for interstitial osmotic pressure and interstitial total pressure (liquid and solid) must be such that the balance is tipped in favor of net outward movement of liquid from the intravascular into the interstitial compartments.

Interstitial Hydrostatic and Osmotic Pressures. There are two schools of thought about interstitial liquid pressure in tissue spaces throughout the body, including the lungs: one school holds that it is slightly positive,[54] and the other, that it is substantially negative.[55] Evidence for and against these views and the implications of negative interstitial pressures for transcapillary liquid exchange have recently been reviewed.[17] The most compelling evidence was summarized earlier in this chapter and indicates that total interstitial pressure surrounding alveolar vessels is slightly negative (minus 3 to 5 cm H_2O) and that total interstitial pressure around extra-alveolar vessels is similar to pleural pressure and varies with lung volume (but probably averages about minus 5 to 10 cm H_2O). Thus, the transmural pressure difference across pulmonary capillaries must be about 13 to 15 mm Hg (10 mm Hg intravascular and minus 3 to 5 mm Hg interstitial). It is important to recognize that if liquid were to accumulate in the interstitial space, interstitial liquid pressure would increase toward positive values and that this process would tend to inhibit further extravasation of liquid by reducing the transmural pressure difference.

Interstitial osmotic pressure is determined by the molecular constituents and their state of chemical binding within the interstitial liquid. Recent experimental studies, in sheep and dogs, of lymph composition, which presumably is a good mirror of interstitial liquid, reveal a substantial protein content (Table 5–4). This indicates, in contrast to previously held concepts, that there is a continuous transcapillary movement of large molecules, which, in turn, contribute to an appreciable interstitial osmotic pressure. Calculations derived from the geometry of sheep lungs and the com-

Table 5–4 Protein Content and Composition of Lung Lymph and Blood Plasma Under Normal Conditions.*†

SPECIES AND ANIMAL NO.	PLASMA			LUNG LYMPH		
	TP	A	G	TP	A	G
Dog						
1	5.2			4.0		
2	6.4	3.6	2.8	3.2	2.4	0.8
3	6.4	3.1	3.3	3.3	1.7	1.6
Cat						
1	7.4			4.9		
Sheep						
1	5.7	2.1	3.6	3.9	1.9	2.0

*Data summarized by Staub.[52]
†Abbreviations: TP = total protein; A = albumin; G = globulin. All in gm/100 ml.

position of lymph obtained from them indicate that effective interstitial osmotic pressure averages about 19 mm Hg throughout the lung.[52] The effect of an extravascular osmotic force is to diminish by an identical amount the effect of an intravascular osmotic force; therefore, the net transcapillary osmotic pressure is only about 6 mm Hg (25 mm Hg intravascular; 19 mm Hg interstitial).

The consequences of abnormal liquid accumulation on interstitial colloid osmotic pressure depend upon the composition of the liquid involved. In the case of extravasation on a hydrostatic basis (e.g., in cardiogenic pulmonary edema), interstitial osmotic pressure would diminish owing to the sieving effect of the endothelial barrier on plasma proteins; this would lower interstitial colloid osmotic pressure and would in turn inhibit additional liquid transudation. However, in the case of increased permeability of the capillary endothelium (e.g., most forms of noncardiogenic pulmonary edema), the leak of plasma proteins would tend to raise interstitial colloid osmotic pressure and eliminate the normal difference between intra- and extravascular osmotic forces; reducing the transcapillary osmotic pressure difference would exaggerate the formation of edema by removing a "protective" force. This may be one reason why noncardiogenic pulmonary edema is often more severe than cardiogenic edema and why the accumulated liquid seems to remain in the lungs for a long time.

Surface tension forces and alveolar pressures exert an unknown effect on transcapillary liquid movement. Of the two forces, the effect of surface tension is probably greater, because surface tension is one of the determinants of pericapillary total interstitial pressure. The higher the surface tension, the lower the interstitial hydrostatic pressure and the greater the tendency for transudation of liquid. Normally, alveolar surface tension is very low, so its effect is minimal; however, in some pathologic conditions (e.g., neonatal respiratory distress syndrome and rapid expansion of the lung following prolonged pneumothorax), abnormal surface forces may contribute to the formation of pulmonary edema. It is possible that in these disorders increased leakiness may also follow injury to cells of the alveolar-capillary membrane.

Alveolar pressure fluctuates above and below atmospheric pressure during breathing. Normally, this change is small, but it may become large in the presence of increased resistance to airflow in the tracheobronchial system (see Chapter 4). Although surface tension forces prevent full transmission of alveolar pressure to interstitial tissues, no matter how high or low alveolar pressure becomes, there must be directional changes of almost equal magnitude in both the interstitial and intravascular spaces of the alveolar-capillary membrane.[56] Thus, the pressure difference *across* the capillary wall is probably only slightly affected by normally occurring changes in alveolar pressure.*

Lymphatic Drainage. The only way that a positive net transcapillary liquid exchange can be maintained without finally flooding the interstitial and alveolar spaces is through an efficient system for removal of substances filtered from the vascular compartment. As mentioned previously, the lung is profusely supplied with lymph capillaries that provide the chief disposal mechanism for H_2O-soluble substances including macromolecules and, at times, even particles.

Recently, it has been demonstrated by several investigators, in conflict with the conclusions from former studies, that albumin instilled into the lungs of experimental animals is absorbed intact by the pulmonary circulation.[57] This observation does not mitigate the statement that under normal physiologic circumstances, although there is undoubtedly liquid and solute exchange in *both directions* across the capillary endothelium, more is filtered than reabsorbed, and the excess is removed by the lymphatic microcirculation.

The volume flow of lymph drained from the human lung is higher than or equivalent to that of other organs and, judging from experimental evidence, is capable of increasing considerably. It is only when the rate of formation of pulmonary interstitial liquid exceeds the removal capacity that abnormal accumulations (i.e., pulmonary edema) can occur. Staub[52] concludes that the lymphatic removal capacity probably can increase up to

---

*This mechanism is misunderstood by advocates of intermittent positive pressure, with or without end-expiratory pressure, in the treatment of acute pulmonary edema. These therapeutic modalities are often useful, but they do not produce their benefits by "damming back" liquid through an increase in alveolar pressure.

ten times above basal rates before significant extravascular liquid retention develops.

Liquid moves along the interstitial space of the alveolar septum toward the peribronchial and perivascular interstitial spaces owing to the hydrostatic pressure gradient created by the differences in the pressures surrounding alveolar and extra-alveolar structures (alveolar pressure being higher than extra-alveolar pressure). Liquid that reaches alveolar spaces or is instilled into them moves along the corners of contiguous alveoli

because surface forces cause liquid to accumulate at the points at which the angle of curvature is least. Once in the neighborhood of the openings into pulmonary lymphatic capillaries, liquid is "sucked" into them by a small pressure difference of unknown origin. Pulmonary lymph flows toward the hilum owing to rhythmic contractions of the smooth muscles in the walls of lymphatic vessels.[58] Undoubtedly, ventilatory movements and circulatory pulsations contribute to the propulsive forces. The unicuspid funnel-shaped valves throughout the lymphat-

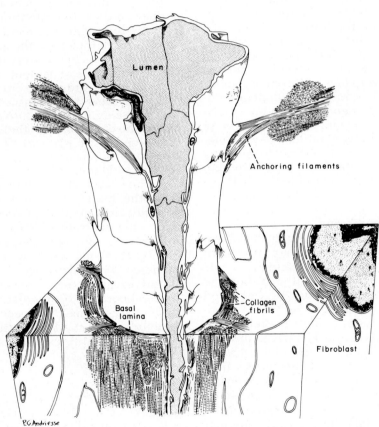

Figure 5-16 A three-dimensional representation of a lymphatic capillary and its surrounding basal lamina and connective tissue elements diagrammed from a series of electron photomicrographs. The lymphatic anchoring filaments appear to originate from the endothelial cells and extend among collagen bundles, elastic fibers, and neighboring cells, thus providing a firm connection between the lymphatic capillary wall and the surrounding connective tissue. (From Leak and Burke.[60] Reprinted by permission from the authors and publisher.)

ic microcirculation ensure a one-way flow of lymph into collecting channels.

It might be expected that in the presence of excess interstitial liquid the resulting increase in pressure in the connective tissue spaces surrounding lymph capillaries would tend to collapse the delicate vessels and thus impair the efficiency of lymph drainage. However, just the opposite occurs. Lymph capillaries actually dilate when interstitial liquid increases owing to the presence of fine fibrillar attachments between the vessel walls and the surrounding tissue.[59] These lymphatic tethers, shown schematically in Figure 5–16, have recently been identified by electron microscopy.[60]

To summarize, although measurements are needed to supply missing information, the best evidence at present indicates that there is a net transcapillary movement of H_2O and solutes from pulmonary capillaries into the pericapillary interstitial space. The intra- and extravascular forces involved are estimated and summarized in Table 5–5 and shown in Figure 5–15. It can be seen that there is a net outward pressure of about 7 mm Hg. As liquid is formed in response to these forces, an equivalent amount is ordinarily removed by the pulmonary lymph capillaries. The lymphatic vessels can actively increase liquid transport considerably and apparently do so when hydrostatic pressure changes or shifts in

blood volume augment the volume of liquid being formed. Thus, the turnover of liquid and solutes in the lungs may increase remarkably; pulmonary edema can only occur when the disposal capabilities of the lymphatics are overwhelmed.

METABOLIC FUNCTIONS

The actual work involved in gas exchange is performed chiefly by the respiratory muscles, which provide the mechanical force required for ventilation, and by the heart, which pumps blood through the pulmonary circulation. Because gas exchange by diffusion is a passive process that does not require energy, virtually the entire metabolic cost of respiration is supplied by organs other than the lung. However, the lung is known to be a metabolically active organ with an O_2 consumption that at times may be appreciable, especially when lung disease is present (e.g., six patients with far-advanced tuberculosis had pulmonary tissue O_2 consumptions that averaged 12 per cent of the total utilization[61]). The metabolic needs of the normal human lung have never been measured precisely but probably are in the range of 4 to 5 per cent of resting whole body O_2 consumption.* Some of the O_2 utilized by the lung is for processes related to respiration, such as the synthesis of surfactant; some is used to satisfy the metabolic requirements of the approximately 40 different cell types that compose the lung; and the remainder of the O_2 is utilized by cells performing nonrespiratory functions, such as the synthesis, storage, release, activation, and inactivation of a variety of chemical substances. Because the major location of many of these biochemical

Table 5–5 Measured and Estimated Variables in the Starling Equation Showing a Net Movement of Liquid from Within the Capillary into the Pericapillary Interstitial Space

$$\dot{Q}_f = K_f[(P_{cap} - P_{is}) - (\pi_{pl} - \pi_s)]$$
$$= K_f[(10 - [-3]) - (25 - 19)]$$
$$= K_f(13 - 6)$$
$$\dot{Q}_f = K_f \times 7$$

*For comparison purposes, the kidney utilizes about 8 per cent and the brain utilizes about 20 per cent of the resting total body O_2 consumption.

activities has been demonstrated to be within or on the pulmonary vascular endothelium,[62] they are considered in the chapter on pulmonary circulation.

VASOACTIVE SUBSTANCES

The fate of several vasoactive substances during a single passage through the pulmonary circulation is presented in Table 5–6. The list is by no means inclusive but contains those substances of pharmacologic importance that have been studied thoroughly. Undoubtedly, the list will lengthen in the future. It should be emphasized that the extent of removal indicated in the table pertains only when the concentration of the substance in pulmonary arterial blood is very low (i.e., in the normal range) and that in various pathologic disturbances when large amounts of the compounds may be released or administered, the capacity of the lung to deal with them may be overwhelmed. Finally, no answer is currently available to the biggest question of all: What happens to the efficacy of these activities in patients with lung diseases?

5-Hydroxytryptamine (5HT) or Serotonin. 5-Hydroxytryptamine may be released from argentaffin cells in the intestine or lung or from platelets. Contrary to original beliefs, it is now known that the major site for inactivation of 5-HT in the body is the lung, and not the liver. Furthermore, the mechanism of inactivation is not by enzymatic degradation but by an uptake and storage process.[63] Some of the 5-HT may be transferred to platelets and some may be retained in the lung and released during anaphylaxis.[64]

Histamine. Histamine is present in tissue mast cells and blood basophils and thus is found both within the parenchyma and connective tissue spaces of the lung and within the pulmonary circulation.[65] This important pharmacologic substance is thought to be one of the chemical mediators of type I (immediate) hypersensitivity reactions, including atopic

Table 5–6 Summary of the Fate of Vasoactive Circulating Substances During a Single Passage Through the Pulmonary Circulation in Experimental Animals*

Amines	
Acetylcholine	Rapidly inactivated
5-Hydroxytryptamine	Almost completely removed
Histamine	Not affected
Epinephrine	Not affected
Norepinephrine	Up to 30% removed
Peptides	
Bradykinin	Up to 80% inactivated
Angiotensin I	Converted to angiotensin II
Angiotensin II	Not affected
Vasopressin	Not affected
Prostaglandins	
Prostaglandins E	Almost completely removed
Prostaglandins F	Almost completely removed
Prostaglandins A	Not affected
Adenine nucleotides	
Adenosine triphosphate	Almost completely removed
Adenosine monophosphate	Almost completely removed

*For details, see text.

asthma. The physiologic significance of the cellular depots of histamine in the lungs of normal man has not been clarified; furthermore, it has not been possible by perfusion studies to demonstrate removal or inactivation of histamine by the lung.[63]

Bradykinin. Kinins are potent endogenous vasodilator substances that probably play a role in inflammatory responses and hereditary angioneurotic edema, and act as a mediator of neonatal circulatory adjustment. Bradykinin has been implicated in the responses to bronchial asthma, pulmonary edema, and anaphylaxis.[63] Bradykinin has not been identified as a secretory product of the lung, although the lungs contain relatively large amounts of precursor. In fact, the pulmonary circulations of many mammals, including man, have been shown to inactivate a large proportion (up to 80 per cent) of an infused dose, presumably by enzymatic activity.[63]

Angiotensin. Angiotensin I is formed in the bloodstream from an L-globulin precursor by the action of the enzyme renin. The decapeptide angiotensin I has relatively little vasomotor potency, but it is rapidly converted to a highly active octopeptide, angiotensin II. The transformation from angiotensin I to angiotensin II is caused by an enzyme that appears to be fixed in the pulmonary circulation. Although other organs also contain converting enzyme, no conversion of angiotensin I to angiotensin II of physiologic significance has been demonstrated in organs other than the lung.[63] Furthermore, the presence of converting activity in the lungs rather than in the blood implies that the renin-angiotensin system has generalized regulatory effects on the circulation rather than just locally on the afferent glomerular arterioles, as proposed originally.

Prostaglandins. These compounds belong to a family that is synthesized and released from different organs under a variety of conditions. The lung appears to have an important role in both the synthesis and the removal of certain prostaglandins. Although the normal lung contains detectable quantities of prostaglandins (principally of the F series), these do not appear to be sufficient to cause systemic effects if released. (They may, of course, have important local actions.) However, in many experimental conditions, and presumably in their clinical analogues as well, prostaglandin synthesis and release by the lung can be accelerated to a rate at which physiologic consequences result. This mechanism may be important in anaphylaxis, mechanical overdistension of the lungs, pulmonary embolism, and pulmonary edema.[66] In general, prostaglandins of the F series cause constric-

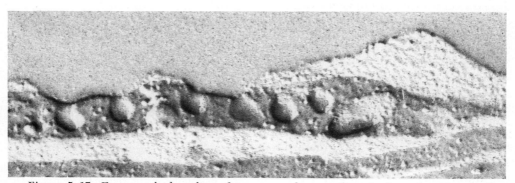

Figure 5–17 Freeze-etched replica of transverse fracture through the pulmonary capillary endothelium of the rat. Particles occur in the cytoplasm, and caveolae intracellulares appear as pits or domes. (× 59,000. Courtesy of Dr. Una S. Ryan.)

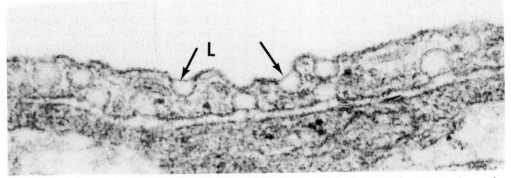

Figure 5-18 Transverse section of pulmonary capillary endothelium of the rat. Several caveolae intracellulares face the capillary lumen (L) and are covered by a delicate diaphragm (arrows) composed of a single lamella. (× 106,000. From Ryan and Smith.[68] Reprinted by permission from the authors and publisher.)

tion of vascular and bronchial smooth muscles; in contrast, prostaglandins of the E series cause smooth muscle dilatation.[67]

As indicated in Table 5-6, the lung inactivates nearly all prostaglandins of the E and F series, but not the A series, that perfuse it. The mechanism of inactivation may be related to the presence of an enzyme capable of metabolizing prostaglandins that has been extracted from the lungs of several species.[63]

LOCUS OF METABOLIC ACTIVITY

The sites at which the various metabolic processes described above are carried out have not been identified with certainty. However, pieces of evidence suggest that the luminal surface of the pulmonary vascular endothelium is specially endowed to participate in the biochemical transformation of at least some circulating vasoactive substances. Electron photomicrographs have revealed ultrastructural specialization that has been linked with the sites of enzymes that metabolize the adenine nucleotides, angiotensin I and bradykinin.[62] As shown in Figure 5-17, the endothelial surface of pulmonary capillaries has a high density of *caveolae intracellulares* that communicate with the bloodstream through a deli-

cate covering layer (Figure 5-18). Cytochemical techniques have revealed that adenine nucleotides are metabolized within the caveolae, and less direct evidence favors a similar location for the metabolism of angiotensin I and bradykinin.[62] Although further details are needed concerning various metabolic pathways and their location within the lung, the studies cited provide an exciting beginning to the structure-function correlations of some of the nonrespiratory activities carried out in the pulmonary circulation.

REFERENCES

1. Heinemann, H. O., and Fishman, A. P.: Nonrespiratory functions of mammalian lung. Physiol. Rev., 49:1–47, 1969.
2. Hellems, H. K., Haynes, F. W., and Dexter, L.: Pulmonary "capillary" pressure in man. J. Appl. Physiol., 2:24-29, 1949.
3. Jenkins, B. S., Bradley, R. D., and Branthwaite, M. A.: Evaluation of pulmonary arterial end-diastolic pressure as an indirect estimate of left atrial mean pressure. Circulation, 42:75-78, 1970.
4. Swan, H. J. C., Ganz, W., Forrester, J., Marcus, H., Diamond, G., and Chonette, D.: Catheterization of the heart in man with use of a flow-directed balloon-tipped catheter. New Eng. J. Med., 283:447-451, 1970.
5. Dock, W.: Apical localization of phthisis; its significance in treatment by prolonged rest in bed. Am. Rev. Turberc., 53:297-305, 1946.

6. West, J. B., and Dollery, C. T.: Distribution of blood flow and ventilation-perfusion ratio in the lung, measured with radioactive CO_2. J. Appl. Physiol., 15:405-410, 1960.

7. Ball, W. C., Jr., Stewart, P. B., Newsham, L. G. S., and Bates, D. V.: Regional pulmonary function studied with xenon. J. Clin. Invest., 41:519-531, 1962.

8. Wagner, H. N., Jr., Sabiston, D. C., Jr., Iio, M., McAfee, J. G., Meyer, J. K., and Langan, J. K.: Regional pulmonary blood flow in man by radioisotope scanning. JAMA, 187:601-603, 1964.

9. Hughes, J. M. B., Glazier, J. B., Maloney, J. E., and West, J. B.: Effect of lung volume on the distribution of pulmonary blood flow in man. Resp. Physiol., 4:58-72, 1968.

10. West, J. B., Dollery, C. T., and Naimark, A.: Distribution of blood flow in isolated lung; relation to vascular and alveolar pressures. J. Appl. Physiol., 19:713-724, 1964.

11. Banister, J., and Torrance, R. W.: The effects of the tracheal pressure upon flow: pressure relations in the vascular bed of isolated lungs. Quart. J. Exp. Physiol., 45: 352-367, 1960.

12. Permutt, S., Bromberger-Barnea, B., and Bane, H. N.: Alveolar pressure, pulmonary venous pressure, and the vascular waterfall. Med. Thorac., 19:239-266, 1962.

13. Howell, J. B. L., Permutt, S., Proctor, D. F., and Riley, R. L.: Effect of inflation of the lung on different parts of pulmonary vascular bed. J. Appl. Physiol., 16:71-76, 1961.

14. Mead, J., and Whittenberger, J. L.: Lung inflation and hemodynamics. In Fenn, W. O., and Rahn, H. (eds.): Handbook of Physiology, Section 3. Respiration. Vol. I. Washington, D. C., American Physiological Society, 1964, pp. 477-486.

15. Fung, Y. C., and Sobin, S. S.: Pulmonary alveolar blood flow. Circ. Res., 30:470-490, 1972.

16. Glazier, J. B., Hughes, J. M. B., Maloney, J. E., and West, J. B.: Measurements of capillary dimensions and blood volume in rapidly frozen lungs. J. Appl. Physiol., 26: 65-76, 1969.

17. Guyton, A. C., Granger, H. J., and Taylor, A. E.: Interstitial fluid pressure. Physiol. Rev., 51:527-563, 1971.

18. Hughes, J. M.: Pulmonary interstitial pressure. Bull. Physiopathol. Resp. (Nancy), 7:1095-1123, 1971.

19. Bruderman, I., Somers, K., Hamilton, W. K., Tooley, W. H., and Butler, J.: Effect of surface tension on circulation in the excised lungs of dogs. J. Appl. Physiol., 19:707-712, 1964.

20. Mead, J., Takishima, T., and Leith, D.: Stress distribution in lungs: a model of pulmonary elasticity. J. Appl. Physiol., 28:596-608, 1970.

21. Cumming, G., Henderson, R., Horsfield, K., and Singhal, S. S.: The functional morphology of the pulmonary circulation. In Fishman, A. P. and Hecht, H. H. (eds.): The Pulmonary Circulation and Interstitial Space. Chicago, University of Chicago Press, 1969, pp. 327-340.

22. West, J. B., Maloney, J. E., and Castle, B. L.: Effect of stratified inequality of blood flow on gas exchange in liquid-filled lungs. J. Appl. Physiol., 32:357-361, 1972.

23. Brody, J. S., Stemmeler, E. J., and DuBois, A. B.: Longitudinal distribution of vascular resistance in the pulmonary arteries, capillaries, and veins. J. Clin. Invest., 47: 783-799, 1968.

24. Schleier, J.: Der Energieverbrauch in der Blutbahn. Pflügers Arch. Gesamte Physiol., 173:172-204, 1919.

25. Maseri, A., Caldini, P., Harward, P., Joshi, R. C., Permutt, S., and Zierler, K. L.: Determinants of pulmonary vascular volume. Recruitment versus distensibility. Circ. Res., 31:218-228, 1972.

26. Warrell, D. A., Evans, J. W., Clarke, R. O., Kingaby, G. P., and West, J. B.: Pattern of filling in the pulmonary capillary bed. J. Appl. Physiol., 32:346-356, 1972.

27. DeFreitas, F. M., Faraco, E. Z., De Azevedo, D. F., Zaduchliver, J., and Lewin, I.: Behavior of normal pulmonary circulation during changes of total blood volume in man. J. Clin. Invest., 44:366-378, 1965.

28. Varnauskas, E.: The effect of physical exercise on pulmonary blood volume. In Muller, C. (eds.): Conference on Pulmonary Circulation. Oslo, Scandinavian University Book, 1965, pp. 105-111.

29. Lee, G. de J.: Regulation of the pulmonary circulation. Brit. Heart J., 33(suppl.):15-26, 1971.

30. Lee, G. de J., and DuBois, A. B.: Pulmonary capillary blood flow in man. J. Clin. Invest., 34:1380-1390, 1955.

31. Morkin, E., Collins, J. A., Goldman, H. S., and Fishman, A. P.: Pattern of blood flow in the pulmonary veins of the dog. J. Appl. Physiol., 20:1118-1128, 1965.

32. Maloney, J. E., Bergel, D. H., Glazier, J. B., Hughes, J. M. B., and West, J. B.: Transmission of pulsatile blood pressure and flow through the isolated lung. Circ. Res., 23:11-24, 1968.

33. Guitini, C., Maseri, A., and Bianchi, R.: Pulmonary vascular distensibility and lung compliance as modified by dextran infusion and subsequent atropine injection in normal subjects. J. Clin. Invest., 45:1770-1789, 1966.

34. Dollery, C. T., and Glazier, J. B.: Pharmacological effects of drugs on the pulmonary circulation in man. Clin. Pharmacol. Ther., 7:807-818, 1966.

35. Roos, A., Thomas, L. J., Jr., Nagel, E. L., and Prommas, D. C.: Pulmonary vascular resistance as determined by lung inflation and vascular pressures. J. Appl. Physiol., 16:77-84, 1961.

36. Borst, H. G., McGregor, M., Whittenberger, J. L., and Berglund, E.: Influence of pulmonary arterial and left atrial pressures on pulmonary vascular resistance. Circ. Res., 4:393-399, 1956.

37. Murray, J. F., Karp, R. B., and Nadel, J. A.: Viscosity effects on pressure-flow relations and vascular resistance in dogs' lungs. J. Appl. Physiol., 27:336–341, 1969.

38. Ingram, R. H., Szidon, J. P., Skalak, R., and Fishman, A. P.: Effects of sympathetic nerve stimulation on the pulmonary arterial tree of the isolated lobe perfused in situ. Circ. Res., 22:801-815, 1968.

39. Kadowitz, P. J., and Hyman, A. L.: Effect of sympathetic nerve stimulation on pulmonary vascular resistance in the dog. Circ. Res., 32:221-227, 1973.

40. Widdicombe, J. G., and Sterling, G. M.: The autonomic nervous system and breathing. Arch. Intern. Med., 126:311-329, 1970.

41. Glazier, J. B., and Murray, J. F.: Sites of pulmonary vasomotor reactivity in the dog during alveolar hypoxia and serotonin and histamine infusion. J. Clin. Invest., 50:2550-2558, 1971.

42. Kazemi, H., Bruecke, P. E., and Parsons, E. F.: Role of the autonomic nervous system in the hypoxic response of the pulmonary vascular bed. Resp. Physiol., 15:245-254, 1972.

43. Harvey, R. M., Enson, Y., Betti, R., Lewis, M. L., Rochester, D. F., and Ferrer, M. I.: Further observations on the effect of hydrogen ion on the pulmonary circulation. Circulation, 35:1019-1027, 1967.

44. Rudolph, A. M., and Yuan, S.: Response of the pulmonary vasculature to hypoxia and H+ ion concentration changes. J. Clin. Invest., 45:399-411, 1966.

45. Fishman, A. P., Fritts, H. W., Jr., and Cournand, A.: Effects of breathing carbon dioxide upon the pulmonary circulation. Circulation, 22:220-225, 1960.

46. Cottrell, T. S., Levine, O. R., Senior, R. M., Wiener, J., Spiro, D., and Fishman, A. P.: Electron microscopic alterations at the alveolar level in pulmonary edema. Circ. Res., 21:783-797, 1967.

47. Staub, N. C., Nagano, H., and Pearce, M. L.: Pulmonary edema in dogs, especially the sequence of fluid accumulation in lungs. J. Appl. Physiol., 22:227–240, 1967.

48. Szidon, J. P., Pietra, G. G., and Fishman, A. P.: The alveolar-capillary membrane and pulmonary edema. New Eng. J. Med., 286:1200-1204, 1972.

49. Mayerson, H. S., Wolfram, C. G., Shirley, H. H., Jr., and Wasserman, K.: Regional differences in capillary permeability. Am. J. Physiol., 198:155-160, 1960.

50. Lauweryns, J. M.: The juxta-alveolar lymphatics in the human adult lung. Am. Rev. Resp. Dis., 102:877-885, 1970.

51. Lauweryns, J. M., and Boussauw, L.: The ultrastructure of pulmonary lymphatic capillaries of newborn rabbits and of human infants. Lymphology, 2:108-129, 1969.

52. Staub, N. C.: Pulmonary edema. Physiol. Rev., 54:678–811, 1974.

53. Chinard, F. P.: The permeability characteristics of the pulmonary blood-gas barrier. In Caro, C. G. (ed.): Advances in Respiratory Physiology. London, Edward Arnold Publishers Ltd., 1966, pp. 106–147.

54. McMaster, P. D.: The pressure and interstitial resistance prevailing in the normal and edematous skin of animals and man. J. Exp. Med., 84:473-494, 1946.

55. Meyer, B. J., Meyer, A., and Guyton, A. C.: Interstitial fluid pressure. V. Negative pressure in the lungs. Circ. Res., 22:263-271, 1968.

56. Robin, E. D., Cross, C. E., and Zellis, R.: Pulmonary edema. New Eng. J. Med., 288:239-246, 292-304, 1973.

57. Dominguez, E. A. M., Liebow, A. A., and Bensch, K. G.: Studies on the pulmonary air-tissue barrier. I. Absorption of albumin by the alveolar wall. Lab. Invest., 16:905-911, 1967.

58. Hall, J. G., Morris, B., and Woolley, G.: Intrinsic rhythmic propulsion of lymph in the unanesthetized sheep. J. Physiol. (Lond.), 180:336–349, 1965.

59. McMaster, P. D.: The relative pressures within cutaneous lymphatic capillaries and the tissues. J. Exp. Med., 86:293-308, 1947.

60. Leak, L. V., and Burke, J. F.: Ultrastructural studies on the lymphatic anchoring filaments. J. Cell. Biol., 36:129-149, 1968.

61. Fritts, H. W., Jr., Richards, D. W., and Cournand, A.: Oxygen consumption of tissues in the human lung. Science, 133:1070-1072, 1961.

62. Smith, U., and Ryan, J. W.: Electron microscopy of the endothelial and epithelial components of the lungs: correlations of structure and function. Fed. Proc., 32:1957-1966, 1973.

63. Vane, J. R.: The release and fate of vaso-active hormones in the circulation. Brit. J. Pharmacol., 35:202-242, 1969.

64. Waalkes, T. P., Weissbach, H., Bozicevich, J., and Udenfriend, S.: Serotonin and histamine release during anaphylaxis in the rabbit. J. Clin. Invest., 36:1115-1120, 1957.

65. Porter, J. F., and Mitchell, R. G.: Distribution of histamine in human blood. Physiol. Rev., 52:361-381, 1972.

66. Said, S. I.: The lung in relation to vasoactive hormones. Fed. Proc., 32:1972-1976, 1973.

67. Fanburg, B. L.: Prostaglandins and the lung. Am. Rev. Resp. Dis., 108:482–489, 1973.

68. Ryan, J. W., and Smith, U.: Metabolism of adenosine 5'-monophosphate during circulation through the lungs. Trans. Assoc. Am. Phys., 84:297–306, 1971.

Chapter Six

DIFFUSION OF GASES, OXYHEMOGLOBIN EQUILIBRIUM, AND CARBON DIOXIDE EQUILIBRIUM

INTRODUCTION

Diffusion causes O_2 molecules to move from alveolar gas into pulmonary capillary blood and also from peripheral tissue capillary blood into contiguous cells. Movement of CO_2 molecules is also governed by diffusion but is normally in the opposite direction to that of O_2. Both gases undergo chemical reactions in the bloodstream at the start and finish of their journeys between the lungs and the peripheral tissues: O_2 reacts solely with hemoglobin, and CO_2 reacts in part with hemoglobin and in part to form HCO_3^-. The reversible chemical reactions between hemoglobin and O_2 and CO_2 are complementary and add considerably to the transport capacity of the blood. This chapter will consider these essential first steps in the process of gas exchange between the inspired air brought into the lungs and distributed through them by ventilation (Chapter 4) and the blood delivered to and removed from the pulmonary capillaries by the circulation (Chapter 5).

DIFFUSION

DEFINITION

Diffusion can be defined as the passive tendency of molecules to move from a region of higher to one of lower concentration.[1] Diffusion is a passive process because no extra energy is required and is caused by molecules moving "by themselves" in an effort to eliminate differences in concentration within the various regions accessible to the molecules.

Exchange of O_2 and CO_2 in the lung takes place in three separable steps, each involving diffusion: (1) diffusion of molecules within the air spaces of the terminal respiratory unit, (2) diffusion of O_2 and CO_2 across the air-blood barrier, and (3) diffusion and chemical reaction within the plasma and red blood cells. The anatomic struc-

tures involved and the barriers to these steps are indicated in the electron photomicrograph in Figure 6-1. Oxygen molecules must diffuse through the alveolar space, cross the air-blood barrier, traverse a plasma layer of variable thickness and the membrane and interior of the red blood cell, and finally combine with hemoglobin.

Gas Phase Diffusion. As indicated in Chapter 4, bulk movement of inspired fresh air proceeds outward in the tracheobronchial tree to about as far as the alveolar ducts. The rate of movement of the inspirate slows progressively until finally it is so slow that it becomes superseded by movement of individual gas molecules owing to their own kinetic energy. Thus, mixing between newly inspired air and residual gas within the terminal respiratory units takes place by diffusion. Given the same differences in concentration, the diffusivity of ordinary respiratory gases in air is about 200,000 times greater than that of the same gases in saline (or presumably in plasma and tissue liquids). With knowledge of these considerations, together with knowledge about the distances from alveolar ducts to alveoli, it is generally agreed that gas phase diffusion does not normally impair the over-all adequacy of diffusion. In other words, movement of newly inspired gas molecules within the residual air of a normal-sized terminal unit is so fast that gas phase diffusion does not limit the total number of molecules that are able to cross the alveolar-capillary membrane and, depending upon the particular gas, combine with hemoglobin. This holds true within the gas volumes encountered in normal lungs; however, when the terminal respiratory units are pathologically enlarged, as in various forms of emphysema, gas phase diffusion may become impaired and, consequently, affect arterial blood composition.[2]

Membrane Diffusion. As mixed venous blood begins to flow through

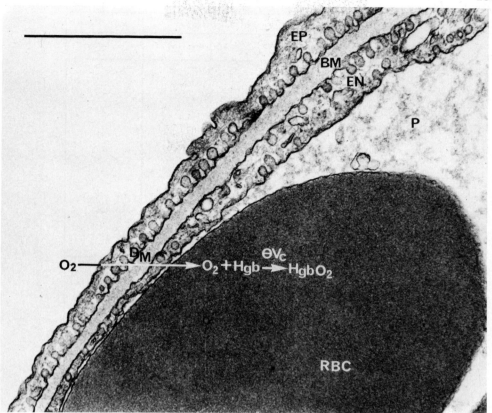

Figure 6–1 Electron photomicrograph showing the pathway for O_2 diffusion across the air-blood barrier in a human lung. An O_2 molecule must cross the epithelium (EP), basement membrane (BM), endothelium (EN), plasma layer (P), and red blood cell (RBC) membrane; resistance to movement through these barriers comprises the membrane component (D_M) of the total resistance to diffusion. After entering the red blood cell, O_2 must combine chemically with hemoglobin (Hgb); this reaction comprises the resistance imposed by the capillary blood volume (Vc) and rate of chemical combination (Θ). For discussion, see text. Horizontal bar = 1 μm. ($\times$ 41,500. Courtesy of Dr. Ewald R. Weibel.)

pulmonary capillaries, the blood becomes exposed to alveolar gas that contains O_2 at a higher concentration and CO_2 at a lower concentration than that which exists within the blood at that moment. Because of the prevailing differences in concentrations, O_2 diffuses from the alveolus into the pulmonary capillary blood and CO_2 diffuses in the opposite direction, as depicted in Figure 6–2. Normally, this exchange takes place rapidly, and equilibrium between the pressures of O_2 and CO_2 within the gas phase and the plasma is

achieved in about 0.25 sec or one third of the total time (0.75 sec) that blood is believed to spend traversing the pulmonary capillary.

Blood Phase Diffusion. The instant that O_2 molecules cross the air-blood barrier and enter the plasma, a new concentration difference for O_2 is established between the plasma and the hemoglobin-combining sites within red blood cells. This difference causes O_2 to move through the plasma and across the cell's membrane and within its interior to the sites of chem-

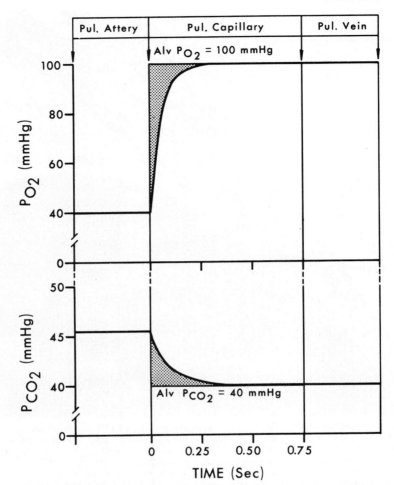

Figure 6–2 Schematic diagram of the changes in PO_2 and PCO_2 from the pressures prevailing in mixed venous blood (pulmonary artery) to those in systemic arterial blood (pulmonary vein) as red blood cells travel through pulmonary capillaries and are exposed to alveolar PO_2 of 100 mm Hg. The mean time available for gas exchange under resting conditions is believed to be 0.75 second. (Adapted from Staub[3] and Hyde, Puy, Raub, and Forster.[4] Reprinted by permission from the authors and publishers.)

ical reaction with hemoglobin. It was originally believed that the combination between O_2 and hemoglobin was virtually instantaneous; however, because of the work of Roughton and Forster,[5] it is now known that the reaction rate is finite and imposes a measurable delay on the diffusion process. This knowledge provided the basis for the development of techniques to subdivide the total resistance to diffusion imposed by the structures within the lung into the resistance to the move-

ment of gases afforded by (1) the air-blood barrier, plasma layer, and red blood cell membrane, and (2) the time required for the chemical combination with hemoglobin in the interior of the red blood cell (see later section).

MEASUREMENT OF DIFFUSING CAPACITY

The diffusing capacity of the lung for any gas (DL_G) indicates the quantity of that gas that diffuses across the air-blood barrier per unit time ($\dot{V}_G$) in response to the difference existing between the mean pressure of the gas in alveolar air ($P\bar{A}_G$) and the mean pressure of the gas in capillary blood ($P\bar{C}_G$):

$$DL_G = \frac{\dot{V}_G}{P\bar{A}_G - P\bar{C}_G}, \text{ ml/min} \times \text{mm Hg.} \quad (1)$$

The quantity of an individual gas that will diffuse in response to a given pressure difference is determined by the solubility and diffusivity of the gas in the alveolar-capillary membrane, the surface area and thickness of the membrane, and in some cases the rate of chemical reaction within the bloodstream. Most inert gases diffuse readily between gas and blood phases, and equilibrium between the concentrations in the alveolar gas and blood is reached rapidly; for example, N_2 achieves 90 per cent equilibration across the air-blood barrier in about 0.005 sec. Therefore, the amount of inert gas that can be taken up or given off by the pulmonary circulation is not detectably limited by the diffusion properties of the lung and its contents but is determined solely by the solubility of the gas and the volume of blood into which it can dissolve. These phenomena prohibit the use of all inert gases for the measurement of pulmonary diffusing capacity but have been taken advantage of by employing certain soluble gases, such as acetylene or N_2O, to measure effective pulmonary blood flow.

The only two gases that can be used to measure the diffusing capacity of the lung are O_2 and CO. These two gases are suitable test substances, owing to their unique ability to combine with hemoglobin. Thus, both have to diffuse across the alveolar-capillary membrane in such large quantities to saturate the available hemoglobin at the gas pressure prevailing in the alveoli that it may not be possible for them to reach complete equilibrium before the hemoglobin-containing red blood cells reach the end of their journeys through pulmonary capillaries. A detectable alveolar-end-capillary pressure difference for O_2 only exists in normal subjects when they exercise heavily or breathe low O_2 mixtures. However, a difference between gas and blood phases always exists for CO under ordinary testing conditions because the capacity of hemoglobin for CO is so high at very low P_{CO} (100 per cent saturation occurs at about 0.5 mm Hg); also, the pressure difference under ordinary testing conditions and the tissue solubility of CO are very low.

Measurement of pulmonary diffusing capacity for O_2 (DL_{O_2}) is complicated and subject to technical difficulties (especially in patients with lung disease) because, as can be seen from Equation 1, it requires simultaneous assessment of mean alveolar and mean pulmonary capillary P_{O_2} values. The former can be approximated by direct measurement, but the latter must be derived mathematically using the technique of Bohr integration. In contrast, CO is ideally suited for the measurement of pulmonary diffusing capacity (DL_{CO}) because its affinity for hemoglobin is 200 times that of O_2. When CO is inhaled in low concentrations, all the molecules that enter the red blood cell are bound by hemoglobin so that for practical purposes the mean capillary P_{CO} is zero. Accordingly, Equation 1 reduces to

$$DL_{CO} = \frac{\dot{V}_{CO}}{P\bar{A}_{CO}}, \text{ ml/min} \times \text{mm Hg.} \quad (2)$$

Several methods using CO are available and widely employed to measure pulmonary diffusing capacity; discussions about the advantages and disadvantages of the different techniques are provided in several sources[1, 6, 7] and will not be reviewed here. Although CO and O_2 are used to measure the same process, it should be remembered that there is a considerable reserve available for O_2 diffusion before limitation (i.e., an alveolar-end-capillary difference) occurs but that CO diffusion is limited normally and may be even further limited by disease before O_2 uptake becomes impaired. The difference in behavior of O_2 and CO accounts for the fact that DL_{CO} usually must be reduced to less than 45 per cent and less than 65 per cent of predicted values in patients at rest and during exercise, respectively, before diffusion impairment for O_2 causes arterial PO_2 to decrease.[8] (See Chapter 7 for further explanation.)

It is theoretically possible to predict DL_{O_2} from DL_{CO}, but simultaneous measurements of DL using the two gases reveal that observed DL_{O_2} is always considerably less than the value predicted from DL_{CO}.[3] Part of the discrepancy undoubtedly relates to uncertainties about the assumptions that underlie the conversion of DL_{CO} to DL_{O_2}. Another part is believed to originate from the random differences in the times individual red blood cells spend traversing pulmonary capillaries; a wide spectrum of exposure times to alveolar gas, and hence regional variations in DL, is implicit in the structure-function models of the alveolar-capillary network that have been developed by several investigators.[9,10] Although regional differences in diffusing capacity on the basis of variations in blood flow can be inferred from studies such as those cited, it is doubtful whether the changes are of sufficient magnitude to result in an alveolar-arterial PO_2 difference in healthy persons breathing ambient air at sea level. This mechanism becomes greatly exaggerated and very likely assumes functional importance in normal subjects breathing air with a low PO_2 (e.g., at high altitude) and in patients with lung diseases. The different behavior of the two molecules, O_2 being a physiologic respiratory gas and CO being an unphysiologic test substance, accounts for the common laboratory combination, mentioned earlier, of a *low* DL_{CO} in the presence of an essentially *normal* alveolar-arterial PO_2 difference. However, tests of DL_{CO} are widely employed and are quite useful in the diagnosis and management of various forms of chronic obstructive pulmonary disease, interstitial pulmonary diseases, and disorders of the pulmonary circulation.[7,11,12]

COMPONENTS OF DIFFUSING CAPACITY

Because the solubility and diffusivity of CO and O_2 in the body tissues and fluids are constant physicochemical properties, barring an extraordinary change in the chemical composition of the alveolar-capillary membrane, the major variables affecting the total diffusion resistance (1/DL) are (1) the resistance to diffusion of the test gas across the alveolar-capillary membrane, capillary plasma, and red blood cell membrane (the membrane component, 1/DM) and (2) the resistance to diffusion within the red blood cells imposed by the chemical reaction of the test gas with hemoglobin (the intravascular component, $1/\theta Vc$). The second factor derives from the volume of blood in the pulmonary capillary (Vc) and the rate (θ) at which the available hemoglobin can combine chemically with the test gas.[5] The total resistance to diffusion can therefore be expressed as the sum of the component resistances[*]:

$$\frac{1}{DL} = \frac{1}{DM} + \frac{1}{\theta Vc}. \qquad (3)$$

Equation 3 not only is useful for conceptual purposes but also can be used in studies of patients to solve graphically for DM and Vc (Figure 6–3). The principle of the method for subdividing DL into its components depends upon the variations in θ that can be determined *in vitro* in a rapid reaction apparatus by changing the

---

[*]If DL, DM, and θVc are viewed as analogues of conductance, a variable that expresses an enhancement of flow, the use of the reciprocal to express their resistances to gas exchange becomes more understandable.

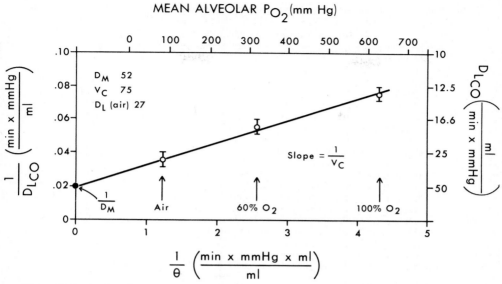

Figure 6–3 A plot demonstrating how experimental values of the diffusing capacity for CO (DL_{CO}) obtained at different alveolar PO_2 values can be analyzed mathematically to obtain the subdivisions of total diffusing capacity: diffusing capacity of the membrane (DM) and pulmonary capillary blood volume (Vc). Changing alveolar PO_2 changes the reaction coefficient (θ) and allows $1/DL$ to be plotted against $1/\theta$. Under these conditions, DM is derived from the value of the Y-intercept and Vc from the slope of the line. For further discussion, see text.

concentrations of O_2 and CO in the test mixture (due to competition between gases for positions in the hemoglobin molecule). Extensive data for θ are limited, especially in pathologic conditions in which the reaction rates may vary. Measurements of DL using gas mixtures similar to those from which θ was measured, and assuming that θ is the same *in vivo* as it is in the reaction chamber, permit derivation of the variables DM and Vc by plotting the results as shown in Figure 6–3. The results differ in normal subjects, mainly in DM, depending upon the method used to measure DL_{CO}. Representative values for DL, DM, Vc, and related morphometric variables in normal persons are shown in Table 6–1.

FACTORS AFFECTING DIFFUSING CAPACITY

As indicated in Table 6–1 and stressed in Chapter 2, 85 to 95 per cent of the alveolar surface of the human lung is normally covered with pulmonary capillaries.[13] The extensive distribution of the alveolar capillary network is vividly displayed in an inflated, injected frog lung (Fig 6–4), and the thinness of the air-blood barrier in man has been demonstrated (Figure 6–1). However, actual measurements of DL are always considerably less than values estimated from morphometric studies of the alveolar-capillary surface. The discrepancy is in part because not all pulmonary capillaries are filled with red blood cells during the DL test, and partly because of the uncertain assumptions that underlie the derivation of DL by both methods.

It is known that DL varies from one mammalian species to another and from one person to another according to body size[15]; consequently, DL will correlate with other indexes of physical dimensions in man such as height, weight, and alveolar volume. The DL

Table 6-1   Morphometric and Physiologic Variables Related to Total Pulmonary Diffusing Capacity (DL), Membrane Diffusing Capacity (DM), and Pulmonary Capillary Volume (Vc) in a Normal Man[*]

Morphometric	
Height, cm	155
Weight, kg	55
Body surface area, m²	1.54
Total lung capacity, L	4500
Alveolar surface area (SA), m²	55
Capillary surface area (SC), m²	52
SC/SA	0.95
Mean thickness air-blood barrier, μm	0.5
Vc, ml	120
Physiologic	
DL_{CO} (single breath, rest), ml/min × mm Hg	24
DL_{CO} (steady state, rest), ml/min × mm Hg	20
DL_{CO} (steady state, exercise), ml/min × mm Hg	59
DL_{O_2} (exercise), ml/min × mm Hg	46
DM_{CO} (single breath, rest), ml/min × mm Hg	52
Vc (single breath, rest), ml	75

[*]Data in part from Weibel[13] and Hamer.[15]

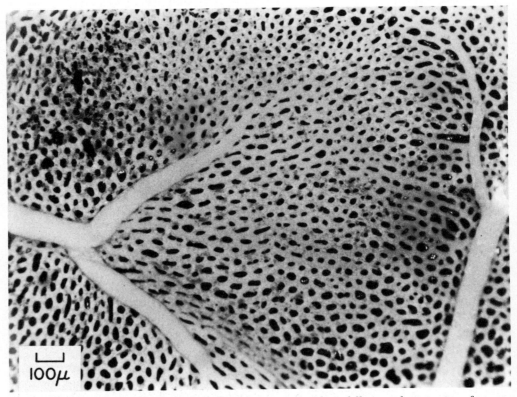

Figure 6-4   Photomicrograph of the capillaries of a frog lung following the injection of opaque material into the vasculature. The arteriole in the upper right supplies part of the capillary network; drainage occurs through the collecting venules on the left. Horizontal bar = 100 μm. (× 78. From Maloney and Castle.[14] Reprinted by permission from the authors and publisher.)

increases during growth and then de- creases gradually with age after matur- ity (Chapter 12), presumably because of the loss of internal surface area, in- cluding pulmonary capillaries, during senescence.[16] The alveolar volume at which the measurements were made affects DL_{CO} values by some methods (breath holding) and not by others (steady state). It also is known that DL may be influenced by changing meta- bolic needs and availability of O_2 (Chapter 2, section on Adaptation). The most conspicuous example of this response in man is the increased DL of natives of high altitude.[17]

Of the two component variables that affect values of DL, the most im- portant by far is Vc; this is true in normal subjects as well as in many pa- tients with pulmonary diseases. Changes in DM are much less common. The DL was shown to vary markedly, as might be expected, when Vc was changed by regulating pulmonary ar- terial and left atrial pressures.[18] When left atrial pressure was low, raising pulmonary artery pressure increased DL substantially (Figure 6–5). The ef- fect was diminished when left atrial pressure was high at the outset. These results can be explained by the effect of changing intravascular pressures on recruitment and distensibility of pulmonary capillaries and hence Vc. An increase in the number and volume of capillaries being perfused prob- ably also accounts for the increase in

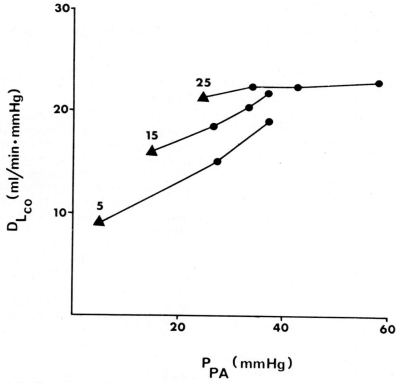

Figure 6–5 The effects of changes in pulmonary arterial pressure (PPA) on single breath diffusing capacity for CO (DL_{CO}) at three different left atrial pressures (5, 15, and 25 mm Hg) in a perfused dog lung. The value at the left of each line (▲) was obtained at zero blood flow; subsequent values (●) were obtained after PPA was raised by increasing flow. (From Karp, Graf, and Nadel.[18] Reprinted by permission from the authors and The American Heart Association, Inc.)

DL_{CO} observed during exercise and when changing from the upright to the supine position. Similarly, the changes in DL induced by certain drugs can be explained as a reflection of the effect of the drugs on Vc.

Because the quantity of O_2 or CO that can be taken up by the bloodstream depends upon the amount of hemoglobin present in the pulmonary capillaries, Vc and hence DL vary proportionately with hemoglobin concentration. To avoid misinterpreting values of DL in patients with anemia and polycythemia, the hemoglobin concentration should be known or determined at the time DL is measured.[19]

Owing to its solubility in water, CO_2 is said to be 20 times more diffusible than O_2. This has led to the generally accepted belief that in pulmonary disorders associated with impaired diffusion O_2 exchange is affected considerably more than CO_2 exchange. Although this is usually true, recent studies using computer analysis of gas exchange have demonstrated that alveolar-end-capillary differences occur for CO_2 as well as for O_2 when the diffusing capacity of the lung is reduced.[20] However, the effects of the changes on O_2 and CO_2 are such that the difference for PCO_2 is approximately one-twentieth that for PO_2 (see also Figure 7-3).

SITE OF GAS EXCHANGE

Throughout the previous section it was implied that the pulmonary capillary is the sole site of gas exchange. This is not necessarily true, because investigators have shown that H_2 and O_2 will diffuse from alveoli into human pulmonary arteries with an internal diameter as large as 3.0 mm.[21] Similarly, Staub[22] noted a color change signifying oxygenation of blood in pulmonary arteries up to 200 μm in diameter in cats breathing 100 per cent O_2. Al-though some of the experimental studies have employed the use of unphysiologic concentration differences between gas and blood phases, it is not surprising that some diffusion of gases into pulmonary arterioles occurs because small blood vessels are often nearly completely surrounded by alveoli, and thus a relatively short diffusion pathway is created (Figure 2-13). Because the quantity of O_2 or CO_2 that diffuses across the air-blood barrier is inversely proportional to the length of the diffusion pathway and directly proportional to the surface area involved, it becomes obvious that virtually all gas exchange must take place across the thin portion of the alveolar-capillary membrane. Similar constraints apply to diffusion across capillaries elsewhere in the body.[23]

OXYHEMOGLOBIN EQUILIBRIUM

OXYHEMOGLOBIN EQUILIBRIUM CURVE

The initial movement of O_2 across the air-blood barrier takes place between alveolar gas and plasma, but as indicated earlier, as soon as O_2 molecules enter and begin to accumulate in plasma, a new concentration difference is established between O_2 in the plasma and that in the interior of the circulating red blood cell. This difference causes O_2 to diffuse into the cells where most of it combines chemically with hemoglobin. Each 1.0 gm of hemoglobin can react with and serve as the carrier for as much as 1.34 ml O_2.[24]* Thus, the O_2 *capacity* of the blood is determined by the concentration of "active" hemoglobin (i.e., the hemoglobin that is chemically able to combine with O_2 [see later section]) in the blood

---

*Some investigators use 1.38, which is the theoretical value based on a hemoglobin Fe content of 0.339 per cent.[25]

Table 6–2 Normal Values for Arterial and Mixed Venous Blood Composition in a 25-year-old Person at Rest*

VARIABLE	ARTERIAL BLOOD	MIXED VENOUS BLOOD
P_{O_2}, mm Hg	100	40
P_{CO_2}, mm Hg	40	46
pH, units	7.40	7.36
Temperature, °C	37.0	37.0
Hemoglobin, gm/100 ml	14.9	14.9
O_2 capacity, ml/100 ml	20.0	20.0
O_2 content, ml/100 ml	19.80	14.62
Combined with hemoglobin	19.50	14.50
Dissolved O_2	0.30	0.12
Hemoglobin saturation, %	97.5	72.5
CO_2 content, ml/100 ml	49.0	53.1
Carbamino CO_2	2.2	3.1
Bicarbonate CO_2	44.2	47.0
Dissolved CO_2	2.6	3.0

*Data in part from Severinghaus[26] and Singer.[27]

and can be computed according to the following equation:

$$O_2 \text{ capacity, ml/100 ml} = \text{hemoglobin, gm/100 ml,} \times 1.34, \text{ml/gm.} \quad (4)$$

Not every O_2 molecule reacts with hemoglobin, and a small quantity of O_2 is present in physical solution in the bloodstream (O_2 dissolved), according to the solubility of O_2 (0.003 ml O_2/100 ml plasma/mm Hg P_{O_2}) and the partial pressure of O_2 in the plasma. The O_2 *content* of the blood is the actual amount of O_2 present in the blood, both chemically combined with hemoglobin and dissolved in plasma.

The relationship between the actual amount of O_2 combined with the hemoglobin contained in a given amount of blood and the O_2 capacity of that quantity of hemoglobin determines the *per cent saturation of hemoglobin* (S_{O_2}):

$$S_{O_2}, \% = \frac{O_2 \text{ content} - O_2 \text{ dissolved}}{O_2 \text{ capacity}} \times 100. \quad (5)$$

Instead of performing the laborious individual measurements necessary to compute percent saturation of hemoglobin according to Equation 5, values are usually obtained directly from spectrophotometric analysis of blood or derived indirectly from simple measurements of P_{O_2}, pH, and temperature.[26]

Values for arterial and mixed venous blood composition in normal adults are given in Table 6–2. About 65 times more O_2 is carried in arterial blood combined with hemoglobin than is dissolved in plasma and cells, thus emphasizing the importance of hemoglobin as an O_2 carrier.

The reversible chemical reaction between O_2 and hemoglobin is defined by the oxyhemoglobin equilibrium curve (Figure 6–6), which relates the percent saturation of hemoglobin to the P_{O_2}. The characteristic feature of the O_2 equilibrium curves of most mammalian hemoglobin is their sigmoid shape, a configuration which indicates that the affinity for O_2 progressively increases as successive molecules of O_2 combine with hemoglobin. The sigmoid shape of the curves is physiologi-

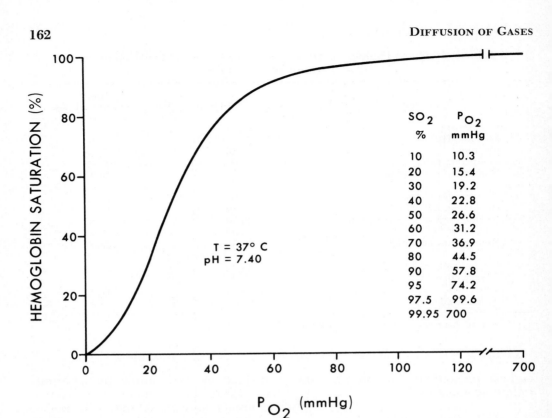

SO$_2$ %	PO$_2$ mmHg
10	10.3
20	15.4
30	19.2
40	22.8
50	26.6
60	31.2
70	36.9
80	44.5
90	57.8
95	74.2
97.5	99.6
99.95	700

T = 37° C
pH = 7.40

Figure 6–6 The normal oxyhemoglobin dissociation curve for man. Values for hemoglobin saturation (SO$_2$) at different PO$_2$ values, under standard conditions of temperature and pH, are indicated. (Data from Severinghaus.[26])

cally advantageous because the flat upper portion allows arterial O$_2$ content to remain high and virtually constant despite fluctuations in arterial PO$_2$, and the middle steep segment enables large quantities of O$_2$ to be released at the PO$_2$ prevailing in the peripheral capillaries. The affinity between O$_2$ and hemoglobin is conventionally expressed as the PO$_2$ at which the available hemoglobin is half saturated (P$_{50}$) under standard conditions of temperature (37° C) and pH (7.40).

The P$_{50}$ of human blood is normally 26.6 mm Hg, but this value is known to vary considerably both in normal subjects under certain conditions and in patients with a variety of diseases. The effects of shifts in the position of the oxyhemoglobin equilibrium curve are depicted schematically in Figure 6–7; note that hemoglobin con-

centration has been arbitrarily set at 14.9 gm/100 ml so that O$_2$ capacity (i.e., 100 percent saturation) is 20.0 ml/100 ml and arteriovenous (or tissue) O$_2$ differences can be easily derived. When the affinity of hemoglobin for O$_2$ increases, O$_2$ is taken up more readily and released less readily at any given PO$_2$; under these circumstances, the equilibrium curve is shifted to the left (curve B) of the normal curve (curve A) and the P$_{50}$ is lower than usual (Figure 6–7). When the affinity of hemoglobin for O$_2$ decreases, the new curve is shifted to the right (curve C) of the normal one and the P$_{50}$ increases. When arterial PO$_2$ is normal, shifts in the curves in either direction influence the release of O$_2$ in the tissues considerably more than the uptake of O$_2$ in the lungs. This phenomenon is also depicted in Figure 6–7 by the convergence of the flat portions (exaggerated for schematic effect) and separation of the steep segments of the three curves. A decrease in O_2 affinity (curve C, $P_{50} = 30.6$ mm Hg) is physiologically useful because it increases the amount of O_2 released at the tissues, where PO_2 is 40 mm Hg, by 1.6 ml/100 ml. In other words, the shift from curve A to curve C increases O_2 release from 4.5 to 6.1 ml/100 ml. In contrast, an increased O_2 affinity (curve B, $P_{50} = 22.6$ mm Hg) is disadvantageous because it reduces the amount of O_2 normally available to the tissues by 1.6 ml/100 ml, or from 4.5 to 2.9 ml/100 ml. When arterial PO_2 is low, as in the hypoxia of high altitude and of severe pulmonary diseases, an increase in P_{50} may not be physiologically useful because it impairs O_2 uptake by arterial blood as much as it facilitates O_2 release by capillary blood.

FACTORS AFFECTING OXYHEMOGLOBIN EQUILIBRIUM

Hemoglobin has probably been studied more thoroughly than any other protein, and a considerable amount of information is now available concerning the relationships between the structure of hemoglobin and its chemical properties. A single molecule of adult hemoglobin consists of two pairs of polypeptide chains: the α-chains containing 141 amino acid residues and the β–chains containing 146. Each chain is twisted into several folds that form a kind of basket into which the Fe-containing heme group fits neatly.[28] The four chains are symmetrically arranged in a tetramer that is held together by chemical contacts, primarily between unlike units ($\alpha_1\beta_1$ and $\alpha_1\beta_2$). Of great importance is the evidence that hemoglobin undergoes conformational

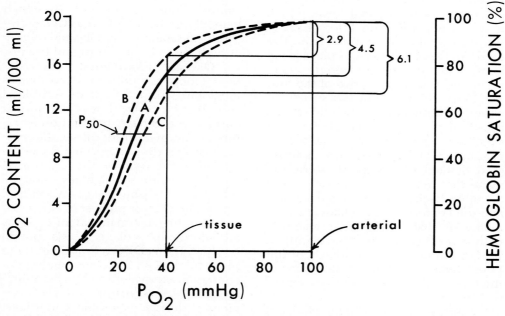

Figure 6–7 Schematic diagram showing the effects of increases and decreases in O_2 affinity on the amount of O_2 available at the PO_2 values prevailing in arterial blood and at the tissues. $P_{50} = PO_2$ at which hemoglobin saturation is 50 per cent. Hemoglobin concentration is assumed for convenience to be 14.9 gm/100 ml; therefore, O_2 content at 100 percent saturation is 20 ml/100 ml. Curve A = normal blood; curve B = blood with increased affinity (decreased P_{50}); curve C = blood with decreased affinity (increased P_{50}). For further discussion, see text.

changes when it reacts with O_2; thus the hemoglobin molecule can be said to breathe because it expands when bereft of O_2 and it contracts when combined with O_2. Shifts in the molecular structure of hemoglobin are also caused by reactions with CO_2, H^+, and certain organic phosphates (particularly 2,3-diphosphoglycerate [DPG]). All the substances that exert an interdependent effect on the chemical bonding properties of hemoglobin are known collectively as ligands. This means that the concentration within red blood cells of any one of the ligands affects the ability of hemoglobin to combine with any of the others. Moreover, this mechanism accounts for many of the physiologically and clinically significant shifts in oxyhemoglobin dissociation relationships.

Two states of hemoglobin with different structural conformations have been distinguished chemically: the *deoxy* form, which occurs when the O_2-combining sites at the heme groups are empty, and the *oxy* form, which occurs when they are filled. Exactly when the change in state from the deoxy to the oxy form takes place is not known, but it seems to require combination by more than two of the four Fe atoms with O_2.[29] The two structures of hemoglobin and the sigmoid O_2 dissociation curve are characteristic for substrate-ligand binding of allosteric enzymes.* The current view is to regard hemoglobin as an allosteric enzyme that reacts with a substrate, O_2; the interactions between α and β chains and the conformational changes of the molecule that result from reactions with other ligands affect the affinity of O_2.[31] A summary of the effects of different ligands and other alterations in the hemoglobin molecule is presented in Table 6–3.

Hydrogen Ion. The O_2 affinity of hemoglobin is strongly influenced by

---

*"An enzyme may possess two separate sites which can bind ligands — the active site, where catalysis occurs, and the allosteric ('other') site where a modifier may bind."[30]

changes in intracellular pH, the so-called *"Bohr effect."* As will be explained in greater detail in Chapters 7 and 8, the addition or removal of CO_2 has a direct effect on H_2CO_3 and hence on H^+ concentration (symbolized $[H^+]$). In the lungs, $[H^+]$ falls as CO_2 is eliminated from pulmonary capillary blood and oxyhemoglobin affinity is increased; in the peripheral capillaries, CO_2 is added to the bloodstream, causing $[H^+]$ to rise and O_2 affinity to decrease. The combined effect is physiologically favorable because it enhances both O_2 uptake in the lungs and O_2 release to the tissues.

Carbon Dioxide. The affinity of hemoglobin is affected by the presence of CO_2 in two ways: first, as noted previously, through the formation of H^+ that reacts, in turn, with hemoglobin, and second, by a direct chemical reaction between CO_2 and hemoglobin with the formation of carbamino compounds. Similar to a rise in $[H^+]$, a rise in carbamino compounds decreases O_2 affinity. Thus, the methods by which hemoglobin handles O_2 and CO_2 reciprocally augment the uptake and release of both gases in the lungs and tissues.

Organic Phosphates. The oxyhemoglobin equilibrium curve of hemoglobin stripped from its red blood cells lies far to the left of the normal curve, even though pH and temperature are normal; furthermore, the position of the displaced curve can be moved to the right by the addition of certain organic phosphates, notably adenosine triphosphate (ATP) and DPG. The DPG is present in only trace amounts in most mammalian cells, as an intermediate of glycolysis, but in red blood cells DPG is four times more plentiful than ATP and has a molar concentration equivalent to hemoglobin.[32] Because the synthesis of DPG increases during anaerobic conditions, red blood cells are equipped with their own inbuilt mechanism for responding to hypoxia in a manner that facilitates O_2 release to the tissues. Figure 6–8 shows the relationship between

Table 6–3   The Effect of Various Influences on Oxyhemoglobin Affinity and P_{50}*

INFLUENCE	O_2 AFFINITY	P_{50}
CO_2 concentration		
Increased	Decreased	Increased
Decreased	Increased	Decreased
pH		
Increased (alkalemia)	Increased	Decreased
Decreased (acidemia)	Decreased	Increased
2,3-Diphosphoglycerate		
Increased	Decreased	Increased
Decreased	Increased	Decreased
CO-hemoglobin, methemoglobin		
Increased	Increased	Decreased
Abnormal hemoglobins		
Chesapeake	Increased	Decreased
Yakima	Increased	Decreased
Rainier	Increased	Decreased
E	Decreased	Increased
Seattle	Decreased	Increased
Kansas	Decreased	Increased

*Data in part from Stamatoyannopoulos et al.[31]

changes in DPG concentration and P_{50} in patients with cardiac disease.[33] The time course of the appearance of changes in intracellular DPG varies with different kinds of anaerobic stress; increased concentrations of DPG have been observed immediately after only ten minutes of vigorous exercise[34] but as long as one to two days after ascent to high altitude.[35] Increased synthesis of DPG appears to be an important component of the adaptive responses in normal persons to an acute need for more tissue O_2; increased DPG concentrations in red blood cells with corresponding increases in P_{50} and decreases in O_2 affinity occur in numerous diseases characterized by reduction in available O_2 (e.g., anemia, right-to-left shunts, congestive heart failure). In contrast, low levels of erythrocyte DPG and increased O_2 affinity have been observed in stored blood and in blood of patients with hypophosphatemia, hexokinase deficiency, and septic shock.

Hemoglobin Concentration. Oxygen affinity has been shown to be dependent upon the concentration of hemoglobin in hemolysates. Because a similar effect has been demonstrated in intact cells, the mean corpuscular hemoglobin concentration should be taken into account when evaluating the position of the oxyhemoglobin equilibrium curve.[36]

Carbon Monoxide Hemoglobin. Carbon monoxide and O_2 compete with each other for combination with hemoglobin, but CO has 200 times greater affinity than O_2. The result of the formation of carboxyhemoglobin is to increase the affinity of the remaining Fe atoms for O_2. Exposure to CO has two dire consequences: it lowers the O_2 capacity of the blood by reducing the amount of hemoglobin that can combine with O_2 and it causes a progressive leftward shift of the oxyhemoglobin equilibrium curve that increasingly impairs the unloading of those O_2 molecules that are able to combine with hemoglobin.[25] Both mechanisms contribute to the production of severe tissue hypoxia and explain why the formation of 50 per cent

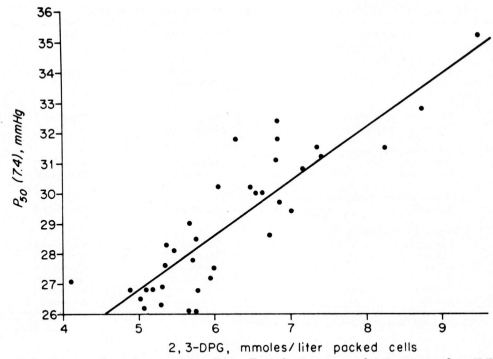

Figure 6–8   Relation between hemoglobin affinity for O_2, expressed as P_{50} measured at pH 7.4, and 2,3-diphosphoglycerate (2,3-DPG) in 39 patients with clinical evidence of cardiac disease. (From Woodson, Torrance, Shappell, and Lenfant.[33] Reprinted by permission from the authors and publisher.)

CO hemoglobin has more serious clinical consequences than when hemoglobin concentration is reduced to half normal by various forms of anemia.[25]

Methemoglobin. Methemoglobin is formed when the Fe atoms are oxidized from the ferrous to the ferric state. As this occurs successively among the four heme groups, the O_2 affinity of the remaining unoxidized Fe atoms increases. The effect of methemoglobin on tissue hypoxia is qualitatively the same but quantitatively less than that produced by equal amounts of CO hemoglobin.[37]

Abnormal   Hemoglobins. Over 100 abnormal hemoglobins have been described, but only about 12 have increased or decreased O_2 affinity.[31] Although altered O_2 affinity is rare and seldom of clinical significance, characterization of the amino acid sequences

of the abnormal hemoglobin species has provided important clues to the location of binding sites and the structure of normal hemoglobin. It is believed that abnormal O_2 affinity is due to conformational changes that effect the interaction between chains and the capability for DPG binding.[30] For example, the decreased P_{50} of fetal hemoblogin can be attributed to the decreased binding of DPG by the γ-chains, which occur in normal fetal hemoglobin instead of β–chains.

CARBON DIOXIDE EQUILIBRIUM

CHEMICAL REACTIONS

Carbon dioxide is similar to O_2 because both are carried by the blood mainly after undergoing reversible chemical reactions rather than in physical solution (Table 6–2). In contrast to O_2, in which combination with hemoglobin is the only (single) process involved, several different chemical reactions play a role in the transport of CO_2 from the tissues to the lungs.[25] Perhaps the best way of describing the mechanisms by which CO_2 is carried in the blood is to examine the various pathways between the sources of CO_2 and its elimination from the body.

Carbon dioxide is one of the end products of aerobic cellular metabolism and thus is being continuously produced virtually everywhere in the body. After CO_2 is formed by cells, it diffuses into the blood plasma owing to a concentration difference between the cell interior and the neighboring capillary blood. Most of the CO_2 that enters the blood passes into red blood cells, where it undergoes one of two possible chemical reactions.

1. The greater part enters into the reversible formation of HCO_3^- through a series of reactions:

$$CO_2 + H_2O \rightleftharpoons H_2CO_3, \text{ and} \quad (6)$$

$$H_2CO_3 \rightleftharpoons H^+ + HCO_3^-. \quad (7)$$

The combination between CO_2 and H_2O is of the molecular type and is comparatively slow. The reaction moves from left to right (hydration) in the tissue capillaries and from right to left (dehydration) in the pulmonary capillaries. The rates of both hydration and dehydration are accelerated several hundred times by the presence of *carbonic anhydrase*, a potent zinc-containing enzyme. Once H_2CO_3 is formed, its transformation into H^+ and HCO_3^- occurs by an extremely rapid ionic reaction. Some of the H^+ and HCO_3^- formed remain within red blood cells, the H^+ combining with hemoglobin and the HCO_3^- combining with K^+ displaced from hemoglobin by the H^+ reaction. More H_2CO_3 can be handled through these pathways by deoxyhemoglobin than by oxyhemoglobin, be-cause the former is a weaker acid and, therefore, a better buffer than the latter (see Chapter 8 for a more complete discussion of buffers).

Some of the HCO_3^- formed by the ionization of H_2CO_3 diffuses out of the red blood cell into the plasma because the membrane is much more permeable to negatively charged anions, such as HCO_3^- and Cl^-, than to positively charged cations, such as K^+ and Na^+. This movement tends to set up an electrostatic difference across the cell membrane that is neutralized by the movement of Cl^- from the plasma into the red blood cell (the *"chloride shift"*).

2. The smaller fraction of CO_2 that enters red blood cells combines reversibly with hemoglobin to form carbamino compounds. As is the case with the capacity of hemoglobin to combine with the H^+ formed from H_2CO_3, more CO_2 is bound in the form of carbamino compounds by deoxyhemoglobin than by oxyhemoglobin.

CARBON DIOXIDE EQUILIBRIUM CURVE

The CO_2 equilibrium curves of oxygenated and deoxygenated blood are shown in Figure 6–9. The curves are nearly linear in the physiologic range (P_{CO_2} 40 to 50), and considerably more, about 6 ml/100 ml, CO_2 is bound at any given P_{CO_2} within that range by deoxy- than by oxyhemoglobin. The shift from the lower to the upper curve in Figure 6–9 occurs during the deoxygenation of blood as it flows through tissue capillaries and adds, in turn, to the capacity of blood to take up CO_2; this enhancement of CO_2 transport is known as the *Haldane effect* and is physiologically of far greater importance than the converse influence of CO_2 (through formation of H^+) on O_2 transport ("Bohr effect," see preceding section). There are two components to the Haldane effect that depend upon chemical differences between deoxy- and oxyhemoglobin: about 70 per cent is due to the augmented capacity of

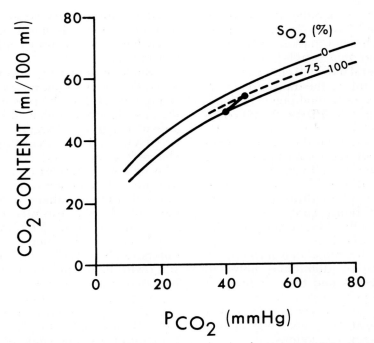

Figure 6–9 Normal CO_2 equilibration (dissociation) curves for whole blood at 0, 75, and 100 per cent oxyhemoglobin saturation (SO_2). The heavy line connecting the two points shows the usual extent of the Haldane effect in arterial and venous blood.

the deoxy-species to form carbamino compounds, and the remainder is due to the enhanced ability of the deoxy-form to absorb H^+ and release base (i.e., buffer the ionization products of H_2CO_3).

To summarize, CO_2 is carried in the bloodstream partly in red blood cells, both as HCO_3^- and bound to hemoglobin as carbamino compounds, and partly in plasma, as HCO_3^-; only a small portion is in physical solution. In the pulmonary capillaries, all of the chemical reactions that occur in tissue capillaries proceed in the reverse direction. Carbonic anhydrase also plays an indispensable role in the lungs by catalyzing the dehydration of H_2CO_3 into CO_2 and H_2O; without the enzyme, or in the presence of carbonic acid inhibitors, the release of CO_2 does not proceed to equilibrium during the time that red blood cells spend

traversing the pulmonary capillary, and a difference develops between the CO_2 concentration in end-capillary blood and that in alveolar gas.

Thus, the normal processes concerned with CO_2 elimination begin with diffusion from the sites of CO_2 production into the bloodstream, include chemical reactions within red blood cells and plasma that greatly increase the carrying capacity of the blood, and end, again, with diffusion of CO_2 out of the blood in pulmonary capillaries into the alveoli.

REFERENCES

1. Forster, R. E.: Exchange of gases between alveolar air and pulmonary capillary blood: pulmonary diffusing capacity. Physiol. Rev., 37:391-405, 1957.
2. Staub, N. C.: Time-dependent factors in pulmonary gas exchange. Med. Thorac., 22: 132-145, 1965.

3. Staub, N. C.: Alveolar-arterial oxygen tension gradient due to diffusion. J. Appl. Physiol., *18*:673-680, 1963.

4. Hyde, R. W., Puy, R. J. M., Raub, W. F., and Forster, R. E.: Rate of disappearance of labeled carbon dioxide from the lungs of humans during breath holding: a method for studying the dynamics of pulmonary CO_2 exchange. J. Clin. Invest., 47:1535-1552, 1968.

5. Roughton, F. J. W., and Forster, R. E.: Relative importance of diffusion and chemical reaction rates in determining rate of exchange of gases in the human lung, with special reference to true diffusing capacity of pulmonary membrane and volume of blood in the lung capillaries. J. Appl. Physiol., *11*:290–302, 1957.

6. Forster, R. E.: Diffusion of gases. *In* Fenn, W. O., and Rahn, H. (eds.): Handbook of Physiology, Section 3. Respiration. Vol. I. Washington, D. C., American Physiological Society, 1964, pp. 839-872.

7. Bates, D. V., Macklem, P. T., and Christie, R. V.: Respiratory Function in Disease. An Introduction to the Integrated Study of the Lung. Philadelphia, W. B. Saunders Co., 1971, pp. 75-90.

8. Gold, W. M., Burgess, J. H., and Nadel, J. A.: Unpublished observations, 1974.

9. Hyde, R. W., Rynes, R., Power, G. G., and Nairn, J.: Determination of distribution of diffusing capacity in relation to blood flow in the human lung. J. Clin. Invest., 46:463–474, 1967.

10. Johnson, R. L., and Miller, J. M.: Distribution of ventilation, blood flow, and gas transfer coefficients in the lung. J. Appl. Physiol., 25:1-15, 1968.

11. Thurlbeck, W. M., Henderson, J. A., Fraser, R. G., and Bates, D. V.: Chronic obstructive lung disease. A comparison between clinical, roentgenologic, functional and morphologic criteria in chronic bronchitis, emphysema, asthma and bronchiectasis. Medicine, 49:81-145, 1970.

12. Burgess, J. H.: Pulmonary diffusing capacity in disorders of the pulmonary circulation. Circulation, 49:541–550, 1974.

13. Weibel, E. R.: Morphological basis of alveolar-capillary gas exchange. Physiol. Rev., 53:419-495, 1973.

14. Maloney, J. E., and Castle, B. L.: Pressure-diameter relations of capillaries and small blood vessels in frog lung. Resp. Physiol., 7:150-162, 1969.

15. Hamer, N. A. J.: The effect of age on the components of the pulmonary diffusing capacity. Clin. Sci., 23:85-93, 1962.

16. Thurlbeck, W. M.: The internal surface area of nonemphysematous lungs. Am. Rev. Resp. Dis., 95:765-773, 1967.

17. Guleria, J. S., Pande, J. N., Sethi, P. K., and Roy, S. B.: Pulmonary diffusing capacity at high altitude. J. Appl. Physiol., *31*:536-543, 1971.

18. Karp, R. B., Graf, P. D., and Nadel, J. A.: Regulation of pulmonary capillary blood volume by pulmonary arterial and left atrial pressures. Circ. Res., 22:1-10, 1968.

19. Forster, R. E.: Interpretation of measurements of pulmonary diffusing capacity. *In* Fenn, W. O., and Rahn, H. (eds.): Handbook of Physiology, Section 3. Respiration. Vol. II. Washington, D. C., American Physiological Society, 1965, pp. 1453-1468.

20. Wagner, P. D., and West, J. B.: Effects of diffusion impairment on O_2 and CO_2 time courses in pulmonary capillaries. J. Appl. Physiol., *33*:62-71, 1972.

21. Sobel, B. J., Bottex, G., Emirgil, C., and Gissen, H.: Gaseous diffusion from alveoli to pulmonary vessels of considerable size. Circ. Res. *13*:71-79, 1963.

22. Staub, N. C.: Gas exchange vessels in the cat lung. Fed. Proc., *20*:107, 1961.

23. Krogh, A.: The Anatomy and Physiology of Capillaries. New York, Hafner, 1959, pp. 22-46, 267-274.

24. Comroe, J. H., Jr., Forster, R. E., II, Dubois, A. B., Briscoe, W. A., and Carlsen, E.: The Lung. Clinical Physiology and Pulmonary Function Tests. 2nd Ed. Chicago, Year Book Medical Publishers, Inc., 1962, p. 141.

25. Roughton, F. J. W.: Transport of oxygen and carbon dioxide. *In* Fenn, W. O., and Rahn, H. (eds.): Handbook of Physiology, Section 3. Respiration. Vol. I. Washington, D. C., American Physiological Society, 1964, pp. 767-825.

26. Severinghaus, J. W.: Blood oxygen dissociation line charts: man. *In* Altman, P. C., and Dittmer, D. S. (eds.): Respiration and Circulation. Bethesda, Md., Federation of American Societies for Experimental Biology, 1971, pp. 204-206.

27. Singer, R. B.: Blood gas variables, factors, and constants: man. *In* Altman, P. C., and Dittmer, D. S. (eds.): Respiration and Circulation. Bethesda, Md., Federation of American Societies for Experimental Biology, 1971, p. 140.

28. Perutz, M. F.: Structure and function of hemoglobin. Harvey Lect., *63*:213-261, 1967-68.

29. Gibson, Q. H., and Parkhurst, L. J.: Kinetic evidence for a tetrameric functional unit in hemoglobin. J. Biol. Chem., *243*:5521-5524, 1968.

30. Harper, H. A.: Review of Physiological Chemistry. 13th Ed. Los Altos, Cal., Lange Medical Publications, 1971, p. 149.

31. Stamatoyannopoulos, G., Bellingham, A. J., Lenfant, C., and Finch, C. A.: Abnormal hemoglobins with high and low oxygen affinity. Ann. Rev. Med., *22*;221-234, 1971.

32. Bunn, H. F., and Jandl, J. H.: Control of hemoglobin function within the red cell. New Eng. J. Med., *282*:1414-1420, 1970.

33. Woodson, R. D., Torrance, J. D., Shappell, S. D., and Lenfant, C.: The effect of cardiac disease on hemoglobin-oxygen binding. J. Clin. Invest., *49*:1349–1356, 1970.

34. Faulkner, J. A., Brewer, G. J., and Eaton, J. W.: Adaptation of the red blood cell to muscular exercise. *In* Brewer, G. J. (eds.): Red Cell Metabolism and Function. New York, Plenum, 1970, pp. 213–227.

35. Lenfant, C., Torrance, J., English, E., Finch, C. A., Reynafarje, C., Ramos, J., and Faura, J.: Effect of altitude on oxygen binding by hemoglobin and on organic phosphate levels. J. Clin. Invest., *47*:2652-2656, 1968.

36. Bellingham, A. J., Detter, J. C., and Lenfant, C.: Regulatory mechanisms of hemoglobin oxygen affinity in acidosis and alkalosis. J. Clin. Invest., *50*:700-706, 1971.

37. Darling, R. C., and Roughton, F. J. W.: The effect of methemoglobin on the equilibrium between oxygen and hemoglobin. Am. J. Physiol., *137*:56-68, 1942.

Chapter Seven

GAS EXCHANGE AND OXYGEN TRANSPORT

INTRODUCTION

The diffusion of O_2 and CO_2 across the air-blood barrier and the chemical reactions of these gases within the bloodstream are two of the chief mechanisms involved in gas exchange and transport of gases between the lungs and the peripheral tissues. But other factors are also important in determining the adequacy of gas exchange and in defining the capacity of the transport system. This chapter considers how O_2 uptake and CO_2 elimina-

171

tion take place under idealized conditions and how deviations from the ideal occur in normal subjects and in patients with pulmonary disorders.

Gas exchange, as mentioned earlier, is the principal function of the respiratory system (i.e., air passages, lungs, muscles of respiration, and nervous pathways and controlling centers); in contrast, O_2 transport is a multisystem process that involves not only the respiratory system but also the circulatory and hemoglobin-regulating systems as well. This chapter describes these components of O_2 transport and how they are interrelated under normal and stressful circumstances.

GAS EXCHANGE

"IDEAL" RELATIONSHIPS

The diffusion of O_2 and CO_2 between alveolar gas and blood in the pulmonary capillaries and the reversible combination of O_2 and CO_2 with hemoglobin are the essential elements of gas exchange. These processes take place continuously in the approximately 100,000 terminal respiratory units in the lung, and the adequacy of respiration in *each gas exchange unit* depends upon the apposition of a thin film of mixed venous blood with just the right amount of fresh air, so that the blood becomes fully oxygenated and part of its CO_2 is eliminated. The local matching of ventilation and perfusion

is the crucial determinant of gas exchange, and a deficiency or excess of ventilation relative to the amount of blood flow leads to either inadequate or wasteful respiration. It is impossible to evaluate the completeness of gas exchange within individual units, but the over-all effectiveness can be assessed through examination of the composition of arterial blood and alveolar gas.

Normal values for the gas pressures prevailing at sea level (barometric pressure 760 mm Hg) for the individual gases, P_{O_2}, P_{CO_2}, P_{N_2}, and P_{H_2O}, in ambient air, conducting airways, gas exchange units, and mixed venous and arterial blood are indicated in Table 7-1. Ambient air consists primarily of N_2 and O_2, all other gases being present in negligible amounts except water vapor, the pressure of which varies considerably depending upon local humidity. As air is inhaled, it is warmed and fully saturated with water vapor at the subject's body temperature (P_{H_2O} at $37°$ C $= 47$ mm Hg); the addition of water vapor in effect dilutes the inspired mixture of N_2 and O_2 and reduces their respective pressures to the values indicated within the conducting airways. After the inspirate reaches the terminal units, gas exchange takes place. More O_2 is removed than CO_2 is added, which causes the volume of each unit to diminish slightly and which raises the concentration and pressure of N_2 within the gas phase slightly. This is known as the respira-

Table 7-1 Normal Gas Pressures (in mm Hg) During Inspiration in Ambient Air, Conducting Airways, Terminal Units (Alveoli), and Arterial and Mixed Venous Blood

	AMBIENT AIR	CONDUCTING AIRWAYS	TERMINAL UNITS	ARTERIAL BLOOD	MIXED VENOUS BLOOD
P_{O_2}	156	149	100	95	40
P_{CO_2}	0	0	40	40	46
P_{H_2O}	15*	47	47	47	47
P_{N_2}	589	564	573	573	573
P_{TOTAL}	760	760	760	755	706

*P_{H_2O} varies according to humidity and has a proportionate effect on P_{O_2} and P_{N_2}.

tory exchange (R) effect. (Under steady state conditions, R is determined by metabolic events, the O_2 consumption [$\dot{V}O_2$]); and the CO_2 production [$\dot{V}CO_2$]); $R = \dot{V}CO_2/\dot{V}O_2$ and normally is about 0.8.)

Before considering the complexities of gas exchange in the normal human lung, it is useful to examine the behavior of the greatly simplified two-compartment lung model shown in Figure 7–1. In this and subsequent figures, the hemoglobin concentration is assumed to be 15.0 gm/100 ml and the arteriovenous difference for O_2 is 4.6 ml/100 ml and for CO_2 is 3.7 ml/100 ml. The large, double-pointed arrows indicate both the magnitude and the distribution of ventilation. The small arrows indicate diffusion of O_2 and CO_2 between alveolar gas and pulmonary capillary blood. The "arterialization"

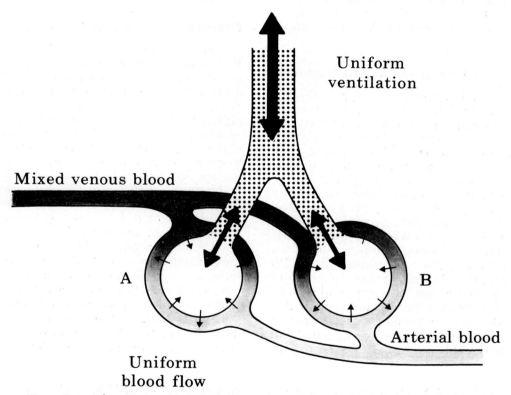

Figure 7–1 Schematic representation of gas exchange in an idealized two-compartment model of the lung in which there is uniform distribution of ventilation and blood flow. (Adapted from Comroe, Forster, Dubois, Briscoe, and Carlsen.[1] Reprinted by permission from the authors and Year Book Publisher, Inc.)

	A	B	A + B	Units
Alveolar ventilation	2.4	2.4	4.8	L/min
Pulmonary blood flow	3.0	3.0	6.0	L/min
Ventilation-perfusion ratio	0.8	0.8	0.8	
Mixed venous PO_2	40	40	40	mm Hg
Mixed venous SO_2	75	75	75	per cent
Mixed venous PCO_2	46	46	46	mm Hg
Alveolar PO_2	101	101	101	mm Hg
Arterial PO_2	101	101	101	mm Hg
Arterial SO_2	97.5	97.5	97.5	per cent
Arterial PCO_2	40	40	40	mm Hg
Alveolar-arterial PO_2 difference	0	0	0	mm Hg

of blood is signified by the change in shading from black (mixed venous blood) to light gray (arterial blood).

In Figure 7-1, alveolar ventilation and blood flow are uniformly distributed to the gas exchange units; normally, there is less alveolar ventilation than pulmonary blood flow and the over-all *ventilation-perfusion ratio* of the lung is 0.8. Because diffusion equilibrium is attained between the blood and gas phases, the values for both P_{O_2} and P_{CO_2} are the same in alveolar gas as in end-capillary and arterial blood.

ALVEOLAR-ARTERIAL DIFFERENCES.

The effectiveness of gas exchange by the lungs is usually assessed through measurements of P_{O_2} and P_{CO_2} in arterial blood. However, as will be shown, additional information about the mechanisms that underlie any abnormalities (if present) is obtained by relating values in blood to those simultaneously present in mean alveolar gas: the *alveolar-arterial* P_{O_2} or P_{CO_2} *difference*. Analysis of arterial blood gas composition is simple and accurate, but measurements of P_{O_2} and P_{CO_2} in continuous or spot samples of expired gas, although readily available, are not representative of *all* alveolar gas; fortunately, mean alveolar gas composition can be calculated with reasonable accuracy using the *alveolar*

air equation; for mean alveolar P_{O_2} (PA_{O_2}):

$$PA_{O_2} = PI_{O_2} - PA_{CO_2} \left[FI_{O_2} + \frac{1-FI_{O_2}}{R} \right],$$
$$(1)$$

where $PI_{O_2} = P_{O_2}$ of inspired gas, $PA_{CO_2} =$ alveolar P_{CO_2} (usually assumed to equal arterial P_{CO_2}), $FI_{O_2} =$ fractional concentration of O_2 in inspired gas, and $R =$ respiratory exchange ratio (see above).

DISTURBANCES OF GAS EXCHANGE.

Measurements of arterial P_{O_2} and P_{CO_2} and calculations of alveolar-arterial P_{O_2} differences provide the best guide to the over-all adequacy of respiration. If abnormal values are obtained, further studies are often necessary to determine which one, or more, of the various processes that contribute to gas exchange is at fault. Normal value use for P_{O_2}, but not P_{CO_2}, vary considerably with age (Chapter 12), and both P_{O_2} and P_{CO_2} are influenced by the altitude at which the subject is living when sampling is performed.

Finding an arterial P_{O_2} value below the range for normal subjects of the same age establishes the presence of *arterial hypoxia.* When defined in terms of P_{O_2}, arterial hypoxia can result *only* from disturbances of respiration or a reduction in the P_{O_2} of inspired air (Table 7-2). *Hypercapnia*, or CO_2 re-

Table 7-2   Causes of Arterial Hypoxia (a Reduction in P_{O_2}) and Their Effect on Alveolar-Arterial P_{O_2} Differences ([A-a]P_{O_2})

CAUSE	EFFECT ON ARTERIAL P_{O_2}	EFFECT ON (A-a)P_{O_2}
Hypoventilation	Decreased	No change
Diffusion abnormality	No change or decreased*	No change or increased*
Ventilation-perfusion imbalance	Decreased	Increased
Right-to-left shunt	Decreased	Increased
Reduction in inspired P_{O_2}	Decreased	No change

*Effects of diffusion abnormalities are infrequently encountered at rest but are more likely to be evident during exercise.

GAS EXCHANGE

175

tention, is defined as an elevation of arterial P_{CO_2} above the normal range; *hypocapnia* is a lower than normal arterial P_{CO_2}.

HYPOVENTILATION

The simplest derangement of gas exchange occurs when insufficient fresh air is inspired (*hypoventilation*) to provide enough new O_2 molecules to raise pulmonary capillary P_{O_2} to normal levels and to allow CO_2 to

leave the bloodstream. When this situation develops, as shown in Figure 7-2, the quantity of O_2 in both arterial and venous blood must decrease, and the amount of CO_2 must increase. Although the blood gas abnormalities that result from hypoventilation may be severe, it should be noted that if ventilation and blood flow remain uniform, as they are in Figure 7-2, no alveolar-arterial difference develops for either O_2 or CO_2.

Pure hypoventilation is a rela-

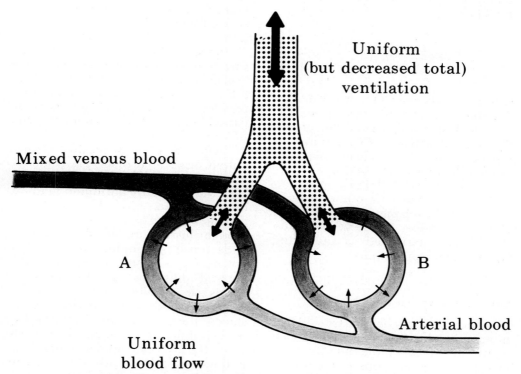

Figure 7-2 Schematic representation of the effects of hypoventilation on gas exchange. Alveolar ventilation is one-half that in Figure 7-1. (Adapted from Comroe, Forster, Dubois, Briscoe, and Carlsen.[1] Reprinted by permission from the authors and Year Book Publisher, Inc.)

	A	B	A + B	Units
Alveolar ventilation	1.2	1.2	2.4	L/min
Pulmonary blood flow	3.0	3.0	6.0	L/min
Ventilation-perfusion ratio	0.4	0.4	0.4	
Mixed venous P_{O_2}	34	34	34	mm Hg
Mixed venous S_{O_2}	64.3	64.3	64.3	per cent
Mixed venous P_{CO_2}	90	90	90	mm Hg
Alveolar P_{O_2}	53	53	53	mm Hg
Arterial P_{O_2}	53	53	53	mm Hg
Arterial S_{O_2}	87.2	87.2	87.2	per cent
Arterial P_{CO_2}	80	80	80	mm Hg
Alveolar-arterial P_{O_2} difference	0	0	0	mm Hg

tively uncommon clinical event; it may be caused by depression of the central nervous system from anesthesia or sedative drugs, by neuromuscular diseases that affect respiratory muscle function, and by thoracic cage injuries (e.g., "flail" chest). In these disorders both the amount of air that is breathed in at the mouth (*minute ventilation*) and the amount that reaches the gas exchange units (*alveolar ventilation*) are reduced. The CO_2 pressures in alveolar gas (PA_{CO_2}), and arterial blood (Pa_{CO_2}) can be expressed by the relationship

$$PA_{CO_2} = Pa_{CO_2} = K \frac{\dot{V}CO_2}{\dot{V}A}, \qquad (2)$$

where $\dot{V}CO_2$ is the CO_2 output (or production), $\dot{V}A$ is the alveolar ventilation, and K is a constant. This equation indicates that if CO_2 production remains constant, halving alveolar ventilation doubles arterial P_{CO_2}.

Although arterial P_{CO_2} may theoretically increase in other disturbances of gas exchange (see below), in clinical practice an elevated value should be interpreted as indicating alveolar hypoventilation.

DIFFUSION ABNORMALITY

The previous chapter stressed that in normal subjects at rest, O_2 and CO_2 equilibrate between the blood and gas phases in only a fraction of the time it takes for red blood cells to travel through the pulmonary capillary network; accordingly, the velocity of blood flow can increase considerably during exercise without causing detectable alveolar–end-capillary differences. In contrast, patients with impaired diffusing capacities can also reach equilibration for O_2 and CO_2 across the air-blood barrier while at rest, but alveolar–end-capillary differences are likely to occur during exercise. The explanation for the en-

hanced effect of exercise in producing arterial hypoxia in the presence of a given abnormality of diffusion from thickening of the air-blood barrier is shown schematically in Figure 7–3. Decreased diffusion (dotted lines) differs from normal (solid lines) in that more time is required for O_2 and CO_2 to achieve equilibrium across a thickened alveolar-capillary membrane. Under resting conditions, blood flow is sufficiently slow that equilibrium (point A) is usually attained even when diffusing capacity is reduced substantially. During exercise, however, the increased velocity of blood flow through pulmonary capillaries shortens the time available for diffusion; when the exposure time of red blood cells to alveolar gas is halved, alveolar–end-capillary differences for O_2 (point B') and CO_2 develop when diffusing capacity is impaired but not when it is normal (point B).

The effect of increasing cardiac output on arterial blood gas composition in the presence of decreased diffusion was originally attributed to thickening of the air-blood barrier, the so-called *alveolar-capillary block*. Although this abnormality has received widespread (and undue) attention, it is not nearly as common a cause of decreased diffusing capacity measurements as a reduction in pulmonary capillary blood volume. In this circumstance, the mechanism of arterial hypoxia is different from that which exists when the alveolar-capillary membrane is thickened; this is also displayed in Figure 7–3. As capillaries are progressively destroyed or obstructed, previously unperfused capillaries are recruited and finally the velocity of blood flow increases. When the disease process is severe, the time available for gas exchange in these patients at rest may be as short as it is in normal subjects during exercise (point B); consequently, during exercise the short pulmonary capillary transit times become even shorter and failure of equilibration occurs (point C).

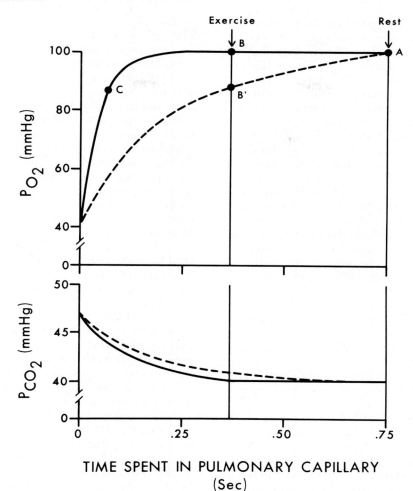

Figure 7–3 Schematic diagram showing the time course of changes in Po_2 and Pco_2 at rest and during exercise in normal subjects and in patients with decreased diffusing capacities from thickened alveolar-capillary membranes and decreased pulmonary capillary blood volumes. At rest, equilibration occurs between the pressures in the blood and gas phases (point A) in both normal subjects (—) and patients with decreased diffusing capacities from a thickened air-blood barrier (- - - -); during exercise, because the time available for gas exchange is shortened, equilibration occurs in normal subjects (point B) but not in patients (point B'). When the capillary bed is destroyed or obstructed, the velocity of blood flow increases in the remaining vessels under resting conditions (point B); during exercise, equilibration is no longer possible (point C).

VENTILATION-PERFUSION IMBALANCE

In contrast to the ideal condition described previously, the distributions of inspired air and pulmonary capillary blood are neither uniform nor proportionate to each other. As emphasized in Chapters 4 and 5, the distributions of ventilation and blood flow can be shown to vary with such common events as changes in body position and changes in lung volume. Thus, there is always some variable degree of ventilation-perfusion imbalance present even in normal subjects. Moreover, increased (above normal) mismatching of ventilation and perfusion is by far the most common cause of arterial hypoxia in patients with disorders affecting the respiratory system. It is worthwhile, therefore, to consider how ventilation-perfusion abnormalities occur, as well as their consequences.

The two-compartment model used to depict ideal gas exchange has been modified to that shown in Figure 7–4. The composition of mixed venous blood, total blood flow, and its distribution are the same as in Figure 7–1. However, the same total alveolar ventilation is now distributed *un*evenly between the two gas exchange units, so that Unit A receives three times more inspired gas than Unit B. Because blood flow is equally distributed to the two units, the *ventilation-perfusion ratios* ($\dot{V}A/\dot{Q}$) differ and cause the alveolar and end-capillary gas compositions to vary as shown. The O_2 and CO_2 contents of the end-capillary blood from each alveolus are determined by the gas pressures in the alveoli, which are in equilibrium with the end-capillary blood, and the respective hemoglobin equilibration curves for the two gases. To derive the final composition of arterial blood after the two effluent vascular pathways mix, it is necessary first to sum algebraically* the contents (or saturations), *not the pressures*, and then to determine the resulting pressures from the oxyhemoglobin and CO_2 equilibrium curves (Figures 6–6 and 6–9); this procedure is required because of the alinear characteristics of both curves.

The final composition of mixed alveolar gas, such as might be measured by recording Po_2 and Pco_2 during expiration at the mouth, is derived by summing the gas tensions and algebraically allowing for the differences in ventilation to the two

units. (In Figure 7–4, [3(116) + 77]/4 = 106, for Po_2.)

An important consequence of a ventilation-perfusion imbalance is evident even in this simplified diagram and analysis: *there must be a difference between the O_2 and CO_2 pressures in mixed alveolar gas and arterial blood.* The alveolar-arterial Po_2 difference is 16 mm Hg, and the arterial-alveolar Pco_2 difference is 2.5 mm Hg in the example chosen. Alveolar-arterial differences occur because the relative overventilation of one unit does not fully compensate— by adding extra O_2 or by eliminating extra CO_2—for the disturbances created by underventilating the other unit. The failure to compensate is greater in the case of O_2 than with CO_2 owing to the flatness of the upper part of the oxyhemoglobin dissociation curve compared with the CO_2 dissociation curve. Increased ventilation raises alveolar Po_2 but adds little "extra" O_2 to the bloodstream; in contrast, the steeper slope of the CO_2 curve provides more CO_2 elimination.

The calculations used to derive the values shown (Figure 7–4) are useful for illustrative purposes but are not completely accurate because mixed venous blood composition is held constant and is not affected, as it would be, by the circulation of arterial blood with reduced O_2 and increased CO_2 through the tissues of the body. A detailed and elegant computer analysis of a ten-compartment lung model, which takes these and other mathematical complexities into account, has been developed by West.[2] Figure 7–5 is reproduced from West's work and shows the effect of increasing ventilation-perfusion inequality on gas exchange, the amount of venous admixture (see below), and the amount of wasted alveolar ventilation (see below). As the inequality increases, arterial Po_2 falls continuously and precipitously, and arterial Pco_2 rises gradually at first and then more swiftly.

---

*In Figure 7–4, simple addition and division by two is all that is required because blood flow is equally distributed; if blood flow to the two alveoli had been uneven, as in the case of ventilation, algebraic weighting would have been necessary.

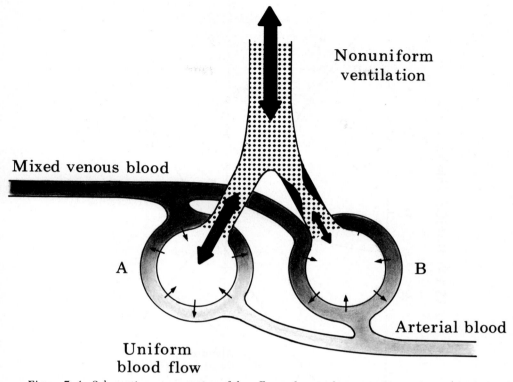

Nonuniform
ventilation

Mixed venous blood

A

B

Arterial blood

Uniform
blood flow

Figure 7–4 Schematic representation of the effects of a ventilation-perfusion abnormality on gas exchange. (Adapted from Comroe, Forster, Dubois, Briscoe, and Carlsen.[1] Reprinted by permission from the authors and Year Book Publisher, Inc.)

	A	B	A + B	*Units*
Alveolar ventilation	3.6	1.2	4.8	L/min
Pulmonary blood flow	3.0	3.0	6.0	L/min
Ventilation-perfusion ratio	1.2	0.4	0.8	
Mixed venous P_{O_2}	40	40	40	mm Hg
Mixed venous S_{O_2}	75	75	75	per cent
Mixed venous P_{CO_2}	46	46	46	mm Hg
Alveolar P_{O_2}	114	77	106	mm Hg
Arterial P_{O_2}	114	77	89	mm Hg
Arterial S_{O_2}	98.2	95.4	96.8	per cent
Arterial P_{CO_2}	36	45	40	mm Hg
Alveolar-arterial P_{O_2} difference	0	0	17	mm Hg

This means, contrary to the usual teaching, that ventilation-perfusion imbalance can be a significant cause of CO_2 retention in patients with pulmonary disease.[3] This statement at first glance may appear to conflict with the common clinical observations that patients with many forms of pulmonary disease (e.g., emphysema and bronchial asthma) may have severe arterial hypoxia caused by ventilation-perfusion abnormalities but also may have arterial P_{CO_2} levels that are normal or, at times, even lower than normal. This apparent discrepancy is explained by the fact that these patients are ventilating more than is normal, and owing to the respective shapes and positions of the equilibrium curves for O_2 and CO_2, hyperventilation of the ventilable units increases CO_2 elimination but does not increase O_2 uptake.[3] Thus, an increase in total ventilation "corrects" the CO_2 retention that would

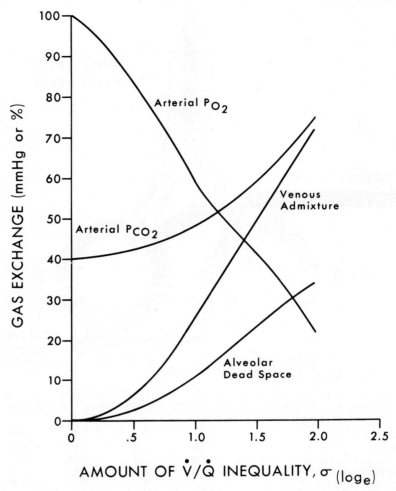

Figure 7-5   Effect of increasing ventilation-perfusion ratio ($\dot{V}/\dot{Q}$) inequality on arterial P_{O_2} and P_{CO_2}, venous admixture, and alveolar dead space in a lung model in which O_2 uptake and CO_2 output are kept constant at 300 and 240 ml/min, respectively. (Adapted from West.[2] Reprinted by permission from the author and publisher.)

otherwise occur, but hypoxia persists.

A new technique was recently described for measuring in man the continuous distributions of ventilation and perfusion.[4] The method is based on the simultaneous steady-state elimination by the lung of six inert gases of markedly different solubilities. Figure 7–6 depicts the distributions of ventilation and blood flow in a normal young man breathing room air in the semirecumbent position. Both distributions are positioned near a ven-

tilation-perfusion ratio of 1 and are narrow and symmetric on a log scale (in the example shown, the log standard deviation was 0.32 for blood flow and 0.29 for ventilation). However, these dispersions, though small, are sufficient to account for an alveolar-arterial P_{O_2} difference of about 5 mm Hg (see also Figure 7–5). The method has been used to study healthy subjects of various ages and in different body positions. The results confirm the long-standing belief that the un-

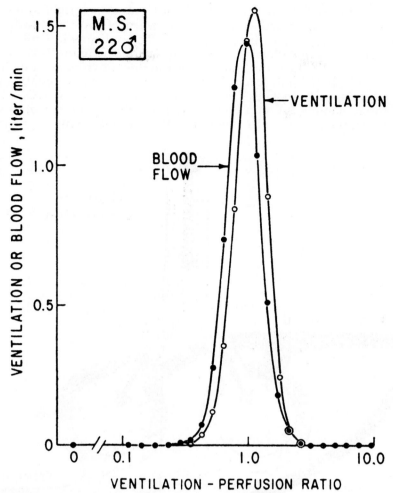

Figure 7–6 The distribution of ventilation and blood flow in a normal 22-year-old man. Both distributions are positioned about a ventilation-perfusion ratio close to 1.0; the curves are symmetrical on a log scale with no areas of high or low ventilation-perfusion ratios and there is no shunt (ventilation-perfusion ratio = zero). (From Wagner, Laravuso, Uhl, and West.[4] Reprinted by permission from the authors and publisher.)

evenness of the distribution of ventilation-perfusion ratios found in young adults worsens with increasing age and that regions of high ventilation-perfusion ratios develop when changing from the supine to the sitting position; the latter findings are consistent with the known effects of posture on the topographic distributions of ventilation, blood flow, and lung volumes discussed in Chapters 4 and 5.

RIGHT-TO-LEFT SHUNTS

Another departure from ideal gas exchange is caused by right-to-left shunts of blood in the lungs; these are found to a slight degree in normal subjects and may be of considerable magnitude in patients with pulmonary disease. A schematic representation of the effects of a right-to-left shunt upon gas exchange is shown in Figure 7–7. Alveolar ventilation, distribution of ventilation, and composition of mixed venous blood are the same as they were under ideal conditions, but distribution of cardiac output is different. The total blood flow remains the same (6 L/min), but only 2 L/min each, instead of 3 L/min each, reaches Units A and B; the remaining 2 L/min flows through the shunt pathway. In other words, there is a right-to-left shunt of one third of the total cardiac output.

Gas exchange in Units A and B is unimpaired (Figure 7–7); in fact, because the individual ventilation-perfusion ratios are high, slightly more O_2 is taken up and more CO_2 eliminated than would occur if the ratios were normal. But this slight augmentation of

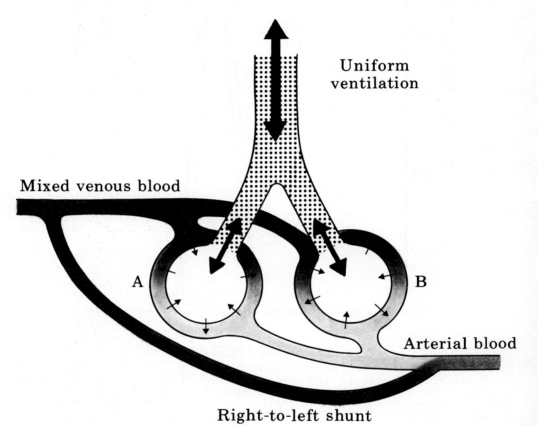

Right-to-left shunt

Figure 7–7 Schematic representation of the effects of a right-to-left shunt on gas exchange. (Adapted from Comroe, Forster, Dubois, Briscoe, and Carlsen.[1] Reprinted by permission from the authors and Year Book Publisher, Inc.)

	$A + B$	Shunt	$A + B$ $+ Shunt$	Units
Alveolar ventilation	4.8	0	4.8	L/min
Pulmonary blood flow	4.0	2.0	6.0	L/min
Ventilation-perfusion ratio	1.2	0	0.8	
Mixed venous Po_2	40	40	40	mm Hg
Mixed venous So_2	75	75	75	per cent
Mixed venous Pco_2	46	46	46	mm Hg
Alveolar Po_2	114	–	114	mm Hg
Arterial Po_2	114	–	59	mm Hg
Arterial So_2	98.2	–	90.5	per cent
Arterial Pco_2	36	–	39	mm Hg
Alveolar-arterial Po_2 difference	0	–	55	mm Hg

gas exchange does not nearly compensate for the deleterious effect of the continuous flow of mixed venous blood through the shunt. The net result from the mixing of blood from the normal and the shunt pathways is analogous to the effects of a ventilation-perfusion inequality: an inevitable reduction of arterial P_{O_2}, an increase in arterial P_{CO_2}, and a creation of alveolar-arterial differences for the two gases.

It should not be surprising that the consequences of a right-to-left shunt are similar to those of a ventilation-perfusion imbalance; a shunt can be viewed as an extreme ventilation-perfusion disturbance: one in which there is perfusion but *no* ventilation at all. Because it is impossible to apportion the contributions to a given alveolar-arterial difference between a ventilation-perfusion disturbance on the one hand and a right-to-left shunt on the other, at least while the subject is breathing ambient air, the effects of each are combined and considered as *venous admixture* or "shunt-like" effect.

EFFECTS OF BREATHING 100 PER CENT OXYGEN

A right-to-left shunt can be differentiated from a ventilation-perfusion inequality in the laboratory and at the bedside by giving the subject 100 per cent O_2 to breathe. Table 7–3 demonstrates how this distinction can be made from examination of the alveolar and arterial gas pressures that result when ideal lungs and lungs with ventilation-perfusion abnormalities or right-to-left shunts breathe 100 per cent O_2; breathing 100 per cent O_2 ultimately replaces all the N_2 with O_2 in ventilable units, leaving only O_2, CO_2, and H_2O in the alveoli. When this occurs,

$$P_{A_{O_2}} = P_{A_{TOTAL}} - P_{A_{CO_2}} - P_{A_{H_2O}}. \quad (3)$$

Because the total pressure and H_2O vapor pressure are the same in all communicating lung units, alveolar P_{O_2} differs from unit to unit only by corresponding differences in alveolar P_{CO_2}. Blood perfusing each unit equilibrates at a high alveolar P_{O_2} that in ideal lungs and lungs with a ventilation-perfusion abnormality is reflected by a high arterial P_{O_2} value. By this mechanism, the administration of 100 per cent O_2 is said to "correct" a ventilation-perfusion disturbance. This must be true if the lung units are ventilated at all, even though they may be ventilated extremely poorly through collateral pathways or only intermittently at high lung volumes when the subject takes a deep breath. When carrying out this study, therefore, it is obviously important to allow enough time and to insist that the subject occasionally take deep breaths to ensure complete N_2 washout and replacement by O_2.

Table 7–3 Effect of Breathing 21 Per Cent and 100 Per Cent O_2 on Mean P_{O_2} Values in Alveolar Gas and Arterial and Mixed Venous Blood in Two-compartment Lung Models with Ideal Gas Exchange (Fig. 7–1), a Ventilation-perfusion Abnormality (Fig. 7–4), and a Right-to-left Shunt (Fig. 7–7)

	IDEAL		VENTILATION-PERFUSION ABNORMALITY		RIGHT-TO-LEFT SHUNT	
	21%	100%	21%	100%	21%	100%
Mixed venous P_{O_2}	40	51	40	51	40	42
Alveolar P_{O_2}	101	673	106	675	114	677
Arterial P_{O_2}	101	673	89	673	59	125
Alveolar-arterial P_{O_2} difference	0	0	17	2	55	552

Alveoli in a lung with a right-to-left shunt also have their N_2 eliminated, and hence blood perfusing those units equilibrates at the elevated alveolar PO_2. The problem in oxygenation is not corrected, however, because mixed venous blood continues to flow through the shunt and mix with blood that has perfused normal units. The poorly oxygenated blood from the shunt lowers the PO_2 of the mixed effluent and perpetuates the alveolar-arterial PO_2 difference. An elevated alveolar-arterial PO_2 difference during a properly conducted 100 per cent O_2 study signifies the presence of a right-to-left shunt, and the magnitude of the difference between the PO_2 value obtained and the normal value can be used to quantify the proportion of cardiac output that is shunted by using the so-called "shunt equation":

$$\frac{\dot{Q}s}{\dot{Q}T} = \frac{Cc' - Ca}{Cc' - C\bar{v}} , \qquad (4)$$

where $\dot{Q}s/\dot{Q}T$ is venous admixture, which is solely due to shunting when 100 per cent O_2 is breathed, and Cc', Ca, and $C\bar{v}$ are the O_2 contents of end-capillary, arterial, and mixed venous bloods, respectively. The Cc' and Ca are derived from alveolar and arterial PO_2 values, which are used to compute dissolved O_2 and percent saturation, and the subject's hemoglobin concentration. Arterial PO_2 is measured directly, and alveolar PO_2 is computed, using Equation 1. Mixed venous O_2 content is measured directly, but if appropriate samples cannot be obtained, it is often estimated by assuming an arteriovenous O_2 difference (normally 4.5 to 5.0 ml/100 ml). In most circumstances, an alveolar-arterial PO_2 difference of 15 mm Hg while breathing 100 per cent O_2 indicates a right-to-left shunt of about 1 per cent of the cardiac output.

SITES OF RIGHT-TO-LEFT SHUNTING

When a normal young subject breathes 100 per cent O_2, an alveolar-arterial PO_2 difference of between 30 and 50 mm Hg can usually be detected; this demonstrates the presence of a right-to-left shunt of approximately 2 to 3 per cent of the cardiac output. Another method of quantifying the magnitude of right-to-left shunts involves the use of insoluble radioactive or other inert gases.[4-6] The results using these techniques differ slightly from those using the O_2 method because insoluble gases only identify shunts of blood from the systemic venous circulation through or around the lungs, whereas the O_2 method is sensitive to venous admixture anywhere proximal to the arterial sampling site. Several studies using insoluble gases have shown virtually no right-to-left shunt (i.e., < 1 per cent) through normal lungs (Figure 7-6); these results, when combined with those from studies of shunts with 100 per cent O_2 breathing, have indicated that most of the small shunt in normal subjects occurs distal to the gas exchange units.[4,6,7] Thus, the normal pathways are not around alveoli, as shown schematically in Figure 7-7, but occur after alveoli, the "*postpulmonary shunt*," as shown in Figure 7-8.

The chief sources of the normal postpulmonary shunt are the bronchial veins and veins from the mediastinum that empty into pulmonary veins and the thebesian vessels of the left ventricular myocardium that empty directly into the left ventricular cavity. However, the right-to-left shunt diagrammed in Figure 7-7 is not purely hypothetic but accurately depicts the pattern of blood flow for shunts in many pathologic conditions. It is important to emphasize that in some instances a discrete abnormal anatomic pathway (as shown) does exist (i.e., intracardiac communications, pulmonary arteriovenous fistulas), but in other instances shunts occur through normal vessels that perfuse regions of lung that are not ventilated at all because the alveoli are filled or closed or the airways leading to the terminal units are completely obstructed (i.e., pneumonia, pulmo-

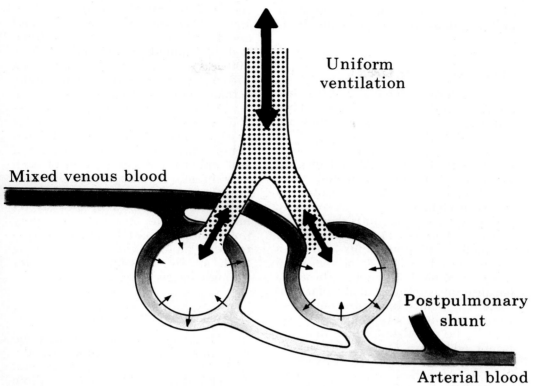

Figure 7–8 Schematic diagram showing the location of the right-to-left shunt present in normal persons. Instead of a pathway that bypasses alveoli (Figure 7–7), the postpulmonary shunt occurs from venous blood that mixes with arterialized blood in the pulmonary veins and left ventricular cavity. (Adapted from Comroe, Forster, Dubois, Briscoe, and Carlsen.[1] Reprinted by permission from the authors and Year Book Publisher, Inc.)

nary edema, atelectasis). When shunts occur in patients with pulmonary disease, they are usually accounted for by the perfusion of nonventilated lung through relatively normal vascular channels.

NORMAL ALVEOLAR-ARTERIAL OXYGEN DIFFERENCE

In healthy subjects 21 to 30 years of age at rest in the seated (slightly reclining) position, a mean alveolar-arterial PO_2 difference of 8 mm Hg was detected.[8] As indicated, the difference is due to the combined venous admixture effect from (1) mismatching of ventilation and perfusion and (2) right-to-left postpulmonary shunting of blood. Each of these mechanisms is responsible for about half of the total alveolar-arterial PO_2 difference in young adult persons. During senescence, the mean value for alveolar-arterial PO_2 difference increases to 16 mm Hg in normal persons 61 to 75 years of age[8]; this effect is mainly caused by increasing ventilation-perfusion inequalities (see Chapter 12 for details). It should be noted that *none* of the normal alveolar-arterial PO_2 difference is caused by failure of diffusion equilibrium to occur. As emphasized in Chapter 6, alveolar-arterial differences for O_2 from diffusion limitation do not develop in normal subjects except during heavy exercise while breathing air with a low

PO_2; this combination may occur at high altitudes or in experimental circumstances.

ALVEOLAR VENTILATION

The terms alveolar volume and alveolar ventilation are misnomers because the phenomena which they are supposed to designate take place in the entire terminal respiratory unit, i.e., alveoli, alveolar ducts, and respiratory bronchioles, not just alveoli. Alveolar volume is the total volume of gas in the gas exchange units at any moment, and alveolar ventilation is the amount of gas that moves into "functioning" terminal respiratory units during a given period. The use of the word functioning has important implications because measurement of alveolar ventilation depends upon the output of CO_2; a terminal respiratory unit may actually be ventilated, but if that unit is not taking up O_2 and eliminating CO_2 (e.g., a unit deprived of its blood flow), it is functionless, and the increment of fresh air it receives does not count as alveolar ventilation.

Alveolar volume is nearly the same as FRC in normal subjects in the recumbent position; the slight difference between measurements of the two variables is due to the *anatomic dead space* (i.e., the volume of the nasopharynx and conducting airways), which is included in most measurements of FRC. About 35 to 40 per cent of the total alveolar volume is contained in the respiratory bronchioles and alveolar ducts, and the remainder is within true alveoli.[9] This value and the fact that all the structures composing the terminal respiratory unit expand and contract proportionately during breathing[10] make possible an estimation of how each breath of fresh air is partitioned among the various anatomic units of the lung. Assuming that a normal adult person has an anatomic dead space of 150 ml and is breathing with a tidal volume of 500 ml, an inspirate is distributed as follows: 150 ml is required to fill the anatomic dead space; the respiratory bronchioles and alveolar ducts increase their volume and accommodate 175 ml (0.35 × 500 ml); and only the remaining 175 ml, or 35 per cent of the inspirate, actually penetrates as far as alveoli.

Although the estimate in the preceding paragraph is crude and is greatly affected by the rate and depth of breathing, it supports the conclusion that only a small proportion of each new breath reaches alveoli by bulk flow through the respiratory system. As indicated in Chapter 6, the gas remaining in the terminal respiratory units after the last breath mixes extremely rapidly with the incoming fresh air by diffusion of molecules through the gas phase.

"WASTED" VENTILATION

Alveolar ventilation cannot be measured directly but must be derived by subtracting the total amount of inspired gas that does not contribute to CO_2 removal, the *wasted ventilation*, from the total amount of gas inhaled through the nose or mouth, the *minute volume*. Wasted ventilation, also known as *physiologic dead space*, is considered to be that volume of each breath that is inhaled but does not reach functioning terminal respiratory units; in other words, the volume that is literally wasted insofar as its contribution to gas exchange is concerned. Wasted ventilation (V_D) is easily determined from the CO_2 pressures of simultaneously collected samples of expired air (PE_{CO_2}) and arterial blood (Pa_{CO_2}), using a modification of the Bohr equation that assumes that arterial PCO_2 is equal to alveolar PCO_2:

$$V_D = \frac{Pa_{CO_2} - PE_{CO_2}}{Pa_{CO_2}} V_E. \qquad (5)$$

Although the assumption of equality between arterial and alveolar PCO_2 is correct in the idealized lung, the two values differ slightly in healthy subjects and may differ considerably in patients with pulmonary disease. Moreover, the notion of wasted ventilation incorporates a drastic oversimplification of the physiologic events that contribute to the values obtained in the measurement. Conceptually, the lung is simply divided into two compartments: (1) an alveolar volume in which alveolar P_{CO_2} is everywhere equal to arterial P_{CO_2} and (2) a wasted ventilation volume in which there is no CO_2 whatsoever. Obviously, what actually occurs is that some terminal respiratory units are over- or underventilated relative to their blood flows; thus, their individual CO_2 outputs and end-capillary P_{CO_2} values vary a great deal. None of these individual variations can be detected by using Equa-

tion 5 because it treats the lung as consisting of only ideal alveoli and a homogeneous dead space.

Wasted ventilation, shown by the stippled regions in Figures 7–1, 7–2, 7–4, and 7–7, can be viewed as being composed of two compartments: (1) the anatomic dead space (defined earlier) and (2) the *alveolar dead space*. The latter volume is contributed to by all those terminal respiratory units that are overventilated relative to their perfusion.[12] As shown in Figure 7–9, wasted ventilation normally increases as end-inspiratory lung volume increases.[13] The observed change is primarily due to an enlargement of the anatomic dead space from the distension of airways that occurs as lung volume and transpulmonary pressure increase. Other changes in breathing

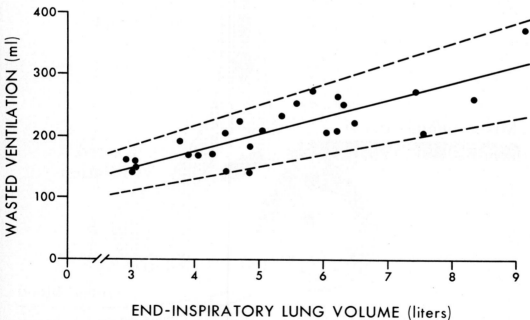

Figure 7–9 Relationship between wasted ventilation (physiologic dead space) and end-inspiratory lung volume in ten healthy young persons breathing with normal tidal volumes and respiratory frequencies. Each point represents a separate measurement. Solid line is the calculated regression line; the hatched lines were drawn by eye to define the "normal range." (Adapted from Lifshay, Fast, and Glazier.[13] Reprinted by permission from the authors and publisher.)

pattern, such as increasing rate and tidal volume, cause the alveolar dead space to increase.[13]

An increase in the alveolar component of wasted ventilation also occurs when regions of the lung are ventilated but unperfused (Figure 7–10). This combination develops in normal persons in the upright position, owing to the effects of gravity on the distribution of pulmonary blood flow, and in patients with pulmonary emboli or with diseases associated with occlusion of pulmonary arteries or capillaries. Alveolus B in Figure 7–10 is stippled to show that inspired air reaching it also contributes to wasted ventilation; gas exchange is obviously impossible because there is no blood supply to the unit. Despite the theoretic challenges about its derivation, wasted ventilation has proved to be one of the most sensitive studies for the physiologic diagnosis of pulmonary vascular disorders.[14]

Wasted ventilation and venous admixture are both commonly employed as indexes of the presence and severity of ventilation-perfusion abnormalities. However, it is important to recognize that the absolute values of both indexes can be shown to vary in the absence of *any* change in the distribution of ventilation and blood flow.[2] Figure 7–11 displays the results of computer analyses of a multicompartment lung model in which the amount of ventilation-perfusion ine-

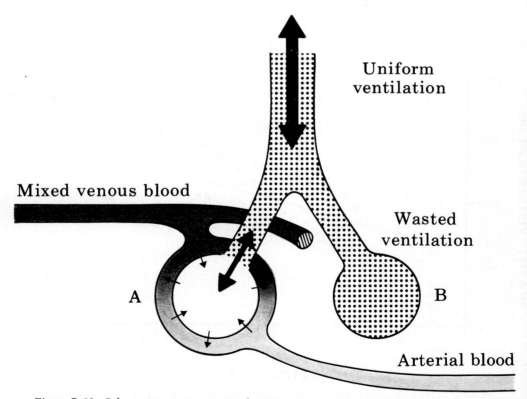

Figure 7–10 Schematic representation of a two-compartment model of the lung showing the effect of pulmonary arterial obstruction on wasted ventilation. When blood flow to Unit B ceases, any ventilation to the unit is wasted because it cannot contribute to gas exchange. Gas exchange in Unit A depends upon the amount of ventilation and blood flow to the unit. (Adapted from Comroe, Forster, Dubois, Briscoe, and Carlsen.[1] Reprinted by permission from the authors and Year Book Publisher, Inc.)

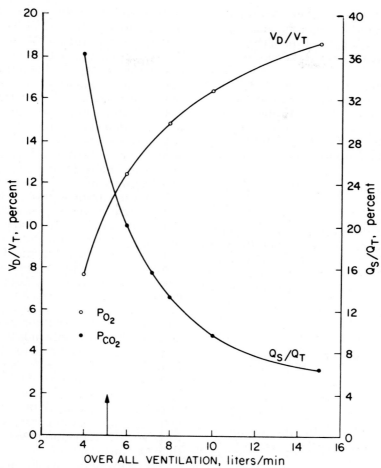

Figure 7–11 Effect of increasing over-all ventilation on alveolar dead space/tidal volume (V_D/V_T) and venous admixture (Q_S/Q_T)/from lung model experiments in which the amount of ventilation-perfusion inequality, O_2 uptake, and CO_2 output were held constant. Note the lack of sensitivity of the two commonly used indexes of ventilation-perfusion inequality when only ventilation is changed. (From West.[2] Reprinted by permission from the author and publisher.)

quality was held constant while ventilation was changed; under these conditions venous admixture ($\dot{Q}s/\dot{Q}T$) decreased and wasted ventilation (V_D/V_T) increased. An increase in total blood flow has opposite effects.[2]

OXYGEN TRANSPORT

DEFINITION AND DETERMINANTS

Oxygen must be continuously supplied to all cells of the body to enable them to carry out their normal metabolic activities; this is true regardless of the specialized function of different cell types, although some cells require more O_2 than others. Without O_2, a human being will lose consciousness in about 20 to 30 seconds and will die in a few minutes. The O_2 demands of a rigorous physical and metabolic existence are met by the integrated responses of the three components of the O_2 transport system: (1) the lungs, which transfer O_2 from environmental air into blood; (2) the heart and blood vessels, which circulate oxygenated blood throughout the body; and (3) the hemoglobin concentration of the blood and the affinity of hemoglobin for O_2.[15]

Systemic O_2 transport (SO_2T), or the amount of O_2 delivered to the tissues of the body per unit time, can be calculated from the cardiac output ($\dot{Q}$) and the arterial O_2 content (aO_2) according to the formula

$$SO_2T, \text{ml/min} = \dot{Q}, \text{L/min}, \times aO_2, \text{ml/L}. \tag{6}$$

Because the arterial O_2 content is determined by the concentration of hemoglobin available for combination with O_2 and the percent saturation of hemoglobin, Equation 6 can be rewritten as follows:

$$SO_2T = \dot{Q} \times (\text{hemoglobin concentration}$$
$$\times 1.34) \times \frac{\text{percent saturation}}{100} \tag{7}$$

or because percent saturation is a function (f) of PO_2 according to the relationship defined by the oxyhemoglobin dissociation curve,*

$$SO_2T = \underset{circulatory}{\dot{Q}} \times$$

$$\underset{erythropoietic}{(\text{hemoglobin concentration} \times 1.34)}$$

$$\times \underset{respiratory}{f(PO_2).} \tag{8}$$

The subtitles in Equation 8 identify the contributions to total O_2 transport of the three organ systems involved: the circulatory system determines cardiac output and peripheral blood flow, the erythropoietic system determines red blood cell mass and hemoglobin concentration, and the respiratory system determines PO_2. In a normal adult

---

*The affinity between O_2 and hemoglobin varies according to the influences discussed in Chapter 6.

at rest, substantially more O_2 is delivered to the tissues (1000 ml/min) than is used by them (250 ml/min). Although at first glance the difference between the O_2 supplied and the O_2 consumed may appear to be an unwarranted luxury, this is not true in the case of individual organs (e.g., the heart, which uses virtually all the O_2 it receives), and the excess provides some leeway during sudden emergencies when more O_2 is needed at once by certain tissues.

Oxygen transport is an important physiologic variable because it sets the upper limit for the quantity of O_2 available to meet the total metabolic needs of the body. Oxygen utilization cannot exceed the supply of O_2 for very long; if it does, the deprived cells must shift from aerobic to anaerobic metabolic pathways to supply their energy needs. One of the consequences of anaerobic metabolism is the production of excess lactic acid. If not relieved, progressive acidosis ultimately disrupts intracellular metabolism and causes cellular death. Under ordinary circumstances, except in severe exercise in which a temporary O_2 debt is tolerated, O_2 transport always is higher than O_2 consumption.

A narrowing of the margin between O_2 supply and demand can develop in several ways: if the demand increases, if the transport system itself is deficient, or both. Regardless of the cause, physiologic adjustments take place in an attempt to improve the balance between the amount of O_2 needed and that available.

ADAPTATIONS TO ACUTE OXYGEN DEMANDS

The numerous vicissitudes of daily life are usually associated with a transient need for more O_2. Undoubtedly, the most common demand for O_2 occurs during physical activity, but increased metabolism may also be induced by fever, food intake, and administration of many drugs. Sudden needs for O_2, as well as the ordinary demands of metabolism occasioned by meals and other factors, are met chiefly by changes in cardiac output. As noted previously, cardiac output may increase three to four times its resting value; therefore, O_2 transport, by this mechanism alone, may increase to 3000–4000 ml/min. In most normal persons, maximal O_2 utilization during exercise is limited ordinarily by maximal cardiac output (see Chapter 10).

Minute volume of ventilation increases during exercise and serves to maintain arterial Po_2 at or slightly above resting values. However, increasing ventilation does not add appreciably to arterial O_2 content owing to the ceiling imposed by the flat portion of the oxyhemoglobin equilibrium curve. Similarly, the slight improvement in ventilation-perfusion relationships that often occurs during exercise may raise arterial Po_2 a few mm Hg from its normal value at rest (about 95 mm Hg in a young healthy adult). However, inspection of the oxyhemoglobin dissociation curve (Figure 6–6) reveals that this change causes the saturation of hemoglobin to increase from 97.2 to 97.5 per cent, and therefore adds only a trivial increment of O_2 to the blood flowing through the lungs. Although the efficiency of gas exchange cannot augment the quantity of O_2 in the bloodstream during increased metabolic needs compared with resting conditions, it should be emphasized that alveolar ventilation must at least keep up with increases in pulmonary blood flow to prevent arterial hypoxia from developing.

A red blood cell lives for about 120 days,[16] and the turnover rate of erythrocytes is nearly 1.0 per cent of the circulating red blood cell mass per day.[15] Accordingly, it is impossible for even a marked acute increase (e.g., doubling or tripling) in red blood cell production to affect noticeably the circulating hemoglobin concentration. However, the hematocrit ratio and the hemoglobin concentration rise slightly in healthy subjects during severe exercise owing to a reduction in circulating plasma volume through extravasation of fluid. In an animal with a large spleen, such as a dog, the release into the circulation of red blood cells that normally are sequestered in the spleen also contributes to a rise in hemoglobin concentration.[17]

The extracellular metabolic acidosis that accompanies heavy exertion presumably also includes an increase in intracellular $[H^+]$; this serves to decrease affinity of hemoglobin for O_2 and, in effect, to increase O_2 transport because the change causes more O_2 to be released to the peripheral tissues. Additional mechanisms by which O_2 transport is increased during exercise are considered in detail in Chapter 10.

ADAPTATIONS TO CHRONIC OXYGEN DEMANDS

Sustained demands for O_2 considerably in excess of ordinary metabolic needs are seldom encountered in normal subjects. However, increased O_2 consumption is a characteristic feature of certain pathologic conditions: thyrotoxicosis, acromegaly, pheochromocytoma, some malignancies, and (probably) Cushing's syndrome.[18] With excesses of thyroid and growth hormones, O_2 supply is increased above normal levels by a combination of mechanisms: an increase in cardiac output and an increase in red blood cell mass. The latter effect is not always evident as a rise in hemoglobin concentration because plasma volume may also increase. (The reason for this paradoxic response of eliminating the beneficial effect of a change in red blood cell mass alone is not well understood; it presumably demonstrates dominance of volume and circulatory compensatory needs over compensation by raising hemoglobin concentration.) An increase in red blood cell DPG has been documented in patients with thyrotoxicosis, but the change is believed to be mediated by a specific effect of the excess thyroid hormone on glycolysis, rather than a response to "relative" hypoxia.[19] Adaptation mechanisms in other hypermetabolic disorders have not been well delineated and whether or not changes in O_2 affinity occur needs to be examined. For the reasons discussed in the previous section, increases in ventilation keep pace with increases in cardiac output but do not add "extra" O_2 to the bloodstream.

ADAPTATIONS TO DEFICIENCIES OF OXYGEN TRANSPORT

Changes may occur in the circulatory, erythropoietic, and respiratory systems that seriously compromise the over-all O_2 transport capabilities. When acute disturbances occur, especially in the cardiovascular system, the body is virtually defenseless, except for shifts in oxyhemoglobin affinity and in redistribution of blood flow to the heart and brain at the expense of perfusion to other organs. Compensation for decreases in O_2 transport is far more adequate in chronic than in acute disorders and in some instances restores delivery to normal. The main mechanisms of adaptation are through an increase in red blood cell mass (*polycythemia*) and a shift in the oxyhemoglobin dissociation curve.

Chronic Circulatory Failure. Oxygen delivery is obviously reduced in conditions in which cardiac output is low. Although an increased red blood cell mass can be demonstrated in chronic disorders, hemoglobin concentration is seldom substantially elevated.[18] The main mechanism of compensation appears to be through a decrease in O_2 affinity caused by an increase in red blood cell DPG concentration. The relationship between the levels of intraerythrocyte DPG and the mixed venous blood O_2 saturation

was described earlier (Chapter 6); it was demonstrated (Figure 6–8) that DPG increased as the circulatory abnormalities, reflected by a reduction in mixed venous blood O_2 saturation, became more severe.[20]

Disturbances of Erythropoiesis. There is an optimum concentration of circulating red blood cells, conveniently measured as the hematocrit ratio, at which systemic O_2 transport is maximum, and not surprisingly, this occurs at the usual hematocrit levels found in the bloodstream of normal subjects (40 to 50 per cent). The relationship between acute changes of hematocrit values and O_2 transport in experimental animals is shown in Figure 7–12; also depicted is the effect of changing hematocrit on the animals' cardiac output.[21] As the hematocrit, and hence hemoglobin, concentration decreases from the normal levels of 45 per cent and 15 gm/100 ml, respectively, cardiac output increases; however, the increase in flow is insufficient to compensate for the reduction in hemoglobin concentration and O_2-carrying capacity, and so O_2 transport decreases. When the hematocrit is increased above about 55 per cent, the effect of viscosity causes a decrease in cardiac output that more than offsets the gain in O_2 capacity of the blood; this combination also leads to a decrease in O_2 transport. The effect of an increase in total circulating blood volume is also demonstrated in Figure 7–12: at any given hematocrit, O_2 transport and cardiac output are always higher when blood volume is expanded than when it is normal.[21] Although comparable experiments have not been performed in man, it is likely that reductions in blood volume account for the failure to demonstrate hemodynamic changes from phlebotomy in patients with polycythemia secondary to arterial hypoxia.[22]

In patients with anemia, regardless of etiology, changes in both cardiac output and O_2 affinity attempt to restore O_2 delivery to normal. With

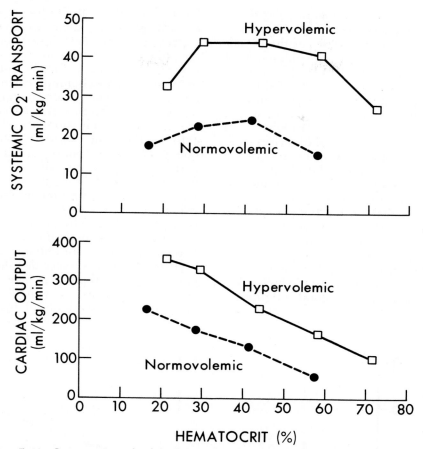

Figure 7–12 Composite graph of the effects of changes in hematocrit ratio on mean values of cardiac output and systemic O_2 transport. Results from experiments in dogs in which blood volume was held constant (normovolemic) or increased (hypervolemic). (Adapted from Murray, Gold, and Johnson.[21] Reprinted by permission from the publisher.)

moderate anemia, an increase in red blood cell DPG with an accompanying decrease in O_2 affinity is the major compensatory mechanism; as anemia increases in severity, cardiovascular adjustments become superimposed upon further decreases in O_2 affinity, and O_2 transport during moderately heavy exercise is surprisingly well maintained.[23]

Most patients with abnormal hemoglobin that is associated with either a high or a low O_2 affinity have normal O_2 transport.[24] Patients whose hemoglobin is characterized by decreased affinity are anemic, and conversely, patients whose hemoglobin reveals increased affinity are polycythemic. In both cases, tissue O_2, an important regulator of red blood cell production (see below), is virtually normal. Customarily, these patients do not have symptoms related to their hematologic disturbances, although defects in O_2 delivery might be demonstrable upon maximal stress.[24]

Arterial Hypoxia. Chronic arterial hypoxia occurs in normal residents of high altitudes who breathe air that has a lower PO_2 than air at sea level. One of the main defenses to high altitude hypoxia is an increase in the O_2-carrying capacity of the bloodstream through the development of polycythemia; moreover, the magnitude of this response is related to the severity of the hypoxia, and thus is determined by the altitude at which the subject resides.[25] Figure 7–13 demonstrates the relationship between red blood cell mass and arterial O_2 saturation compiled from studies of healthy subjects living at varying altitudes[25-29] and recalculated with appropriate corrections for trapped plasma and total body hematocrit.[30] The changes in circulating red blood cell mass induced by arterial hypoxia are a straightforward demonstration of the regulatory system through which available O_2 controls red blood cell production. The O_2-sensitive receptors are located mainly in the kidneys and, although there is some evidence to suggest that the juxtaglomerular cells are involved in the response, the exact cellular site(s) for the detection of hypoxia and elaboration of the regulating hormone, *erythropoietin*, is unknown; the hormone, in turn, leads to increased production of red blood cells by the bone marrow.[31] The adequacy of the response depends, in part, upon the availability of Fe for the synthesis of hemoglobin. An increase in circulating hemoglobin concentration means that more O_2 is carried in the bloodstream at the same PO_2, so that the receptors are "satisfied" and stop producing excess erythropoietin. It is clear that the presence of polycythemia is one of the chief mechanisms by which natives and long-term residents of high alti-

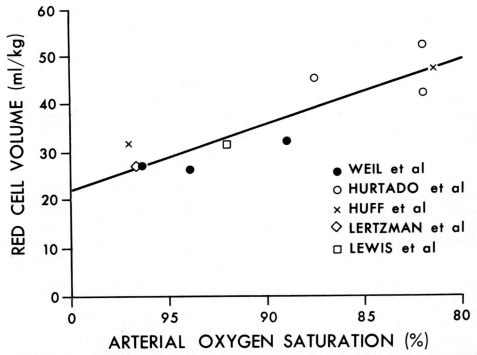

Figure 7–13 Composite graph showing results from several published studies of red cell volume and arterial oxygen saturation in normal acclimatized subjects living at various altitudes. The solid line is the regression line. The effect of hypoxia from residence at altitude is to increase red cell volume. (Adapted from Murray.[30] Reprinted by permission from the publisher.)

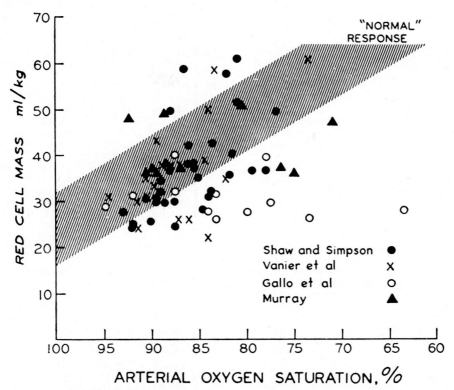

Figure 7–14 Composite graph showing results from several published studies of red cell mass (volume) and arterial oxygen saturation in patients with pulmonary disease. The shaded area delineates the normal range (mean ± two standard deviations) obtained by analysis of data in Figure 7–13. (From Murray.[18] Reprinted by permission from the publisher.)

tude maintain O_2 transport at rest and during exercise despite severe arterial hypoxia.[32] A decrease in O_2 affinity through an increase in red blood cell DPG also occurs at high altitude; however, the contribution of this mechanism is limited because when alveolar PO_2 is low, O_2 loading may be impaired as much as O_2 release is enhanced.[23]

Arterial hypoxia is a commonly seen consequence of many pulmonary diseases, but both the polycythemic and the DPG responses of patients are often substantially less evident than they are in healthy subjects living at high altitudes with the same degree of hypoxia. The poor relationship between red blood cell mass and percent arterial O_2 saturation, using data collected from several studies, is shown in Figure 7–14[18,34-36]; the wide scatter of the results is obvious, as is the fact that most of the points lie below the normal range. No one knows why erythropoietic compensation in patients with hypoxia caused by pulmonary disease fails to be as good in restoring O_2 delivery as that in normal subjects at high altitudes. It may be either the effect of the disease itself on the bone marrow and/or red blood cell metabolism or a variety of secondary influences that impair normal responses. Clearly, these processes need to be explored further to provide more understanding than is currently available about an important aspect in the pathophysiology of pulmonary disease.

REFERENCES

1. Comroe, J. H., Jr., Forster, R. E., II, Dubois, A. B., Briscoe, W. A., and Carlsen, E.: The Lung. Clinical Physiology and Pulmonary Function Tests. 2nd Ed. Chicago, Year Book Medical Publishers, Inc., 1962, pp. 1-390.
2. West, J. B.: Ventilation-perfusion inequality and overall gas exchange in computer models of the lung. Resp. Physiol., 7:88-110, 1969.
3. West, J. B.: Causes of carbon dioxide retention in lung disease. New Eng. J. Med., 284:1232-1236, 1971.
4. Wagner, P. D., Laravuso, R. B., Uhl, R. R., and West, J. B.: Continuous distributions of ventilation-perfusion ratios in normal subjects breathing air and 100% O_2. J. Clin. Invest., 54:54-68, 1974.
5. Fritts, H. W., Jr., Hardewig, A., Rochester, D. F., Durand, J., and Cournand, A.: Estimation of pulmonary arteriovenous shunt-flow using intravenous injections of T-1824 dye and Kr^{85}. J. Clin. Invest., 39:1841-1850, 1960.
6. Mellemgaard, K., Lassen, N. A., and Georg, J.: Right-to-left shunt in normal man determined by the use of tritium and krypton 85. J. Appl. Physiol., 17:778-782, 1962.
7. Davidson, F. F., Glazier, J. B., and Murray, J. F.: The components of the alveolar-arterial oxygen tension difference in normal subjects and in patients with pneumonia and obstructive lung disease. Am. J. Med. 52:754-762, 1972.
8. Mellemgaard, K.: The alveolar-arterial oxygen difference: its size and components in normal man. Acta Physiol. Scand., 67:10-20, 1966.
9. Weibel, E. R., and Gomez, D. M.: Architecture of the human lung. Use of quantitative methods establishes fundamental relations between size and number of lung structures. Science, 137:577-585, 1962.
10. Klingele, T. G., and Staub, N. C.: Alveolar shape changes with volume in isolated, air-filled lobes of cat lung. J. Appl. Physiol., 28:411-414, 1970.
11. Bouhuys, A.: Respiratory dead space. In Fenn, W. O., and Rahn, H. (eds.): Handbook of Physiology, Section 3. Respiration. Vol. I. Washington, D. C., American Physiological Society, 1964, pp. 699-714.
12. Severinghaus, J. W., and Stupfel, M.: Alveolar dead space as an index of distribution of blood flow in pulmonary capillaries. J. Appl. Physiol., 10:335-348, 1957.
13. Lifshay, A., Fast, C. W., and Glazier, J. B.: Effects of changes in respiratory pattern on physiological dead space. J. Appl. Physiol., 31:478-483, 1971.
14. Nadel, J. A., Gold, W. M., and Burgess, J. H.: Early diagnosis of chronic pulmonary vascular obstruction. Value of pulmonary function tests. Am. J. Med., 44:16-25,1968.
15. Finch, C. A., and Lenfant, C.: Oxygen transport in man. New Eng. J. Med., 286:407-415, 1972.
16. Berlin, N. I., Waldmann, T. A., and Weissman, S. M.: Life span of the red blood cell. Physiol. Rev., 39:577-616, 1959.
17. Gold, P. M., and Murray, J. F.: Changes in red cell distribution, hemodynamics, and blood volume in acute anemia. J. Appl. Physiol., 26:589-593, 1969.
18. Murray, J. F.: Classification of polycythemic disorders. With comments on the diagnostic value of arterial blood oxygen analysis. Ann. Intern. Med., 64:892-902, 1966.
19. Snyder, L. M., and Reddy, W. J.: Mechanism of action of thyroid hormones on erythrocyte 2,3-diphosphoglyceric acid synthesis. J. Clin. Invest., 49:1993-1998, 1970.
20. Woodson, R. D., Torrance, J. D., Shappell, S. D., and Lenfant, C.: The effect of cardiac disease on hemoglobin-oxygen binding. J. Clin. Invest., 49:1349-1356, 1970.
21. Murray, J. F., Gold, P., and Johnson, B. L., Jr.: The circulatory effects of hematocrit variations in normovolemic and hypervolemic dogs. J. Clin. Invest., 42:1150-1159, 1963.
22. Segel, N., and Bishop, J. M.: The circulation in patients with chronic bronchitis and emphysema at rest and during exercise, with special reference to the influence of changes in blood viscosity and blood volume on the pulmonary circulation. J. Clin. Invest., 45:1555-1568, 1966.
23. Sproule, B. J., Mitchell, J. H., and Miller, W. F.: Cardiopulmonary physiological responses to heavy exercise in patients with anemia. J. Clin. Invest., 39:378-388, 1960.
24. Stamatoyannopoulos, G., Bellingham, A. J., Lenfant, C., and Finch, C. A.: Abnormal hemoglobins with high and low oxygen affinity. Ann. Rev. Med., 22:221-234, 1971.
25. Weil, J. V., Jamieson, G., Brown, D. W., and Grover, R. F.: The red cell mass-arterial oxygen relationship in normal man. Application to patients with chronic obstructive airway disease. J. Clin. Invest., 47:1627-1639, 1968.
26. Hurtado, A., Merino, C., and Delgado, E.: Influence of anoxemia on the hemopoietic activity. Arch. Intern. Med., 75: 284-323, 1945.
27. Huff, R. L., Lawrence, J. H., Siri, W. E., Wasserman, L. R., and Hennessy, T. G.: Effects of changes in altitude on hematopoietic activity. Medicine, 30:197-217, 1951.
28. Lewis, C. S., Jr., Samuels, A. J., Daines, M. C., and Hecht, H. H.: Chronic lung disease, polycythemia and congestive heart failure. Cardiorespiratory, vascular and

renal adjustments in cor pulmonale. Circulation, 6:874-887, 1952.

29. Lertzman, M., Frome, B. M., Israels, L. G., and Cherniack, R. M.: Hypoxia in polycythemia vera. Ann. Intern. Med., 60:409-417, 1964.

30. Murray, J. F.: Arterial studies in primary and secondary polycythemic disorders. Am. Rev. Resp. Dis., 92:435-449, 1965.

31. Krantz, S. B., and Jacobson, L. O.: Erythropoietin and the Regulation of Erythropoiesis. Chicago, University of Chicago Press, 1970, pp. 25-46.

32. Lenfant, C., and Sullivan, K.: Adaptation to high altitude. New Eng. J. Med., 284:1298-1309, 1971.

33. Lenfant, C., Torrance, J. D., and Reynafarje, C.: Shift of the O_2-Hb dissociation curve at altitude: mechanism and effect. J. Appl. Physiol., 30:625-631, 1971.

34. Shaw, D. B., and Simpson, T.: Polycythaemia in emphysema. Quart. J. Med., 30:135-152, 1961.

35. Vanier, T., Dulfano, M. J., Wu, C., and Desforges, J. F.: Emphysema, hypoxia and the polycythemic response. New Eng. J. Med., 269:169-178, 1963.

36. Gallo, R. C., Fraimow, W., Cathcart, R. T., and Erslev, A. J.: Erythropoietic response in chronic pulmonary disease. Arch. Intern. Med., 113:559-568, 1964.

Chapter Eight

ACID-BASE EQUILIBRIUM

INTRODUCTION

Acid-base equilibrium was once an esoteric topic reserved for the laboratory specialist. Now, however, it is widely recognized that acid-base disorders are an important component of the physiologic disturbances associated with numerous common diseases. Furthermore, rapid and accurate instruments for the measurement of pH and related variables are available in most hospitals and are being increasingly utilized for the determination of the presence and severity of acid-base abnormalities. Therefore, the subject has assumed great practical significance.

Despite the importance of understanding the concepts and the mechanisms that regulate acid-base balance, most physicians have at best a superficial "working" knowledge of the fac-

199

tors that contribute to acid-base equilibrium in health and disease. Part of the difficulty in mastering the subject lies in its inherent complexity, although it is no more confusing than other more readily assimilated topics. Another, perhaps greater, source of mystery stems from the puzzling terminology used to describe the pathophysiology of acid-base disorders; the clinical terms are vague and ambiguous, and the more precise chemical terms bewilder because they originate in the unfamiliar language of thermodynamics and are usually "explained" by frightening equations. These pitfalls are for the most part unnecessary and avoidable.

Maintenance of acid-base equilibrium is considered in this book on the normal structure and function of the lung for two reasons. First, the lungs are the chief organ for the elimination of CO_2 and hence govern the amounts of H_2CO_3 in the body. Second, changes in both Pco_2 and acid-base equilibrium exert a profound effect on the control of breathing; this interrelationship, which is considered in greater detail in Chapter 9, provides a physiologic safeguard against acid-

base imbalances, which would be more severe in the absence of changes in ventilation. This chapter examines the main variables that contribute to acid-base equilibrium and how the system responds to changes.

DEFINITIONS

ACIDS

An acid is a proton or an H^+ donor. A fundamental property of an acid (HB) is that it dissociates wholly or partly into its component ions, so that

$$HB = H^+ + B^-, \qquad (1)$$

where B^- is the conjugate base of the acid (described later).

The strength of an acid is determined by the degree to which it dissociates in solution. Correspondingly, the acidity or pH depends upon the concentration of active H^+ in a given amount of solution. The conventional symbols of H, H^+, $[H^+]$, HB, B^-, and pH are defined in Table 8–1; these definitions are used throughout this chapter and the remainder of the text.

Table 8–1   Definition of the Common Symbols Used to Describe the Properties of Acids and Bases in Physiologic Solutions*

SYMBOL	DESIGNATION	DEFINITION
H	Hydrogen	An atom of H existing in a combined state
H^+	Hydrogen ion Proton	The free and chemically active ionization product of H
$[H^+]$	Hydrogen ion concentration	The molar concentration of H^+ in a solution
HB	Acid	General designation of the chemical combination of H and its conjugate base
B^-	Conjugate base (general) H^+ acceptor Proton acceptor	General designation of the base paired with a given acid after ionization
pH	Intensity factor	Measurement of activity of $[H^+]$

*Further explanations are provided in the text.

Table 8–2   Comparison of the Chemical Properties of 0.1 N Solutions of a Strong
Acid and a Weak Acid

ACID	DISSOCIATION CONSTANT (UNITS)	IONIZED H$^+$ (mEq/L)	pH (UNITS)	TOTAL H° (mEq/L)
Strong				
Hydrochloric acid	∞	0.1	1	0.1
Weak				
Acetic acid	1.8×10^{-5}	0.0013	2.9	0.1

°Titratable acidity to pH 7.0

Because a strong acid dissociates into its component ions considerably more than a weak one, a solution of a strong acid has more free H$^+$ available for immediate chemical reactions than a solution of a weak acid. But it is important to realize that if the concentrations of the two solutions (expressed as their normality) are equal, they have exactly the same *total* number of H atoms in the mixture. Thus, the principal difference between the two kinds of acids is that H is ionized and "freed" for possible reactions in the strong acid but combined and unreactive (until ionized) in the weak acid.

A distinction must be made, therefore, between the ionic and combined forms of H that determine, respectively, the *intensity* with which the H in the solution will react and the *total quantity* of H available in the mixture.[1] The intensity factor, also called the "actual acidity," is the concentration of active H$^+$ in solution, or [H$^+$], and is measured as pH. The quantity factor, also called the "titratable acidity," is the amount of H$^+$ in solution *plus* the H available for ionization and is measured by titration against a base.[2] The different chemical properties of a representative strong acid and weak acid are shown in Table 8–2.

The acids present in biologic solutions behave the same as those in test tubes, and it is of considerable significance that most of the acids normally present in the body are weak acids. This implies that there is a great deal of combined H in body liquids but little free H$^+$.

BASES

A base is a proton-binder, or H$^+$ acceptor. There are strong and weak bases, depending on how much H$^+$ the base will bind; the stronger the base, the greater the affinity for H$^+$. As noted in Equation 1, to describe an acid (HB) and its ionization products H$^+$ and B$^-$, the B$^-$ moiety is known as the *conjugate base* of that acid. Weak acids have strong conjugate bases that bind most of the available H so that little is in the free ionized form. This condition exists in most of the acid-base pairs of the body and is one of the reasons why the pH of intracellular and extracellular liquids is nearly neutral.

pH

The term pH was introduced by Sörensen[3] in 1909 as a convenient means of describing certain properties of chemical solutions. Although the modern definition has changed since Sörensen's time, the distinction he made between H$^+$ activity and the total quantity of available H is physiologically meaningful. Within well-defined chemical limitations, pH is the negative logarithm of H$^+$ activity (aH$^+$):

$$pH = -\log (aH^+). \qquad (2)$$

Equation 2 adds a new constraint to the measurement of acidity: not only is the number of H$^+$ ions important but so is the designation of their chemical activity. Because the activity may vary under certain conditions, the relationship is expressed as

$$aH^+ = \gamma H^+[H^+], \qquad (3)$$

where γH^+ is the activity coefficient and $[H^+]$ is the molar concentration of H.

A few years ago, the physiologic utility of pH was questioned, and proposals were made to substitute $[H^+]$, derived from pH using Equations 2 and 3, and to ignore the activity coefficient. These efforts resulted in a controversy over the relative usefulness of pH vs. $[H^+]$ to quantify the acidity of biologic systems.[4] The chief argument for $[H^+]$ was that it is an arithmetic function and, therefore, easier to deal with than a negative logarithm. However, of overriding importance is the fact that the behavior of a substance in a chemical system is proportional to its energy (chemical potential), and this, in turn, is a logarithmic function of the activity of the substance. A pH electrode responds to the chemical potential of H^+, and thus the instrument provides a precise and readily obtained measurement of the chemical behavior of H^+ in the system.[4] This information is precisely what the clinician, physiologist, and chemist need to know. Moreover, other substances can be shown to behave physiologically in logarithmic relationships to their activities, and as pointed out in Chapter 7, a logarithmic distribution seems to be the best method for describing the distributions of ventilation and perfusion in normal lungs (Figure 7–6). Nature may not recognize a logarithm but certainly seems to respond in a manner that is accurately defined by logarithmic functions.

BUFFER SOLUTION

A buffer solution is a mixture of substances, usually a weak acid with its salt of a strong base, that resists a change in $[H^+]$, and therefore in pH.[2] When a strong acid or base is added to a solution containing a buffer, the change in pH is minimized compared with that which would occur if the buffer were not present. The buffers present in body liquids are extremely important because they serve to maintain pH within the fairly narrow limits required by most cells to function normally.

The action of a buffer may be illustrated by showing what happens when a strong acid (e.g., HCl) or strong base (e.g., NaOH) is added to a buffer of the usual variety, consisting of a mixture of a weak acid (e.g., H_2CO_3) and its salt with a strong base (e.g., $NaHCO_3$). The buffer mixture would be as follows:

$$Na^+ + HCO_3^- + H_2CO_3 \rightleftharpoons Na^+ +$$

$$H^+ + 2HCO_3^- + \text{some } H_2CO_3. \quad (4)$$

When a strong acid (HCl) is added, the H^+ reacts with HCO_3^- in the buffer mixture:

$$H^+ + HCO_3^- \longrightarrow H_2CO_3. \quad (5)$$

Equation 5 shows that the reaction product from the addition of H^+ to the buffer mixture is a weak acid (H_2CO_3). In other words, the strong acid is converted to an equivalent concentration of a weak one. In the process, free H^+ is "mopped up" as it is added to the buffer mixture, and the resulting change in pH is minimal. When a strong base (NaOH) is added,

$$H^+ + OH^- \longrightarrow H_2O. \quad (6)$$

Equation 6 shows that the product of the addition of OH^- to the buffer mixture is H_2O. Thus OH^- is mopped up by H^+ and converted to harmless H_2O in the process.

BLOOD BUFFERS

The amount of change in the pH of blood during a given acute alteration in acid-base equilibrium depends upon the buffering capacity of the blood. Furthermore, as implied in the general discussion of buffer solutions, large quantities of acid or base may be added to the body without producing a life-threatening alteration in pH. It is important to understand how pH is stabilized, not only to appreciate how the process operates but also to be able to identify the presence of different kinds of abnormalities and to measure their severity.

The body has several buffer systems within its extracellular and intracellular liquids. Although the extent to which each buffer contributes to the defense of body pH varies with differing kinds of acid-base disturbances (see subsequent sections), the chief buffering systems in approximate order of their importance are (1) HCO_3^- in plasma, interstitial, and intracellular water, (2) intracellular protein, (3) intraerythrocyte hemoglobin, (4) plasma proteins, and (5) bone carbonate, collagen, and other body solids.

The HCO_3^- system heads the list because HCO_3^- is present in appreciable quantities in nearly all body liquids and is readily available to stabilize pH. This huge reservoir of HCO_3^- has aptly been named the "alkali reserve" of the body to signify its role in the maintenance of pH.

Bicarbonate differs from other body buffers in that the product of its reaction with H^+ is a *volatile acid,* H_2CO_3. A volatile acid can be excreted in the gas with which it is in equilibrium, in this case CO_2; thus, H_2CO_3 can be viewed as having an "escaping tendency" because CO_2 leaves the body through the lungs.[1] These processes can be expressed by the following equation:

$$H^+ + HCO_3^- \longrightarrow H_2CO_3 \xrightarrow{\text{CA}}$$

$$H_2O + CO_2 \uparrow , \tag{7}$$

where CA indicates carbonic anhydrase, and $\uparrow$ indicates that CO_2 is eliminated by the lungs.

Equations 5 to 7 can be used to describe the changes in HCO_3^- levels, particularly plasma HCO_3^- (symbolized as $[HCO_3^-]$), when nonvolatile (sometimes called fixed) acids or bases are added to the body.* In general, the addition of nonvolatile acids lowers $[HCO_3^-]$, and the addition of bases raises $[HCO_3^-]$; moreover, the severity of the acid-base derangement is reflected in the amount by which $[HCO_3^-]$ deviates from normal values. The chief pathways of production and disposal of CO_2, H^+, and HCO_3^- are shown schematically in Figure 8–1.

TYPES OF ACID-BASE DISORDERS

Acid-base disturbances are traditionally differentiated into those of respiratory origin and those of nonrespiratory (metabolic) origin. These two types of disorders are fundamentally different but frequently coexist. As a result, three variables (directly measured or derived) are required to describe the conditions and how they interact: arterial P_{CO_2} defines the respiratory component; $[HCO_3^-]$, buffer base, or base excess defines the nonrespiratory component; and pH assesses the net result of the combined effects of respiratory and nonrespiratory disorders on acid-base equilibrium.[6]

Respiratory Origin. Respiratory acid-base disorders occur when the primary cause is excessive retention or elimination of P_{CO_2}. As emphasized in Chapter 6, arterial P_{CO_2} is determined by the relationship between CO_2 production ($\dot{V}_{CO_2}$) and alveolar ventilation ($\dot{V}_A$) so that

$$Pa_{CO_2} = K \frac{\dot{V}_{CO_2}}{\dot{V}_A}. \tag{8}$$

Hyperventilation and *hypoventilation* are defined as an excess or de-

*It is important to specify nonvolatile acids in contrast to volatile (i.e., H_2CO_3) acids because, as will be shown, the addition and removal of these two types of acids have opposite effects on $[HCO_3^-]$.

SOURCES

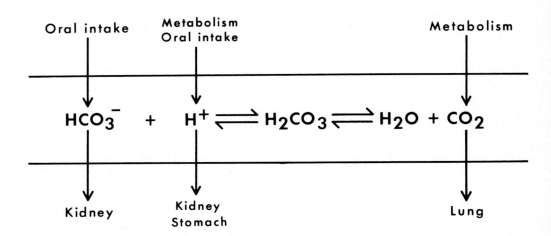

REMOVAL PATHWAYS

Figure 8–1   Schematic representation of the chief sources and removal pathways of H^+, HCO_3^-, and CO_2.

ficiency, respectively, of alveolar ventilation in relation to metabolism; according to Equation 8, therefore, arterial blood Pco_2 must increase during hypoventilation and decrease during hyperventilation. *Hyperpnea* means increased breathing that may or may not be related to metabolism, and hence the term carries no implication about Pco_2. The presence and magnitude of a respiratory acid-base imbalance can be simply recognized and quantified by measuring arterial Pco_2. The level of Pco_2 is important because it directly determines the concentration of H_2CO_3 present in the blood according to the following relationship:

$$H_2CO_3 = Pco_2 \times 0.0301, \qquad (9)$$

where H_2CO_3 is in mM/L or mEq/L, Pco_2 is in mm Hg, and 0.0301 is the solubility coefficient (α) of CO_2 in plasma at body temperature (37° C). Although H_2CO_3 is a weak acid, it dis-

sociates to a limited extent and produces H^+ and HCO_3^- as follows:

$$H_2CO_3 \rightleftharpoons H^+ + HCO_3^-. \qquad (10)$$

This reaction is an important one, not only because it provides HCO_3^- for buffering and other chemical reactions but also because it shows that respiratory disturbances *per se*, by changing the amount of H_2CO_3 in the bloodstream, also change the level of $[HCO_3^-]$.

Nonrespiratory (Metabolic) [*] *Origin.* Nonrespiratory acid-base disorders occur when the primary cause is excessive retention or elimination of nonvolatile acid or base by the body.

---

[*] "Metabolic" is a poor term to describe all nonrespiratory causes of acid-base disturbances; for example, excessive administration of acid or alkali affects acid-base equilibrium but has nothing to do with "metabolism." The designation "nonrespiratory" will be used throughout.

The definition is straightforward, but in contrast to respiratory acid-base derangements, which are readily recognized and quantified by changes in arterial P_{CO_2}, identification of the kind and severity of a nonrespiratory disturbance is more complex. As mentioned previously in the discussion of blood buffers, $[HCO_3^-]$ must decrease or increase when nonvolatile acids or bases (respectively) are added to the body, and therefore changes in $[HCO_3^-]$ serve as a useful guide to the presence or absence of nonrespiratory acid-base disorders. However, the level of $[HCO_3^-]$ fails to be a completely satisfactory indicator of these conditions for two reasons: (1) other buffers of the body, though quantitatively less important than HCO_3^-, are variably involved in the defense of pH, and so the effect of adding nonvolatile acid or base is not reflected solely in the HCO_3^- system, and (2) nonrespiratory acid-base disorders frequently cause ventilation to increase or decrease, which, as just discussed (Equations 9 and 10), changes P_{CO_2} and H_2CO_3 and, therefore, the level of $[HCO_3^-]$. (For example, if nonvolatile acid is added to the body, it "consumes" HCO_3^-; it also stimulates ventilation, which by lowering P_{CO_2} has the added effect of further reducing $[HCO_3^-]$.)

These factors have led to attempts to derive a variable that would reflect the impact of a nonrespiratory disorder on all the buffering systems of the body and would also correct for the influence of any secondary changes on HCO_3^- from the respiratory effects of the primary disturbance; in other words, it would be a "pure" indicator of the nonrespiratory component of an acid-base derangement. The most commonly used indexes and their normal values are listed in Table 8–3.

Plasma Carbon Dioxide Content. The plasma CO_2 content, in mEq/L or mM/L, is the total amount of CO_2 that can be evolved from the plasma of a blood specimen that has been col-

Table 8–3 Commonly Used Indexes of the Metabolic (Nonrespiratory) Component of Acid-base Disorders and Their Normal Values in Arterial Blood

INDEX	NORMAL VALUES (mEq/L)	
	MEAN	RANGE
Plasma CO_2 content	25	25–29
Plasma HCO_3^-	24	20–28
Standard HCO_3^-	23	21–25
Buffer base	50	45–55
Base excess	0	−2.3–2.3

lected and centrifuged under anaerobic conditions.[7] Because the volatile H_2CO_3 has been retained, the total plasma CO_2 content ([total CO_2]) consists of

$$[Total\ CO_2] = [HCO_3^-] + [H_2CO_3], \quad (11)$$

or substituting from Equation 9,

$$[Total\ CO_2] = [HCO_3^-] + [PCO_2 \times 0.0301]. \quad (12)$$

A derivative measurement, which is now of historical interest only, is the CO_2-combining power.[8] If a blood specimen is not obtained and processed anaerobically, the volatile H_2CO_3 will escape; however, the plasma can be approximately "arterialized" in the laboratory by equilibrating it with 5.5 per cent CO_2 so that the P_{CO_2} is raised to about 40 mm Hg. The CO_2-combining power differs from the total plasma CO_2 content not only if the patient's P_{CO_2} differs from that which is artificially restored in the laboratory, but also because of differences between *in vivo* and *in vitro* buffering capabilities of blood.

Plasma Bicarbonate Ion Content. The actual level of $[HCO_3^-]$, also expressed in mEq/L or mM/L, can be either determined by direct measurement or derived from the familiar Henderson-Hasselbalch equation

$$pH = pK + \log \frac{[HCO_3^-]}{[H_2CO_3]}, \quad (13)$$

or by substitution from Equation 9,

$$pH = pK + \log \frac{[HCO_3^-]}{[PCO_2 \times 0.0301]}, \quad (14)$$

where pK, the dissociation constant, is 6.10 for plasma at 37° C. If pH and either PCO_2 or CO_2 content are known, HCO_3^- can be calculated mathematically or obtained from nomograms or diagrams.[5,6]

Standard Bicarbonate Ion. Neither the plasma CO_2 content nor the $[HCO_3^-]$ is a pure metabolic index because both are affected by secondary respiratory adjustments that may accompany the primary disorder. Standard HCO_3^-, in mEq/L, has been proposed as a means of correcting $[HCO_3^-]$ for the respiratory component of a mixed acid-base disorder and is derived from a nomogram by adjusting (graphically) the PCO_2 of the specimen from its original value to 40 mm Hg.[9] There are some theoretic disadvantages implicit in the derivation of standard HCO_3^- that have caused it to be abandoned in favor of other indexes of nonrespiratory disorders.

Buffer Base. Buffer base is the total quantity of all bases in whole blood that are capable of binding H^+ at the prevailing pH, expressed in mEq/L. For practical purposes, the chief buffer bases of plasma are HCO_3^- (normally about 24 mEq/L) and protein (normally about 17 mEq/L) and to a much lesser extent HPO_4 (Figure 8–2). In contrast, cells (Figure 8–2) have a different composition of buffer bases than plasma, with protein, particularly hemoglobin in red blood cells, predominating over HCO_3^-.[5] Other anions besides HCO_3^- and protein may at times behave chemically as

bases but not at the pHs customarily encountered in the body.

A precise measurement of the value of whole blood buffer base in individual cases is virtually impossible to obtain because it requires analysis of the ionic constituents of plasma and erythrocytes. However, a clinically useful number can be obtained by graphic solution of the Singer and Hastings[5] or Siggaard-Andersen[6] nomograms; these can be solved if two of the three variables, PCO_2, pH, and $[HCO_3^-]$, are known, and hemoglobin or hematocrit has been measured.

The utility of buffer base lies in the fact that it does not change when PCO_2 is added or removed from the bloodstream. Any change in $[HCO_3^-]$ induced by a variation in PCO_2 is offset by an equal and opposite change in the other buffers* (Figure 8–3). Furthermore, because buffer base decreases or increases according to the addition of nonvolatile acids or bases to the body, it serves as a useful index of the severity of metabolic acid-base disorders.

Base Excess. Although the derived values of buffer base have practical application, there are some inherent drawbacks in the concept that can be avoided by using base excess. Base excess (BE) means the change in buffer base (ΔBB) between the normal level (NBB) and the derived one (BB) for the given subject, corrected for hemoglobin concentration, so that

$$BE = \Delta BB = NBB - BB. \quad (15)$$

An absolute value for BB is not required because the procedure involves either actually titrating the blood specimen with acid to a pH of 7.40

---

*Equal but opposite effects occur because any change in $[HCO_3^-]$ from the addition or subtraction of PCO_2 (H_2CO_3) must be associated with an equivalent change in $[H^+]$, which, in turn, subtracts or adds (respectively) to the non-bicarbonate buffers.[5]

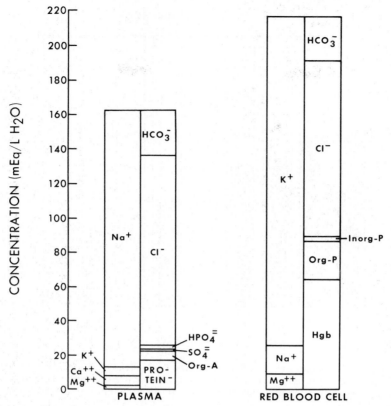

Figure 8–2 Composition of blood plasma and red blood cell intracellular liquid. Concentrations are in mEq/L of plasma and cell H_2O. The total heights of the two sets of columns differ owing to differences in the amount of H_2O in plasma (93 per cent) and in red blood cells (70 per cent).

while the P_{CO_2} is held constant at 40 mm Hg or determining BB with the aid of graphs. A small correction is then made to adjust for the different buffering capacities of oxyhemoglobin and deoxyhemoglobin; the results are expressed in mEq/L.[10] Positive values indicate a base excess (or a deficit of acid) because acid must be added to the blood to restore its pH to 7.40. Similarly, negative base excess values indicate an excess of acid (or a deficiency of base) because acid must be withdrawn from (or base added to) the blood to restore its pH to 7.40.

Much effort has been directed toward deriving the ideal index of nonrespiratory acid-base disorders, and a great deal has been learned in the process. From a practical point of view, however, except when P_{CO_2} is enormously elevated, knowledge of base excess and buffer base values seldom helps the clinician more than the information provided from HCO_3^- levels alone. The results of analysis of $[HCO_3^-]$ are nearly always available from studies of "electrolytes" that have been carried out separately; these have the added value of serving as a rough guide to the accuracy of P_{CO_2} and pH measurements, because the three variables should agree within reasonable limits when fitted into the Henderson-Hasselbach equation (Equation 14), or derived from graphs

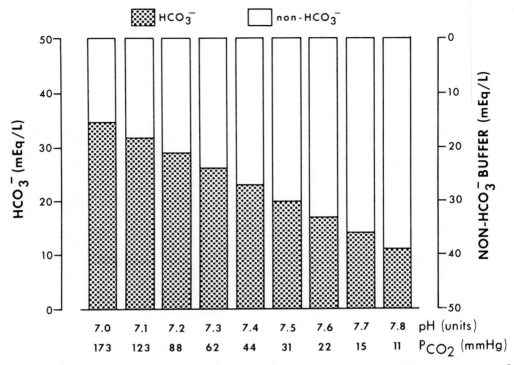

Figure 8–3 Demonstration of the effect of varying P_{CO_2} on HCO_3^- and non-HCO_3^- components of buffer base. However, total buffer base, the sum of the two components, does not change as P_{CO_2} is increased or decreased. (Adapted from Singer and Hastings.[5] Reprinted by permission from the authors and publisher.)

that relate the three variables (Figure 8–4). It is more important to become familiar with one of the nonrespiratory indexes and to know its limitations and its usefulness than to argue about which one is best. In the subsequent graphic analysis of acid-base disorders, the HCO_3^- system is used because it is easier to understand and display than either buffer base or base excess.

ACIDOSIS-ALKALOSIS

Acidosis and alkalosis are abnormal processes that result from the excessive production or elimination of acids or alkali (base) by the body and that tend to raise or lower pH.[1] But it is important to recognize that the pH is not necessarily above or below normal values; whether or not it changes de-

pends on the adequacy of compensatory mechanisms and on the presence of associated disorders.

ACIDEMIA-ALKALEMIA

Acidemia and alkalemia describe the state of the arterial blood pH when it is less than 7.36 or greater than 7.44, respectively.[1] The arterial blood pH during the evolution of acidosis and alkalosis represents the net result of the interaction of all the various abnormal processes and the compensatory mechanisms that affect the amount of H^+ in the bloodstream.

EXTRACELLULAR-INTRACELLULAR pH

Owing to the permeability of H^+ across endothelial barriers, the pH of capillary and venous blood (about 7.36)

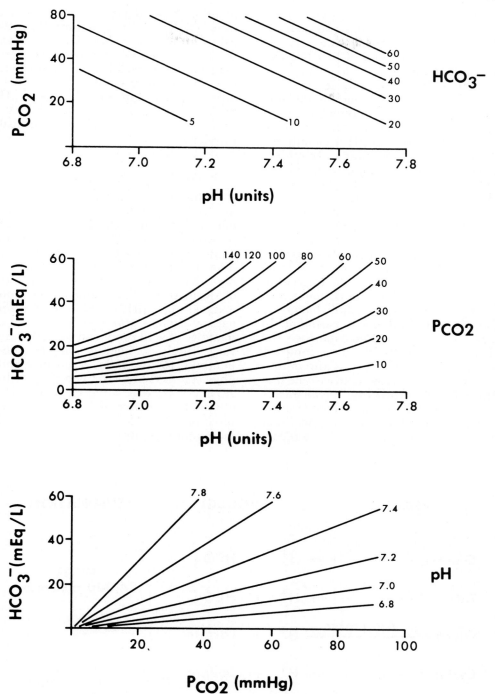

Figure 8–4 Graphic solutions to the Henderson-Hasselbalch equation. Three different ways of expressing the relationships among pH, P_{CO_2}, and HCO_3^- are shown. The method shown in the bottom panel is used in subsequent figures.

is virtually identical with that of most of the remainder of the extracellular fluid; the important exception is the pH of cerebrospinal fluid (CSF) because a relatively impermeable membrane, the blood-brain barrier, is involved (see Chapter 9). Cell membranes are also not as readily permeable to the movement of H^+ as vascular endothelium, so intracellular pH is usually not the same as extracellular and capillary blood pH. Intracellular pH, though difficult to determine, has been measured by a variety of techniques and has been found to be approximately 7.0 in most animal tissues under normal conditions.[11] Although the factors that control intracellular pH are poorly understood, it is recognized that changes in pH in either the intracellular or extracellular compartment may not be reflected by parallel changes in the pH of the other compartment. In fact, in some circumstances the changes in pH in the two compartments may be in opposite directions.

It seems reasonable to assume that physiologic regulatory mechanisms are geared to the maintenance of intracellular pH rather than extracellular pH; in this context, it should be recognized that blood pH is at best only an indirect measurement of the more critical intracellular value. However, in the discussions that follow about normal acid-base equilibrium and respiratory and nonrespiratory acid-base disorders, the pH considered is blood pH because that is the variable customarily measured in the analysis of clinical problems.

NORMAL ACID-BASE EQUILIBRIUM

The chief by-products of cellular metabolic activities are water and various acids, mainly H_2CO_3 and acids of phosphate and sulfates (Figure 8–5). Under normal conditions, these residues are disposed of by the body at a rate that closely parallels their rate of formation, and intracellular and extracellular pHs are held within narrow limits. Moreover, because the quantity of acid produced by cells may vary widely in healthy subjects, depending, for example, upon diet and physical activity, regulatory mechanisms exist that serve to govern H^+ elimination so that it keeps pace approximately with H^+ production and maintains equilibrium. Thus, the body

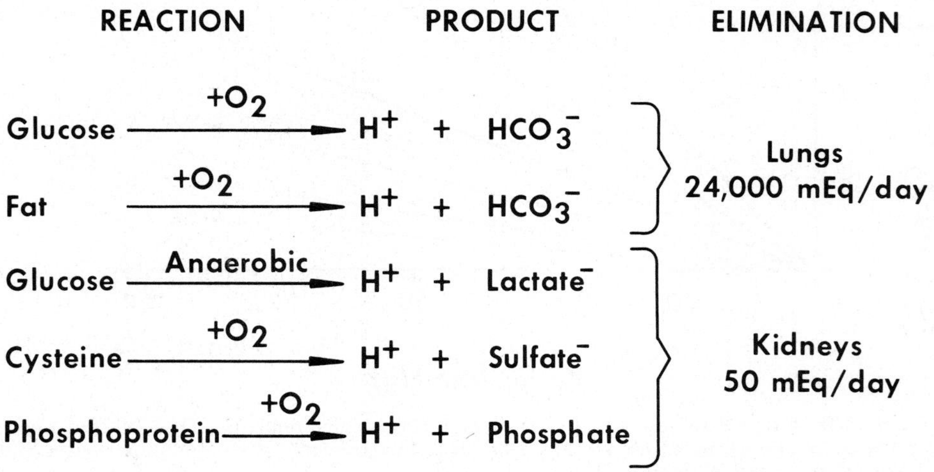

Figure 8–5 Condensed chemical reactions depicting the products of several important metabolic pathways and the routes by which H^+ is eliminated.

is able to cope adequately with the usual daily vicissitudes of acid production, and it is only during abnormal circumstances that acidosis or alkalosis occurs.

Although newly produced H^+ is ultimately disposed of by the mechanisms described below, it is important to emphasize that the various responses of the body are actuated according to markedly differing time sequences. The first defense against an accumulation of H^+ and consequent lowering of pH is virtually instantaneous and consists of the sequestration or "mopping up" of H^+ by the various buffer systems throughout the body. The next defense is by the lung, which responds within seconds to minutes to a stimulus to change CO_2 elimination. Finally, hours to days are required for completion of adjustments in the renal handling of acids. Thus, acid-base "balance" must be viewed as a dynamic condition, and the factor of *time* must be considered when analyzing the acid-base status of a patient.

VOLATILE ACIDS

The only volatile acid produced by the body in significant quantities is H_2CO_3. Furthermore, because CO_2 is the end product of normal oxidative metabolism, large amounts of H_2CO_3 are formed, and the rate of its production is nearly 500 times that of all other acids combined. Additional H_2CO_3 besides that from aerobic metabolism may be generated by the reaction of H^+ from nonvolatile acids with HCO_3^- buffers (Equation 5); H_2CO_3 from both sources is disposed of through the elimination of CO_2 by the lungs (Equation 7). Removal of CO_2 obviously does not affect the total quantity of H in the body, but the process is an effective means of defending pH because during the chemical reactions that release CO_2 (Equation 7), active H^+ is converted to harmless H in molecules of body water.

The mechanisms by which CO_2 is transported in the bloodstream and eliminated from the lungs are reviewed in Chapter 6. The intimate relationship between the control of breathing and the level of P_{CO_2} in arterial blood is considered in Chapter 9. This relationship can be summarized by saying that the minute volume of alveolar ventilation is closely regulated by a rapidly responding system that normally holds arterial P_{CO_2} constant within narrow limits, 38 to 43 mm Hg at sea level. However, many peripheral and central stimuli are known to influence the control of breathing, with the result that under both normal and pathologic conditions, ventilation, and hence P_{CO_2} and acid-base equilibrium, can be disturbed (see subsequent section).

NONVOLATILE ACIDS

Nonvolatile acids are not in equilibrium with gases, so they must be removed from the body in solution by the kidneys instead of by the lungs. (Lactate and other organic acids are in part excreted in the urine and in part metabolized to CO_2 and water.) In addition to the excretion of H^+ formed by the production of nonvolatile acids, the kidneys also significantly influence acid-base equilibrium by regulating body stores of HCO_3^-. Bicarbonate conservation and H^+ elimination can be considered separate functions because they occur in different parts of the nephron; however, they are interrelated processes because both involve H^+ secretion by tubule cells, and together they constitute the main renal contribution to acid-base equilibrium. (The collective handling of other ions also affects acid-base balance but indirectly through effects on H^+ secretion.)

The regulation of HCO_3^- stores is fairly straightforward because it involves simply the reabsorption and return to the bloodstream of virtually all the HCO_3^- present in the glomerular filtrate. Because approximately 180 L of filtrate are formed each day, with a $[HCO_3^-]$ nearly equal to that in plasma, over 4000 mEq of HCO_3^- could be lost from the body in 24 hours, which would rapidly and severely deplete the HCO_3^- stores and buffering capacity of the body; however, excessive loss is prevented by reabsorption of most of the HCO_3^- from the filtrate as it passes through the tubular system. Bicarbonate ions and/or Cl^- are selectively reabsorbed as the principal anions that accompany Na^+ as it is actively transported from the glomerular filtrate back into the bloodstream. However, HCO_3^- is not a very diffusible ion, so it is removed from the filtrate after being transformed into the more diffusible CO_2 molecule by the process illustrated in Figure 8–6. Note that Na^+ from within the tubular lumen is exchanged for H^+ secreted by the tubule

cell. The H^+ is one of the ionization products of H_2CO_3 that are formed by the hydration of CO_2 in a reaction catalyzed by carbonic anhydrase. The CO_2 and water involved may come either from metabolism within the cells or from movement into them from capillary blood or tubular filtrate. Figure 8–6 also shows that the HCO_3^- that reaches the capillary blood is another ionization product of H_2CO_3, and hence is not the original HCO_3^- that was present in the glomerular filtrate (encircled in Figure 8–6).

The reabsorption of HCO_3^- appears to be governed in part by a threshold mechanism that serves to regulate the level of $[HCO_3^-]$. The process operates by the selective reabsorption of either HCO_3^- or Cl^- as the attendant anion of Na^+, depending upon whether HCO_3^- is to be conserved or wasted.

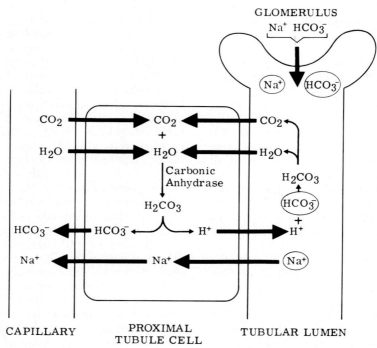

Figure 8–6 Schematic representation of the excretion of H^+ in the proximal tubules of the kidney. The Na^+ and HCO_3^- present in the glomerular filtrate are identified as (Na⁺) and (HCO₃⁻) The (Na⁺) is reabsorbed in exchange for H^+; the H^+ then reacts with the (HCO₃⁻) to form H_2O and CO_2 that diffuse into the tubular cell. The arrows depict the direction of movement. For further details, see text.

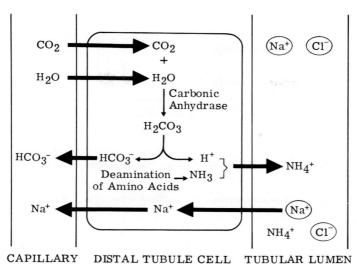

Figure 8-7 Schematic representation of the excretion of H^+ in the distal tubule of the kidney. The Na^+ and Cl^- present in the glomerular filtrate are identified as Na^+ and Cl^- Within the cell, H^+ combined with NH_3, formed by deamination of amino acids, to form NH_4^+ that is exchanged for Na^+ that is returned to the bloodstream.

Thus, there is a reciprocal and equivalent relationship between the amount of HCO_3^- and Cl^- reabsorbed and the amount rejected. Although the HCO_3^- threshold may vary widely under different conditions and although the factors that control the threshold are incompletely understood, it is clearly responsive to changes in arterial P_{CO_2}. This relationship is an important one because it appears to underlie the renal compensation for primary respiratory (i.e., P_{CO_2}-dependent) acid-base changes.

Although HCO_3^- reabsorption depends upon H^+ secretion, the H^+ involved is not lost from the body but can be viewed as moving from cell to filtrate and back again (as H in H_2O). The excretion of surplus H^+ takes place mainly in the distal tubules. The H^+ is also formed there by the hydration of CO_2 under the influence of carbonic anhydrase and ionization of H_2CO_3. The H^+ is then secreted into the tubular lumen in exchange for Na^+ and in the process reacts with one of three substrates, depending upon which is available in the filtrate. (1)

Hydrogen ions may combine with HCO_3^- to form water and CO_2, as discussed earlier (Figure 8-6). Under ordinary conditions, about half the filtered HCO_3^- is reabsorbed in the proximal tubules, and the remainder is absorbed in the distal system. (2) They may combine with NH_3, produced by the deamidization of protein, to form NH_4^+, either in the cell itself or in the filtrate (Figure 8-7). Ammonia is a strong binder of H^+, and increased NH_3 production is an important pathway of H^+ binding and elimination in states of acidosis. (3) They may combine with $HPO_4^=$ to form $H_2PO_4^-$ (Figure 8-8). The extent of this reaction is measurable as titratable acidity. Thus, in order to quantify all the H^+ secreted in the urine ($[Total\ H^+]u$), it is necessary to know the total amount of H^+ excreted in the urine as titratable acid ($[TA]u$) and ammonium ($[NH_4^+]u$):

$$[Total\ H^+]u = [TA]u + [NH_4^+]u.\ \textbf{(16)}$$

To determine *net* renal acid loss, any HCO_3^- that appears in the urine must be subtracted from $[Total\ H^+]u$

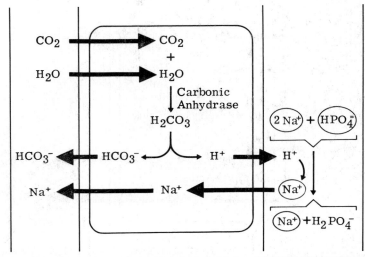

CAPILLARY   DISTAL TUBULE CELL   TUBULAR LUMEN

Figure 8–8   Schematic representation of the excretion of H^+ in the distal tubule of the kidney. The Na_2HPO_4 present in the glomerular filtrate ionizes into 2 Na^+ and $HPO_4^=$. The H^+, formed within the cell, is exchanged for one Na^+ that is returned to the bloodstream. Thus the urine contains NaH_2PO_4.

because excreted HCO_3^- represents loss of base, an effect that offsets loss of an equivalent amount of acid.[12] The excretion of surplus H^+ serves to conserve additional Na^+, but more importantly, as shown in Figures 8–7 and 8–8, an amount of HCO_3^- is generated and added to the body stores that is exactly equal to the amount of H^+ excreted. If 100 mEq of HCO_3^- are consumed by the 100 mEq of nonvolatile acids produced by the body each day, the kidneys not only excrete 100 mEq of H^+ but also generate 100 mEq of HCO_3^- in the process. Thus, the buffers of the body that were depleted in the original defense against the H^+ are completely restored and homeostasis is preserved.

RESPIRATORY ACID-BASE DISORDERS

RESPIRATORY ACIDOSIS

The hallmark of respiratory acidosis is an increased arterial P_{CO_2}.

Retention of CO_2 may occur in patients with normal lungs owing to faulty regulation of ventilation by the central nervous system or to impairment of respiratory muscle function. Retention of CO_2 also develops in patients with a variety of pulmonary diseases. Some of the most common causes are listed in Table 8–4.

Failure to eliminate CO_2 may occur within seconds or minutes in patients undergoing anesthesia or receiving sedative drugs. A sudden depression of ventilation leads to rapid CO_2 retention and *acute* respiratory acidosis. The consequences of acute hypercapnia have been studied experimentally by exposing normal subjects to high concentrations of CO_2 in the inspired air.[13] The results of these studies are represented as line A in Figure 8–9, which extends rightward from the point of normality (P_{CO_2} 40 mm Hg, $[HCO_3^-]$ 24 mEq/L, and pH 7.40) and demonstrates that as P_{CO_2} increases, there is only a slight rise in $[HCO_3^-]$, and pH falls.

However, the acidosis that de-

Table 8–4   Common Causes of CO_2 Retention and Respiratory Acidosis

With normal lungs
  Anesthesia
  Sedative drugs
  Neuromuscular disease (poliomyelitis, myasthenia gravis, Guillain-Barré
    syndrome)
  Obesity (Pickwickian syndrome)
  Brain damage
  Idiopathic
With abnormal lungs
  Chronic obstructive pulmonary disease (chronic bronchitis, emphysema)
  Diffuse infiltrative pulmonary diseases (advanced)
  Kyphoscoliosis (severe)

velops is less severe than that which would occur in the absence of intracellular buffering mechanisms. Figure 8–10 demonstrates how acute respiratory acidosis was defended in dogs given 20 per cent CO_2 to breathe.[14]

Entry of Cl^- into cells in exchange for HCO_3^- accounted for 29 per cent of the buffering; similarly, exchange for intracellular Na^+ and K^+ for extracellular H^+ accounted for 51 per cent; smaller increments of buffering were

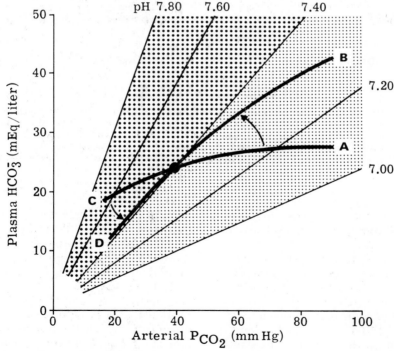

Figure 8–9   Respiratory acid-base disorders. Pooled results from several studies of the effects of acute and chronic variations in arterial P_{CO_2} on plasma HCO_3^- and pH. When P_{CO_2} is raised acutely (*acute respiratory acidosis*), HCO_3^- and pH values lie along line A. After compensation by retention of HCO_3^- is complete (*chronic respiratory acidosis*), values lie along line B. When P_{CO_2} is lowered acutely (*acute respiratory alkalosis*), resulting HCO_3^- and pH values lie along line C. After compensation by rejection of HCO_3^- is complete (*chronic respiratory alkalosis*), values lie along line D. For further details and references, see text.

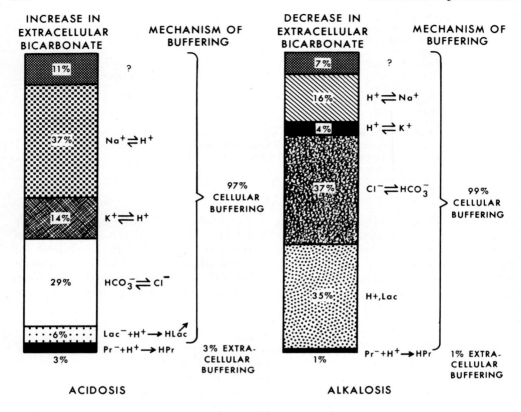

RESPIRATORY DISTURBANCES

Figure 8–10 Diagrammatic representation of the mechanisms of buffering in dogs with acute respiratory acidosis (breathing 20 per cent CO_2) and acute respiratory alkalosis (mechanical hyperventilation). Lac = lactate; Pr = protein. (Adapted from Pitts.[14] Original data from Swan, R. C., and Pitts, R. F.: J. Clin. Invest. 34:205, 1955, and Swan, R. C., Axelrod, D. R., Seip, M., and Pitts, R. F.: J. Clin. Invest. 34:1795, 1955. Reprinted by permission from the author and Year Book Publishers, Inc.)

contributed by reactions involving lactate, plasma proteins, and an unidentified source.

If CO_2 retention persists for several days, the relationship between Pco_2 and $[HCO_3^-]$ depicted by line B (Figure 8–9) is encountered.[15-18] In patients with *chronic* respiratory acidosis, therefore, $[HCO_3^-]$ is considerably higher than in those with acute conditions, and pH is consequently also higher (i.e., closer to normal values). The elevation in $[HCO_3^-]$ occurs through an alteration in the renal threshold with subsequent retention of HCO_3^- and loss of an equivalent

amount of Cl^-. As shown by the results depicted in Figure 8–11, it takes five to seven days for compensation by the kidney to become maximal in experimental animals[19]; accordingly, the shift from line A to line B in man, shown by the arrow in Figure 8–9, probably also develops over a period of several days. Although patients with chronic CO_2 retention appear to be better off with their blood pHs raised *toward* normal by renal compensation, the question still remains why pH is not returned *to* normal levels in view of the kidney's demonstrable capacity to retain additional HCO_3^- when arterial

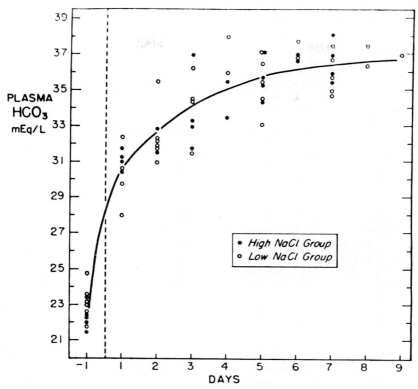

Figure 8-11 Time course of the changes in plasma HCO_3^- in response to respiratory acidosis induced in dogs constantly breathing an atmosphere containing 11 to 13 per cent CO_2. Plasma HCO_3^- continues to increase until about the fifth day after exposure. The amount of NaCl in the diet did not affect the response. (From Polak, Haynie, Hays, and Schwartz.[19] Reprinted by permission from the authors and publisher.)

PCO_2 is raised even higher. Because intracellular pH has been shown to be normal in patients with chronic hypercapnia despite persistent extracellular acidosis, it is tempting to suggest that the answer to the question lies in the effect of intracellular rather than extracellular pH on the renal HCO_3^- threshold.[20]

RESPIRATORY ALKALOSIS

Hyperventilation quickly lowers arterial PCO_2 and produces *acute* respiratory alkalosis. Hyperventilation, which is defined by a lower than normal arterial PCO_2, is a common clinical finding in patients with normal lungs

and may even occur in patients with pulmonary diseases. Some of the many causes of excessive CO_2 elimination are listed in Table 8-5. The effects of acute hyperventilation on arterial PCO_2, $[HCO_3^-]$, and pH have been examined in anesthetized patients[21]; the results from these studies have led to the relationship defined by line C in Figure 8-9. Although $[HCO_3^-]$ falls somewhat, the rise in pH becomes progressively more severe as PCO_2 is lowered.

The defenses against a severe change in pH during acute respiratory alkalosis, like those during acute respiratory acidosis, are nearly all attributable to intracellular reactions (Figure 8-10). The two main mechanisms

Table 8-5 Common Causes of Excessive CO_2 Elimination and Respiratory Alkalosis

With normal lungs
  Anxiety
  Fever
  Drugs (e.g., aspirin)
  Central nervous system lesions (tumors, inflammation)
  Endotoxemia
With abnormal lungs
  Pneumonia
  Diffuse infiltrative pulmonary diseases (early)
  Acute bronchial asthma (early)
  Pulmonary vascular diseases
  Congestive heart failure (early)

are production of lactate to reduce the HCO_3^- content of extracellular liquids (35 per cent) and exchange of intracellular Cl^- for extracellular HCO_3^- (37 per cent). The pH is also protected by exchanges of Na^+ and K^+ for H^+ and an unidentified reaction.[14]

When a state of hyperventilation persists, renal mechanisms are actuated and compensation occurs by selective loss of HCO_3^- and retention of Cl^-. In *chronic* respiratory alkalosis, as occurs in normal subjects at high altitude, the relationship between arterial PCO_2 and $[HCO_3^-]$ represented by line D in Figure 8-9 is observed.[22-24] Line D is extremely close to the pH 7.40 line, indicating that compensation (renal and possibly other mechanisms) is almost perfect, and blood pH is restored to within normal values. The transition from acute to chronic respiratory alkalosis, signified by the arrow from line C to line D, is quite similar to the time course of the adjustments in chronic CO_2 retention since it requires several days to be fully developed.

NONRESPIRATORY ACID-BASE DISORDERS

NONRESPIRATORY ACIDOSIS

Either an increase in nonvolatile acids or excessive loss of bases from the body produces nonrespiratory acidosis. A clinical classification of these two basically different varieties is given in Table 8-6. In either case, the process results in a deficit of buffer base, base excess, and $[HCO_3^-]$. A reduction of these components means that pH must fall and $[H^+]$ must rise. Acidosis, as mentioned, is also a potent stimulus to increased ventilation, and as a consequence PCO_2 also falls. Three possible relationships between $[HCO_3^-]$ and PCO_2, depending upon the rapidity with which the acidosis develops and the magnitude of the ventilatory response, are shown by lines A, B, and C in Figure 8-12.*

Note that in Figure 8-12 the axes are reversed compared with those in Figure 8-9; this is because the primary change in nonrespiratory acid-base disturbances is an alteration in $[HCO_3^-]$. Therefore, $[HCO_3^-]$ is shown as the independent variable on the abscissa in Figure 8-12. In contrast, the primary change in respiratory disorders is reflected in PCO_2. Therefore, PCO_2 occupies the abscissa in Figure 8-9.

Nonrespiratory acidosis is almost immediately "sensed" by peripheral chemoreceptors, with the result that ventilation increases and PCO_2 falls.

---

*It should be emphasized that the lines in Figures 8-9 and 8-12 are chiefly for clarification. They are drawn from composite data in the literature, but have been adjusted, when necessary, for uniformity of presentation. Moreover, they should not be used for clinical purposes without knowledge about the range of variation (confidence bands) that may be encountered.

Table 8–6 Common Causes of Nonrespiratory ("Metabolic") Acidosis

Increase in nonvolatile acids
    Diabetes (betahydroxybuteric, acetoacetic acids)
    Uremia (phosphoric, sulfuric acids)
    Severe exercise, hypoxia, shock, idiopathic (lactic acid)
    Methyl alcohol ingestion (formic acid)
    Aspirin ingestion (salicylic acid)
Excessive loss of bases (usually $NaCO_3$ from lower gastrointestinal tract)
    Severe diarrhea (e.g., cholera, diarrhea in infants)
    Fistulas (e.g., pancreatic, biliary)

The distinction between acute (line A) and chronic (line B) nonrespiratory acidosis is determined by the magnitude of the ventilatory response, which depends in turn upon the adjustments that must take place in the extracellular environment of the central chemoreceptors. As explained in detail in the next chapter, this process is reflected in the composition of cerebrospinal fluid (CSF) and requires up to one to two days for completion; until then, the ventilatory response is not fully developed owing to the presence of a gradually lessening inhibitory influence that offsets part of the

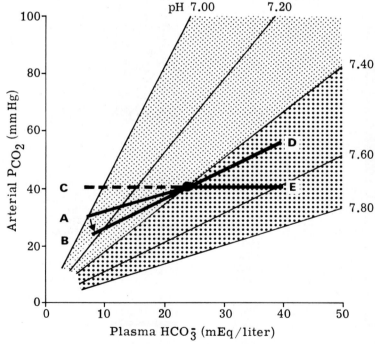

Figure 8–12 Nonrespiratory acid-base disorders. Pooled results from several studies of the effects of variations in plasma HCO_3^- on arterial P_{CO_2} and pH. When HCO_3^- is lowered acutely (*acute nonrespiratory acidosis*), P_{CO_2} and pH values lie along line A. After CSF adjustments allow ventilation to increase further (*chronic nonrespiratory acidosis*), values lie along line B. Line C depicts the pH changes that would result from a given reduction in HCO_3^- if no increase in ventilation occurred (i.e., P_{CO_2} remained at 40 mm Hg). Two patterns of ventilation occur in response to HCO_3^- increase (*chronic respiratory alkalosis*): one with hypoventilation (line D) and one with no change (line E). For further details and references, see text.

stimulating effect of the systemic acidosis. Line A in the figure shows the consequences of a fall in [HCO_3^-] plus the immediate stimulus to respiration; hyperventilation serves to compensate partially for a reduction in [HCO_3^-], but the effect becomes progressively less able to prevent pH from decreasing.

In addition to extracellular buffering by HCO_3^- and elimination of CO_2 by increasing ventilation in acute nonrespiratory acidosis, intracellular reactions also participate in the defense of body pH. As shown by the experimental results depicted in Figure 8–13, buffering in acute nonrespiratory

acidosis is also achieved by exchange of intracellular Na^+ (36 per cent) and K^+ (15 per cent) for extracellular H^+.[14]

Line B in Figure 8–12 depicts the relationship between [HCO_3^-] and P_{CO_2} when the ventilatory response is maximal[25]; in chronic nonrespiratory acidosis, the added compensatory effect of the secondary increase in ventilation, which is signified by the arrow, is evident in the position of line B in comparison with line A (i.e., at any given [HCO_3^-], P_{CO_2} is lower but pH is nearer to normal after compensation occurs). Line C shows the effect of lowering [HCO_3^-] on pH if there was no respiratory compensation at all and

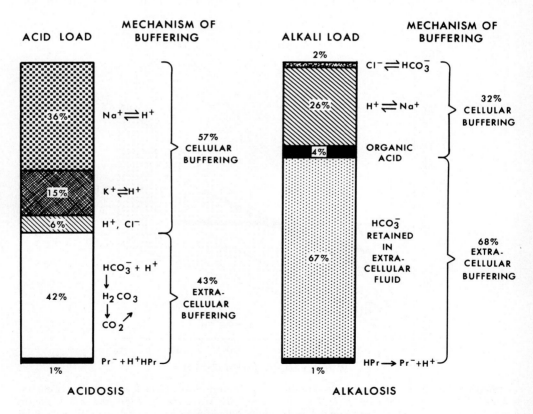

NONRESPIRATORY DISTURBANCES

Figure 8–13 Diagrammatic representation of the mechanisms of buffering in dogs with acute nonrespiratory acidosis (intravenous HCl) and acute nonrespiratory alkalosis (intravenous $NaHCO_3$). (Adapted from Pitts.[14] Original data from Giebisch, G., Berger, L., and Pitts, R. F.: J. Clin. Invest. 34:231, 1955. Reprinted by permission from the author and Year Book Publishers, Inc.)

arterial P_{CO_2} remained at 40 mm Hg. It is obvious that pH changes more with a given reduction in $[HCO_3^-]$ along line C than along either line A or B. Line C is a broken line to emphasize that it is artificial and has no clinical analogue except perhaps in rare patients who develop nonrespiratory acidosis but cannot augment their ventilation because of neuromuscular paralysis or severe coexisting pulmonary disease.

NONRESPIRATORY ALKALOSIS

Excessive elimination of nonvolatile acids or accumulation of bases produces nonrespiratory alkalosis. Although the common causes of nonrespiratory alkalosis may involve both these processes, they are classified according to their basic pathogenesis in Table 8–7. The mechanisms by which the body defends itself against an increase in pH in acute nonrespiratory alkalosis have been studied in dogs given large amounts of HCO_3^-. The results of these experiments are shown in Figure 8–13. Of the total infused HCO_3^-, two-thirds remained in the extracellular spaces; P_{CO_2} (and hence H_2CO_3) doubled owing to alveolar hypoventilation. One-third of the buffering was produced by intracellular reactions, predominantly (26 per cent) an exchange of intracellular H^+ for extracellular Na^+.[14]

The conditions causing chronic nonrespiratory alkalosis all produce increases in $[HCO_3^-]$, buffer base, and base excess; however, despite similarities in $[HCO_3^-]$, the various disorders

Table 8–7 Common Causes of Nonrespiratory Alkalosis

Increase in bases
    Hypochloremic alkalosis (diuretics)
    Alkali administration
Excessive loss of nonvolatile acids
    Vomiting or gastric aspiration
    Hypokalemic alkalosis

differ in their influence on ventilation, and hence on arterial P_{CO_2} and pH. At least two patterns of response have been demonstrated in man and are shown in Figure 8–12.[26] Line D shows that under some circumstances, such as the administration of HCO_3^- or other buffers, P_{CO_2} rises, which minimizes the pH change at any given level of $[HCO_3^-]$. In contrast, line E shows the presence of alkalosis from the administration of thiazide diuretics or aldosterone in which there is no respiratory "compensation." Alveolar hypoventilation failed to occur (line E) when extracellular alkalosis was accompanied by losses of K^+ and presumed shifts of H^+ into the intracellular phase, but it is not known whether the absence of a ventilatory response was due to the accumulation of H^+ in the cells of the respiratory center or to the effects of low serum K^+ on respiratory neuronal activity, or to some other mechanism; subjects who received ethacrynic acid also had high P_{CO_2} values, but ones that tended to fall between lines D and E, though closer to D.[26] These observations suggest strongly that a continuum of ventilatory responses is likely to develop in nonrespiratory alkalosis, depending upon the relative magnitude of the losses and shifts of H^+ on the one hand and K^+ on the other.

MIXED ACID-BASE DISORDERS

An understanding of acid-base disorders is facilitated by considering them as "pure" entities. However, this is seldom the case in clinical circumstances in which they are often found to coexist. Furthermore, the factor of time and the influence of therapy must always be included when interpreting data from patients with acid-base disturbances. Detailed consideration of these important problems is beyond the scope of this chapter, and good reviews are available elsewhere.[6,12,14]

This chapter has emphasized the inter-relationships between respiration and acid-base equilibrium and has provided background for discussion of the control of respiration that is continued in the next chapter.

REFERENCES

1. Filley, G. F.: Acid-Base and Blood Gas Regulation. Philadelphia, Lea & Febiger, 1971, pp. 1–213.
2. Harper, H. H.: Review of Physiological Chemistry. 14th Ed. Los Altos, Calif., Lange Medical Publications, 1973, pp. 505-510.
3. Sörensen, S. P. L.: Enzymstudien. II. Mitteilung. Über die Messung und die Bedeutung der Wasserstoffionen-konzentration bei enzymatischen Prozessen. Biochem. Z., 21:131-304, 1909.
4. Davis, R. P.: Editorial: Logland: A Gibbsian view of acid-base balance. Am. J. Med., 42:159-162, 1967.
5. Singer, R. B., and Hastings, A. B.: An improved clinical method for the estimation of disturbances of the acid-base balance of human blood. Medicine, 27:223-242, 1948.
6. Siggaard-Andersen, O.: The acid-base status of the blood. Scand. J. Clin. Lab. Invest., 15(Suppl. 70):1-134, 1963.
7. Van Slyke, D. D., and Neill, J. M.: Determination of gases in blood and other solutions by vacuum extraction and manometric measurement. I. J. Biol. Chem., 61:523-573, 1924.
8. Van Slyke, D. D., and Cullen, G. E.: Studies of acidosis. I. The bicarbonate concentration of the blood plasma; its significance, and its determination as a measure of acidosis. J. Biol. Chem., 30:289-346, 1917.
9. Jørgensen, K., and Astrup, P.: Standard bicarbonate, its clinical significance, and a new method for its determination. Scand. J. Clin. Lab. Invest., 9:122-132. 1957.
10. Astrup, P., Jørgensen, K., Siggaard-Andersen, O., and Engel, K.: The acid-base metabolism. A new approach. Lancet, 1:1035-1039, 1960.
11. Waddell, W. J., and Bates, R. G.: Intracellular pH. Physiol. Rev., 49:285-329, 1969.
12. Hills, A. G.: Acid-Base Balance. Chemistry, Physiology, Pathophysiology. Baltimore, Williams and Wilkins Company, 1973, pp. 115-126.
13. Brackett, N. C., Jr., Cohen, J. J., and

14. Schwartz, W. B.: Carbon dioxide titration curve of normal man. Effect of increasing degrees of acute hypercapnia on acid-base equilibrium. New Eng. J. Med., 272:6-12, 1965.
14. Pitts, R. F.: Physiology of the Kidney and Body Fluids. An Introductory Text. 3rd Ed. Chicago, Year Book Medical Publishers, Inc., 1944, pp. 198-241.
15. Refsum, H. E.: Acid-base status in patients with chronic hypercapnia and hypoxaemia. Clin. Sci., 27:407-415, 1964.
16. Van Ypersele de Strihou, C., Brasseur, L., and de Coninck, J.: The "carbon dioxide response curve" for chronic hypercapnia in man. New Eng. J. Med., 275:117-122, 1966.
17. Dufano, M. J., and Ishikawa, S.: Quantitative acid-base relationships in chronic pulmonary patients during the stable state. Am. Rev. Resp. Dis., 93:251–256, 1966.
18. Brackett, N. C., Jr., Wingo, C. F., Muren, O., and Solano, J. T.: Acid-base response to chronic hypercapnia in man. New Eng. J. Med., 280:124-130, 1969.
19. Polak, A., Haynie, G. D., Hays, R. M., and Schwartz, W. B.: Effects of chronic hypercapnia on electrolyte and acid-base equilibrium. I. Adaptation. J. Clin. Invest., 40:1223-1237, 1961.
20. Robin, E. D., Bromberg, P. A., and Tushan, F. S.: Carbon-dioxide in body fluids. New Eng. J. Med., 280:162-164, 1969.
21. Arbus, G. S., Hebert, L. A., Levesque, P. R., Etsten, B. E., and Schwartz, W. B.: Characterization and clinical application of the "significance band" for acute respiratory alkalosis. New Eng. J. Med., 280:117-123, 1969.
22. Severinghaus, J. W., and Carcelen, B. A.: Cerebrospinal fluid in man native to high altitude. J. Appl. Physiol., 19:319-321, 1964.
23. Pugh, L. G. C. E., Gill, M. B., Lahiri, S., Milledge, J. S., Ward, M. P., and West, J. B.: Muscular exercise at great altitudes. J. Appl. Physiol., 19:431–440, 1964.
24. Lahiri, S., and Milledge, J. S.: Acid-base in Sherpa altitude residents and lowlanders at 4880 M. Resp. Physiol., 2:323-334, 1967.
25. Lennon, E. J., and Lemann, J., Jr.: Defense of hydrogen ion concentration in chronic metabolic acidosis. A new evaluation of an old approach. Ann. Intern. Med., 65:265-274, 1966.
26. Goldring, R. M., Cannon, P. J., Heinemann, H. O., and Fishman, A. P.: Respiratory adjustment to chronic metabolic alkalosis in man. J. Clin. Invest., 47:188-202, 1968.

Chapter Nine

REGULATION
OF
RESPIRATION

INTRODUCTION

The demands of the body for uptake of O_2 and elimination of CO_2 vary considerably in normal persons during their usual daily life; O_2 consumption may increase tenfold, from a "basal" level while asleep to a maximal level during strenuous exercise. Remarkably, over this range arterial blood P_{O_2} remains constant within narrow limits. This constancy is made possible by a series of control mechanisms that regulate ventilation in accordance with metabolic demands and

223

roughly in proportion to the associated increases in cardiac output.

Respiration is also governed, as discussed in Chapter 8, by alterations in the concentration of nonvolatile acids in the blood; the changes in ventilation that occur under these conditions serve to restore arterial blood pH toward a more normal value and are a principal means by which the body compensates for nonrespiratory acid-base imbalances. Reflex hyperventilation occurs in normal persons upon ascent to high altitudes and in patients with various pulmonary diseases. Variations in the rate and depth of breathing that are not directly attributable to changes in the composition of arterial blood or to reflexes originating within the lung are encountered in patients with a variety of common clinical disorders, such as fever, metabolic diseases, and psychiatric disturbances. Besides the changes in the pattern of ventilation that occur in response to clinical or environmental abnormalities, specially coordinated respiratory movements are required for talking, singing, sniffing, coughing, hiccuping, sneezing, vomiting, and breath holding.

The multiple and diverse influences that affect breathing and gas exchange are mediated by an intricate control system that incorporates peripheral and central receptors and a complex network of nerve pathways and integrating "centers" in the brain and spinal cord. The purpose of this chapter is to examine the structure, function, and organization of the various components of the system that controls respiration in healthy man. In addition, the mechanisms by which breathing is regulated during common physiologic stresses are also considered.

ORGANIZATION

Early studies of the neurophysiologic organization of respiratory control employed the gross methods of transection, ablation, and electrical stimulation of specific parts of the brain; these experiments led to the concept that there are various localized centers that govern rhythmic respiration and the pattern of breathing.[1] More recent experimental investigations using the techniques of recording respiratory neuron activity by microelectrodes have produced results that have relocated the sites of respiratory activity within the medulla.[2] Certainly, the neurophysiologic behavior of the central nervous system is considerably more complex than originally believed, and generally accepted explanations for many phenomena are simply not available.[3] However, certain foci of activity and levels of organization can be demonstrated in the laboratory, and these have their counterparts in the "experiments of nature" that occur in patients with various forms of damage to the central nervous system.

MEDULLA

The medulla appears to be the main headquarters for spontaneous respiration in all mammals studied to date, including man. This statement is based on two observations. (1) Rhythmic respiration continues, although the pattern of breathing is likely to change, following transection of the brain at the pontomedullary junction; this indicates that higher centers are not necessary to maintain ventilatory efforts. Moreover, transection below the medulla eliminates respiratory movements. (2) Most of the neurons with respiratory periodicity that have been located are found in the medulla. Figures 9–1 and 9–2 are schematic diagrams of a dorsal projection and cross section of the medulla showing the locations of respiratory neurons. Although there is considerable overlap among neurons showing primarily inspiratory activity and those showing mainly expiratory activity, some ana-

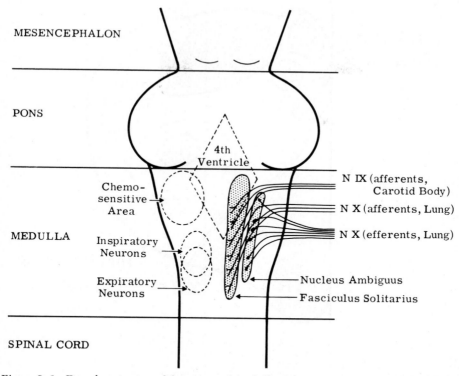

MESENCEPHALON

PONS

4th
Ventricle

Chemo-
sensitive
Area

MEDULLA

Inspiratory
Neurons

Expiratory
Neurons

N IX (afferents,
          Carotid Body)

N X (afferents, Lung)

N X (efferents, Lung)

Nucleus Ambiguus

Fasciculus Solitarius

SPINAL CORD

Figure 9–1   Dorsal projection of the pons and medulla showing the approximate locations of the cranial nerves (N) and centers involved in the control of breathing.

tomic separation of these functions can be seen in the dorsal projection in which the inspiratory units lie slightly rostral (i.e., cephalad) to the expiratory units.

Most of the respiratory neurons within the medulla are found surrounding the nucleus ambiguus (the motor nucleus of the vagus and glossopharyngeal nerves); if these neurons are damaged or destroyed (e.g., in patients with bulbar poliomyelitis), death from respiratory failure usually results.[4] Another smaller collection of respiratory neurons lies ventromedial to the fasciculus solitarius (Figure 9–2).

Even though the aggregates of respiratory neurons are no longer believed to comprise discrete homogeneous centers and the units are located in a region different from the one originally supposed, the identification of two different functional populations of neurons still provides a plausible (and the best) explanation for the genesis of rhythmic respiration.[5] According to the hypothesis, the two groups of neurons are self-reexciting and mutually inhibitory; this provides a mechanism for rhythmic discharge that, in turn, may be modified by influences from higher centers or by incoming afferent signals. However, little is known about the connecting pathways of the respiratory neurons, both those from other regions in the brain and those to respiratory muscles, and how the neurons respond to respiratory and nonrespiratory sensory stimuli.

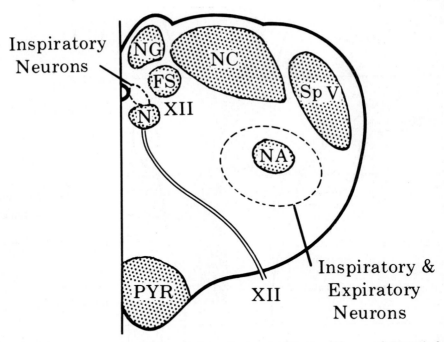

Inspiratory
Neurons

NG
FS
N XII
NC
Sp V
NA
PYR   XII

Inspiratory &
Expiratory
Neurons

Figure 9-2 Cross section of the medulla at the level of the twelfth cranial (N XII) showing the approximate locations of inspiratory and expiratory neurons. NG = nucleus gracilis; FS = fasciculus solitarius; NC = nucleus cuneatus; Sp V = spinal tract fifth cranial nerve; NA = nucleus ambiguus; PYR = pyramid.

PONS

Neurons with respiratory activity have also been identified in the pons, although they are less numerous than in the medulla. In contrast, neurons showing both inspiratory and expiratory activity (phase-spanning), rather than solely inspiratory or expiratory activity, are relatively more numerous in the pons than in the medulla. It seems clear that these neurons and other pontine structures may exert a profound influence on respiration in certain experimental preparations, but the pathways by which these phenomena are mediated are uncertain.

Figure 9-3 shows schematically the effect on the pattern of breathing of transection of the upper, middle, and lower levels of the pons.[6] (1) Transection at the junction between the pons and midbrain does not affect normal breathing (eupnea) if the vagi are intact; bilateral vagotomy plus transection at this level causes a deepening and slowing of breathing (the usual result of vagotomy in most mammalian species except man). (2) Midpontine transection in animals with intact vagi causes spontaneous breathing with a slow and regular pattern; however, important respiratory abnormalities can be demonstrated in recordings from peripheral nerves if the animal is mechanically ventilated. A striking change in respiratory pattern to apneustic breathing (characterized by a sustained inspiratory spasm) immediately follows cutting the vagi in the midpontine-transected animal. (3) Transection at the pontomedullary junction does not affect spontaneous respiration, but breathing is likely to become irregular in rate or depth (gasping), ataxic, or both.

These results plus those found

when using electrical stimulation have led to the conclusion among many neurophysiologists that the pons contains two important regulatory centers: the *apneustic center* and the *pneumotaxic center*. These aggregates of neurons, presumably located in the lower and upper pons, respectively, are believed to act upon the medullary neurons to maintain and control rhythmic respiration. The tonically active pontine apneustic center continually excites the medullary inspiratory center and thus facilitates inspiration. Signals from the periodically active pneumotaxic center as well as afferent impulses from the vagus nerves actuate the expiratory center and cause it to "turn off" inspiration. Several variations on this basic theme have been proposed.

Newer theories have incorporated evidence that the respiratory neurons are not consolidated into discrete centers but are intermingled and apparently connected and also that pontine impulses are not required for the respiratory oscillator to function. The numerous respiratory neurons in the pons with *both* inspiratory and expiratory activities are thought to play a role in smoothing the transition from one respiratory phase to the next.[7] Evidence indicates that the lower pons level is involved in the Hering-Breuer inflation reflex because the response

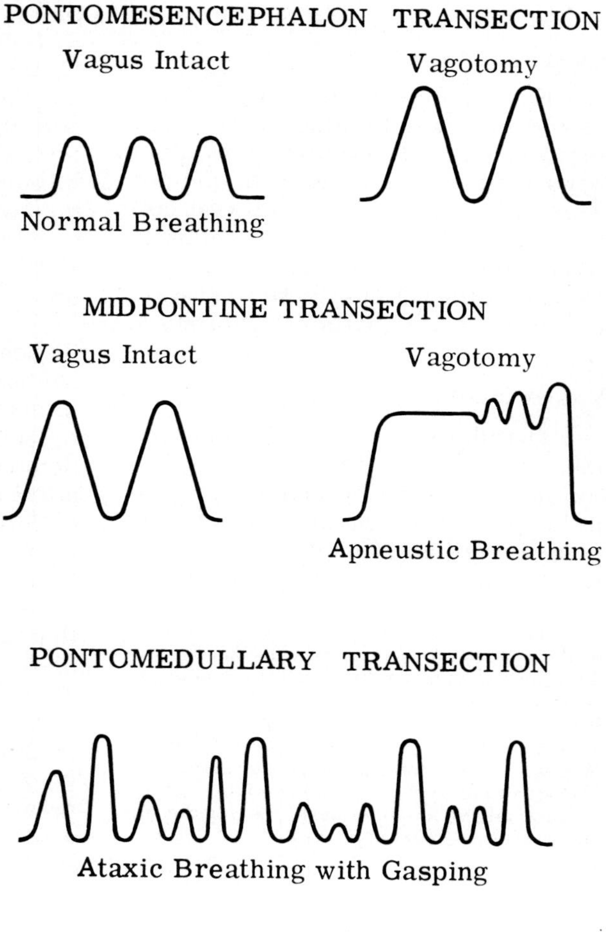

PONTOMESENCEPHALON TRANSECTION

Vagus Intact   Vagotomy

Normal Breathing

Figure 9–3 Breathing patterns resulting from pontomesencephalon, midpontine, and pontomedullary transections with the vagus nerves intact and after vagotomy. (Adapted from Campbell, Agostoni and Davis.[6] Reprinted by permission from the authors and Lloyd-Luke [Medical Books] Inc.)

MIDPONTINE TRANSECTION

Vagus Intact   Vagotomy

Apneustic Breathing

PONTOMEDULLARY TRANSECTION

Ataxic Breathing with Gasping

disappears after pontomedullary transection and because lung inflation has a marked inhibitory effect on pontine respiratory neuron activity.[8]

MESENCEPHALON AND DIENCEPHALON

Electrical stimulation and transection experiments have provided evidence that the mesencephalon (midbrain) and diencephalon (e.g., hypothalamus, thalamus) contain structures that when activated serve to augment tidal volume, respiratory rate, or both.[6] Stimulation of the reticular-activating system* is probably responsible for the pattern of behavior that characterizes the general "arousal" reaction; the arousal response not only alerts the organism but also prepares it for immediate muscular activity.[10]

CEREBRAL CORTEX

Stimulation of some parts of the cerebral cortex inhibits respiratory movements, but stimulation of other parts increases respiratory frequency. The pathways from the cerebral cortex to the origin of respiratory muscle motoneurons in the spinal cord appear to be distinct from those pathways concerned with rhythmic respiration.

VAGUS NERVE

Distribution of the afferent and efferent endings of the vagus nerves in the larynx, tracheobronchial tree, and pulmonary parenchyma has already been described (Chapter 3), and the main central vagal motor and sensory

---

*The reticular-activating system is located in the reticular formation, which extends from the upper cervical cord through the brain stem into the diencephalon. The reticular formation is composed of relatively long mono- or polysynaptic paths that receive input from and transmit output to both rostral and caudal sites. The reticular-activating system is believed to perform vital integrative functions besides being the site of the arousal response.[9]

pathways are depicted schematically in Figure 9–1. Most of the vagal afferent fibers from the lung turn caudally after they enter the medulla and synapse in the fasciculus solitarius. From the fasciculus solitarius, there appear to be extensive connections within the medulla and to a lesser extent with higher regions of the brain.

The importance of the contributions of vagal activity to the patterns of breathing is evident in Figure 9–3; the results of transections at different levels in the pons and medulla are strikingly different, depending upon whether or not the vagi are intact.[6] The effect of vagotomy in these experiments is primarily owing to removal of afferent impulses from the lung that affect the rate and depth of breathing. As stated previously, there are three principal receptor systems in the lung: pulmonary stretch receptors, irritant receptors, and J receptors (Chapter 3). Of these, pulmonary stretch receptors are tonically active in most mammals and increase their impulse rate during normal inspiration; removal of the inhibitory action on inflation of vagally mediated sensory reflexes (e.g., by vagotomy or nerve block) slows respiratory rate and increases tidal volume.

Judging from the results of studies in healthy persons, the level of vagal control of normal tidal ventilation in man is trivial because no change in the rate and depth of breathing was detected after bilateral vagal blockade.[11] (It is of interest that the absence of control contrasts with the presence of impulses in the vagus during inflation.) However, it was shown in the same type of blocking experiments that the inhibitory reflex to inflations of the lung above tidal volume was abolished, and of considerable interest was the finding that the ventilatory response to CO_2 was modified by vagotomy.[12] These observations have been interpreted as demonstrating that a vagally mediated stretch reflex is present during deep breaths in normal subjects and that the hyperpnea from CO_2 may depend in part upon vagal afferents. As mentioned (Chapter 3), vagal inhibition of normal tidal breathing is present in man during the newborn period.

There is good clinical and experimental evidence that the tachypnea and hyperventilation that accompany many common pulmonary diseases, such as asthma, pneumonia, and pulmonary embolism, are caused by abnormal afferent vagal input.[13] Although much has been learned by complete vagal blockade about the vagal contribution to the abnormal breathing patterns in these conditions, differential block by direct current[14] and inhalation of local anesthetics[15] should provide additional important information about the specific pathways involved.

SPINAL CORD

The final common pathway to the skeletal muscles involved in ventilatory movements is the *alpha motoneuron* (Figure 9–4). The signals transmitted along this nerve represent the integrated result of all the neural impulses that originate at supraspinal levels (e.g., hindbrain, midbrain, diencephalon, and cortex) plus those that originate from segmental sensory stimuli (e.g., muscle spindle and tendon organ afferents).

Skeletal muscles contain different types of contractile elements: the

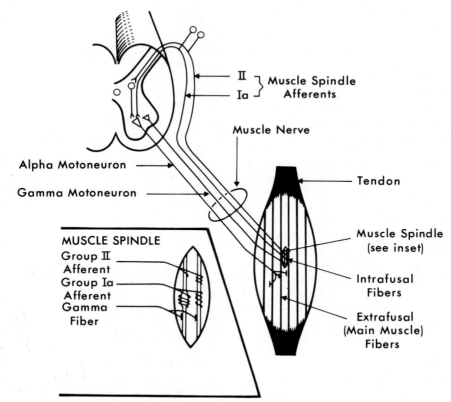

Figure 9–4 Schematic representation of the proprioceptive and motor innervation of skeletal muscle. For discussion, see text. (Adapted from Campbell, Agostoni, and Davis.[6] Reprinted by permission from the authors and Lloyd-Luke [Medical Books] Inc.)

main muscle (extrafusal) fibers, whose shortening performs voluntary movements, and the specialized organs of proprioception called *muscle spindles,* which contain two types of muscle fibers in addition to sensory endings. The main muscle fibers are innervated by alpha motoneurons, and the fibers within the muscle spindles are innervated by *gamma motoneurons* (also called fusimotor fibers). The afferent and efferent nerves to skeletal muscles and muscle spindles are shown schematically in Figure 9–4.[6]

Stretching a muscle causes its muscle spindles to discharge and this, in turn, stimulates the alpha motoneuron. Consequently, the main muscle contracts, which counteracts further stretch. Similarly, because the afferent signals from the muscle spindles are widely distributed, synergistic muscle groups are activated, and antagonist groups are inhibited. All these events increase opposition to the stretch that actuated the response in the first place.

Although the precise role of muscle spindles in the regulation of breathing is not certain, studies following deafferentation in man and other animals by dorsal root section clearly establish their contribution to normal ventilation. It has been suggested that the function of muscle spindles may be to provide a mechanism by which the main muscle mass compensates, by adjusting its force of contraction, to changes in the load upon it. Whether the system is designed to cope with sudden unanticipated loads or to control the accuracy of respiratory muscle movement against predicted loads (such as in singing or playing a wind instrument) is debatable.

SUMMARY

In the central nervous system, many regions have been identified that are involved in the normal control of respiration. The integrative

focus of nerve traffic from higher centers and the cranial nerves and the source of rhythmic respiration are in the medulla, although pontine structures are necessary for smooth regular breathing. Nerve impulses from the brain descend in the anterolateral portion of the spinal cord to the segmental level where the supraspinal messages are integrated with additional afferent information from proprioceptors in the respiratory muscles. The net result of all these processes is a signal to the main muscle via its alpha motoneuron and a subsequent relaying of the message to synergistic and antagonistic muscle groups.

Although many of the concepts described here were derived from animal experiments, additional supporting evidence is available in studies of patients with selective neurologic damage.[12,16] Table 9–1 lists the alterations in breathing that have been described in patients and correlated with specific lesions in the central nervous system. The disturbances range from changes in the pattern of breathing to forgetfulness of the need to breathe (Ondine's curse) to total or selective paralysis of respiratory muscle function. These observations strongly suggest that the general plan of the organization of the central nervous system is the same in man as in other mammals and demonstrate the debt owed by neurophysiology to clinical medicine.

PERIPHERAL CHEMORECEPTORS

Chemosensitive cells are the receptors for many physiologic phenomena: taste, smell, and the reactions to changes in blood gas and H^+ composition. The chemoreceptors in the kidney that regulate red blood cell mass by secreting erythropoietin and the chemosensitive mechanisms that cause pulmonary arterial vasocon-

Table 9–1 Alterations in Breathing Pattern Observed in Patients with Lesions Localized (Mainly) to Various Regions of the Central Nervous System*

LOCATION OF LESION	BREATHING PATTERN
Cerebral cortex	
Temporal lobe	Apnea (transient)
Diffuse	Cheyne-Stokes respiration
Diencephalon	
Pyramidal tracts	Cheyne-Stokes respiration
Mesencephalon and upper pons	
Medial reticular formation	Central neurogenic hyperventilation
Lower pons and medulla	
Around nucleus ambiguus	Apnea (permanent)
Medial reticular formation	Ondine's curse (loss of automaticity)
Spinal cord	
Anterolateral C$_2$ (reticulospinal pathway from cordotomy)	Ondine's curse
Dorsal root section (deafferentation)	Temporary muscle paralysis

*See also Guz[12] and Plum.[16]

striction in response to alveolar hypoxia to maintain a balance between ventilation and perfusion have already been discussed (Chapters 5 and 7). Additional groups of chemosensitive cells have been identified in various organs of the body by the use of chemical stimulants, such as phenyl diguanide, nicotine, and lobeline. However, these neurons are not necessarily chemoreceptors, and they probably subserve other physiologic functions (e.g., vagal sensory receptors). This section and the next will consider two well-defined chemosensitive systems that regulate breathing: the peripheral chemoreceptors in the carotid and aortic bodies that communicate with the brain via afferent nerves and the central chemoreceptors that are located within the brain itself. Both systems are vitally important in governing the physiologic responses to acute and chronic alterations in the concentration of O_2, CO_2, and H^+ in the bloodstream.

CAROTID AND AORTIC BODIES

Hyperventilation is one of the principal compensatory responses to acutely induced hypoxia. This reaction, which appears in all mammalian species, depends on specialized chemoreceptors that are strategically located to "taste" the chemical composition of circulating blood. Heymans and Heymans[17] discovered the chemoreceptor activities of the *carotid bodies* and later Comroe[18] established that the *aortic bodies* have similar functions.

The carotid bodies are nestled in the bifurcation of the common carotid arteries. They are well vascularized and their blood flow is high relative to their size. The carotid bodies contain two main cell types that surround the abundant blood vessels: type I cells (also called glomus cells, chief cells, or enclosed cells), which contain cytoplasmic vesicles with dense cores, and type II cells (also called supporting cells, sheath cells, enclosing cells, or sustentacular cells), which have thin cytoplasmic extensions that ensheath the type I cells. Interspersed among these cells are numerous axons and their terminals (Figure 9–5). There has been a controversy about the innervation of the carotid body and how nerve stimuli affect the function of the organ. Based on new information about the ultrastructure and neurophysio-

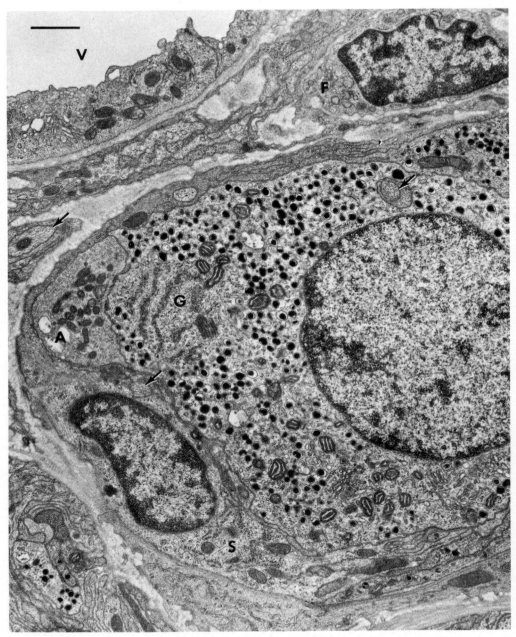

Figure 9–5 Electron photomicrograph of the carotid body of a cat. G = glomus cell (Type I cell) with abundant large dense-cored vesicles; S = sheath cell (Type II cell); A = afferent nerve ending with numerous synaptic vesicles; V = blood vessel; F = fibroblast (probable); and arrows = axons. Horizontal bar = 1 μm. (× 12,800. Courtesy of Dr. Donald McDonald.)

logic responses of the carotid body, previous concepts have had to be revised; it is now believed (Figure 9–6) that virtually all the nerve endings in contact with glomus cells are axons of afferent nerves that travel in a branch of the carotid sinus nerve. The few terminals on glomus cells that appear to be efferent (<5 per cent of the total) are from sympathetic fibers that reach the carotid body from the superior cervical ganglion. Other sympathetic nerves from the same source innervate blood vessels within the carotid body. The only efferent nerves that travel with the afferent axons in the sinus nerve are preganglionic parasympathetic fibers that innervate blood vessels.[19]

The structure of aortic chemore-

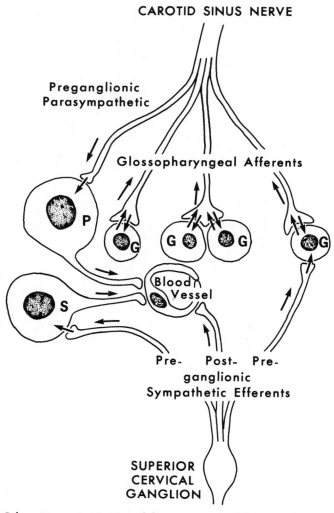

Figure 9–6 Schematic representation of the innervation of the carotid body. Afferent fibers of the glossopharyngeal (IX) nerve form reciprocal synapses with glomus cells (G); blood vessels are innervated by postganglionic fibers of parasympathetic (P) and sympathetic (S) origin; occasional preganglionic sympathetic fibers synapse with glomus cells. Arrows indicate the direction of impulses. (Adapted from information supplied by Dr. Donald McDonald.)

ceptors appears to vary in different species; remarkably little is known about them in man.[20] In cats, there are a few discrete organs that resemble tiny carotid bodies; however, in dogs, loose aggregates of glomus cells are often distributed in diffuse and irregular strands along branches of the vagus nerves and in the connective tissue below the aortic arch between the aorta and the pulmonary artery as shown in Figure 9–7.[21] The aortic chemoreceptors receive a systemic arterial blood supply from small branches of the aorta and brachiocephalic arteries; despite early reports to the contrary, recent studies of both newborn and adult dogs using dissection and injection techniques failed to reveal any glomus cells supplied by branches of the pulmonary artery; however, a pulmonary arterial blood supply to aortic bodies has been demonstrated in the human fetus and in the fetal and newborn kitten.[21] Afferent nerve impulses from the aortic chemoreceptors travel to the brain by way of the vagus nerve.

PHYSIOLOGIC FUNCTION

The chief stimulant to peripheral chemoreceptor activity is a reduction

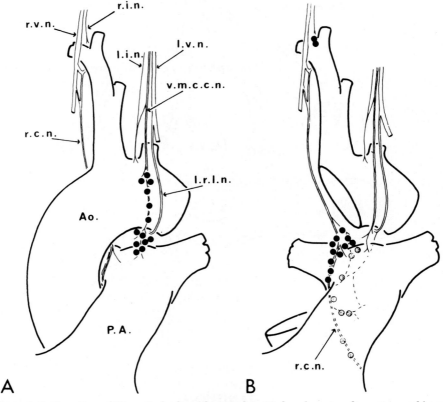

Figure 9–7 Location of 34 aortic bodies identified in 23 dogs by microdissection and histologic examination. *A*, Bodies innervated by the left vagus; *B*, bodies innervated by the right vagus. Ao = aorta; P.A. = pulmonary artery; r.v.n., l.v.n. = right and left vagus nerves; r.i.n., l.i.n. = right and left innominate nerves; l.r.l.n. = left recurrent laryngeal nerve; r.c.n. = recurrent cardiac nerve; v.m.c.c.n. = ventromedial cervical cardiac nerve. (From Coleridge, Coleridge, and Howe.[21] Reprinted by permission from the authors and The American Heart Association, Inc.)

in arterial P_{O_2}; however, the carotid and aortic bodies also respond to variations in arterial pH. The effects of changes in P_{CO_2} are controversial, but the results of experiments in which arterial P_{CO_2} was varied but pH was held constant (Figure 9–8) suggest that the influence of changes in arterial P_{CO_2} is mainly through its effect on pH.[22] When two stimuli affect the peripheral chemoreceptors simultaneously, the resulting change in ventilation is greater than the sum of the two independent responses added together. In other words, the response is synergistic.

Normally, a fall in arterial P_{O_2}, or other physiologic stimulus, affects all peripheral chemoreceptors at virtually the same time, and the ventilatory and circulatory responses represent the net effect of all the afferent impulses from the various receptors involved. However, the effects from stimulating one set of chemoreceptors are not necessarily the same as those from another, and in some circumstances the reactions may be mutually antagonistic. For example, when delay paths are interposed between the aortic and carotid chemoreceptors of the dog so that the responses from each can be examined separately, carotid body stimulation caused hyperpnea, bradycardia, and hypotension, in contrast to aortic body stimulation, which caused hyperpnea, tachycardia, and hypertension.[23]

Furthermore, there appear to be considerable species differences in the relative contributions from the

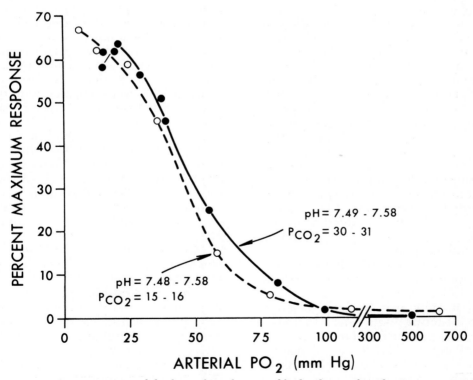

Figure 9–8   Average neural discharge from the carotid body of a cat, plotted as percent maximum activity, showing response to changing arterial P_{O_2} at two different values of P_{CO_2}; pH was kept nearly constant. (Adapted from Hornbein and Roos.[22] Reprinted by permission from the authors and publisher.)

two sets of peripheral chemoreceptors. The experiments performed on dogs and cats indicate that stimulation of both the aortic and carotid bodies increases the minute volume of ventilation; in contrast, studies in patients who have had their carotid bodies removed surgically in an effort to relieve bronchial asthma have failed to reveal an effect on ventilation of stimulating the remaining aortic bodies by induced mild to moderate hypoxia.[24] It appears, therefore, that in man the chemoreceptors in the carotid body are far more important in governing the physiologic responses, at least to hypoxia, than are those in aortic bodies.

All experiments on the chemical control of ventilation are bedeviled by the fact that any ventilatory response causes a new change in the chemical environment of both the central and peripheral chemoreceptors, which, in turn, also affects ventilation. This complicates attempts to sort out the separate contributions from peripheral and central chemoreceptor drives to a given respiratory stimulus; part of the difficulty can be avoided when studying acute hypoxia, by keeping arterial PCO_2 constant because only the peripheral chemoreceptors respond to sudden changes in PO_2. However, there is no completely satisfactory way of dissociating the effect of an induced change in PCO_2 from that of the resulting change in PO_2 and pH, although efforts have been made to take advantage of differences in the time of onset of the responses from peripheral and central receptors.[25]

The peripheral chemoreceptors are tonically active in normal persons breathing ambient air at sea level, and this activity can be suppressed by administering high concentrations of O_2. Whereas the effect of hyperoxia on ventilation is small and difficult to demonstrate, the effects of hypoxia are usually considerable and readily demonstrable. Breathing gas mixtures with steadily decreasing O_2 concentration produces a progressively increasing ventilatory response. Furthermore, as shown in Figure 9–9, less hyperventilation results from acute hypoxia when end-tidal PCO_2 is allowed to fall, as it normally does when ventilation increases, compared with when PCO_2 is not allowed to fall so low or is held constant by adding CO_2 to the inspired gas mixture.[26] The flattest ventilatory response curve occurs because the normal reduction in PCO_2 acts through the central chemoreceptors to depress ventilation and thus to offset much of the stimulating effect of acute hypoxia *per se* on the peripheral chemoreceptors. The suppressive effect of the fall in PCO_2 on ventilation is reduced or eliminated when CO_2 is added to the inspired gas mixture (Figure 9–9).

No one knows how the peripheral chemoreceptors respond to changes in their chemical environment, but changes in blood flow are an important modulating influence. The abundant vascular supply of the carotid bodies has already been mentioned, but how much of this blood flow actually bathes the sensory elements and how much is "wasted" through shunts is unknown. A large blood flow compared with the metabolic demands of an organ means that the arteriovenous difference "across" the organ is small and that the O_2 requirements of the cells may even be satisfied by the small amount of O_2 dissolved in arterial plasma. Sensitivity to PO_2 rather than to O_2 content (see Chapter 5) may explain why chemoreceptors are *not* stimulated in the presence of either anemia or CO-hemoglobin, conditions in which O_2 content is reduced but arterial PO_2 is normal.

The relationship between the blood flow to and the function of the carotid body can be shown by experiments in which a reduction in carotid artery perfusion pressure caused an increase in afferent nerve activity.[27] The clinical implication of these studies is that carotid body stimulation occurs during hypotension or shock or both, and presumably contributes to

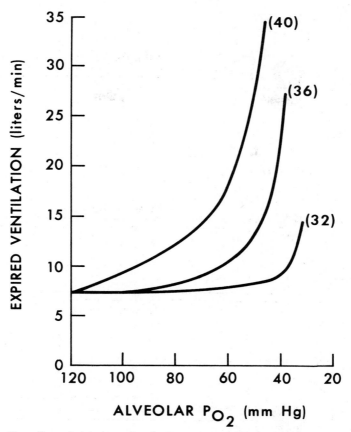

Figure 9–9   The effect of changing alveolar P_{O_2} on expired ventilation, while alveolar P_{CO_2}, was held constant at 40, 36, and 32 mm Hg. (Replotted from data of Weil, Byrne-Quinn, Sodal, Friesen, Underhill, Filley, and Grover.[26])

the cardiopulmonary responses that accompany these disorders. Stimulation of the sympathetic nerve fibers emerging from the superior cervical ganglion caused vasoconstriction of the carotid body and a small increase in afferent nerve traffic in the sinus nerve.[28] This response is analogous to the one that occurs in hypotension because both depend upon a reduction in the chemoreceptor blood flow.

Originally (Figure 9–10), it was believed that the glomus cells were the sensory elements of the carotid body and that they relayed their afferent messages to the brain through a branch of the glossopharyngeal nerve.

Biscoe[29] subsequently concluded from a series of neurophysiologic experiments that the fibers in the carotid body nerve were not all afferents but a mixture of afferents and efferents; furthermore, it was proposed that free nerve terminals and not glomus cells were the sensors of hypoxia (or other stimuli) and that the glomus cells served to modulate the interaction between afferent and efferent nerves. Thus, stimulation of efferent fibers leading to glomus cells causes the cells to degranulate and release a transmitter (possibly dopamine) that, in turn, depresses afferent nerve traffic. However, McDonald and Mitchell[19]

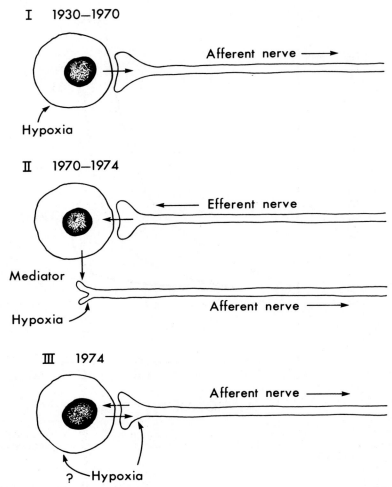

I   1930–1970

Afferent nerve ⟶

Hypoxia

II   1970–1974

Efferent nerve

Mediator

Hypoxia

Afferent nerve ⟶

III   1974

Afferent nerve ⟶

? Hypoxia

Figure 9–10 Schematic representation of the evolution of theories about carotid body innervation and site of stimulation by hypoxia. For details, see text.

were unable to identify efferent nerves leading to the carotid body but did find ultrastructural evidence of reciprocal synapses between the glomus cells and the adjacent afferent nerve terminal. A reciprocal synapse is a junction between two cells across which impulses travel in both directions (instead of the customary one-way path of most synapses): thus, the glomus cells and adjacent nerves appear capable of both receiving and transmitting information and constitute a local feedback system. Accord-

ingly, McDonald and Mitchell proposed that the nerve terminals are the chemosensitive elements and, in addition to sending afferent impulses to the brain, release transmitter that causes the neighboring glomus cell to depolarize and release its own transmitter (possibly dopamine) that depresses the initial response. The chief difference between the Biscoe and McDonald-Mitchell theories is that the presence of reciprocal synapses eliminates the need for efferent nerves to complete the feedback loop.

Evidence to support the position that the nerve terminals of afferent axons are the sensory receptors was also provided by Mitchell and co-workers.[30] These investigators found that neuromas could be made to develop at the central end of the severed sinus nerves of cats and that the neuromas responded to changes in PO_2, PCO_2, and cyanide in a way similar to that of the carotid body despite the absence of glomus cells.

Although there is no doubt that carotid bodies mediate the normal respiratory responses to acutely induced hypoxia in man, they do *not* play a role in regulating the usual ventilatory adjustments to exercise.[24] Moreover, carotid bodies are not essential for the adaptive responses to *chronic* hypoxia, as shown by studies in persons known to have a blunted or absent chemoreceptor response and in animals whose chemoreceptors have been denervated or removed.[25]

CENTRAL CHEMORECEPTORS

Total denervation of the peripheral chemoreceptors abolishes the hyperpnea of acutely induced hypoxia but does not eliminate, although it modifies, the ventilatory responses to changes in PCO_2 or pH. This early demonstration of the existence of respiratory chemoreceptors that are anatomically distinct from the carotid and aortic bodies was followed by numerous experiments that have established the location of chemosensitive regions within the central nervous system. Furthermore, there is abundant evidence that the activity of these chemoreceptors is closely reflected in and presumably indirectly governed by the chemical composition of CSF.

LOCATIÓN

Chemosensitive areas in the central nervous system have been searched for by directly applying or injecting certain chemicals in various locations and then observing whether ventilation is stimulated or depressed. Many of the early experiments indicated that the neuronal structures that were directly affected by drugs were located mainly in the same areas from which respiratory activity could be evoked by electrical stimulation, i.e., the "respiratory center" in the ventromedial portion of the medulla. However, it is now believed that the hyperpnea produced by the injection of chemicals into the brain substance in the ventromedial reticular formation is nonspecific and that neurons with respiratory periodicity, the "true" centers, are located more laterally and dorsally (Figure 9–2).

The results of early studies were not entirely consistent, and it was also observed that ventilatory responses could be elicited by injection of HCO_3^- into regions of the medulla other than those that were responsive to electrical stimulation.[31] These and other related observations raised the possibility that there were multiple chemosensitive regions in the brain. The location and behavior of central chemoreceptors were considerably clarified by the significant contributions of Leusen,[32,33] who showed that changes in the composition of artificial CSF used to perfuse the brain from the third or lateral cerebral ventricles to the cisterna magna (ventriculocisternal perfusion) had a marked influence on ventilation: increasing $[H^+]$ stimulated ventilation, whereas lowering $[H^+]$ depressed it. These results have been confirmed and extended by many investigators and form the basis of the belief that the chemosensitive elements of the central nervous system are within "reach" of the CSF.

Chemosensitive areas have been identified in the ventrolateral regions[34] and elsewhere[35] on the surface of the medulla. However, there is no morphologic evidence of specialized receptor cells in these locations, and it is likely that the effects of applied chemical substances and changes in the CSF itself are directly sensed by neurons that, in turn, influence breathing. Just how superficial the chemosensitive structures are is a matter of dispute: according to some, they are located close to (within 1 to 2 mm) the surface of the medulla,[36] but others believe they may be more deeply situated but still affected by the diffusion of substances from the CSF.[37]

PHYSIOLOGIC FUNCTION

Experiments carried out in the 1920s revealed that intravenous administration of HCl caused hyperpnea, and although blood pH decreased, CSF pH rose. Similarly, administration of $NaHCO_3$ caused a rise in arterial pH but a fall in CSF pH. The change in CSF and arterial pHs in *opposite* directions during infusion of nonvolatile acids or bases differed strikingly from the demonstration that pHs from the two sites change in the *same* direction when P_{CO_2} is altered.[38]

An explanation for these phenomena was provided by the even earlier experiments by Jacobs[39,40] on the relative diffusibility of CO_2, H^+, and HCO_3^- across biologic membranes. Jacobs demonstrated that CO_2 diffused readily across cell membranes and, consequently, immediately lowered intracellular pH. In contrast, H^+ and HCO_3^- are poorly diffusible ions, so adding them to the bloodstream has a small and very delayed effect on intracellular pH. The rapid diffusion of CO_2 and slow diffusion of H^+ and HCO_3^- account for the different ventilatory stimuli that reach the central chemoreceptors in patients with respiratory and nonrespiratory acid-base disorders. It should be pointed out that even though CSF is an extracellular fluid, it is separated from the bloodstream by a biologic membrane, the blood-brain barrier. Thus, CO_2 has rapid access to CSF and affects its pH, but H^+ and HCO_3^- are excluded temporarily.

It is now agreed that $[H^+]$ and $[HCO_3^-]$ in the CSF change slowly after changes in blood pH in patients with nonrespiratory acidosis or alkalosis, and the slowness of response stands in marked contrast to the immediate change in CSF pH that accompanies alterations in blood P_{CO_2} in such patients. These observations also indicate that the ventilatory responses in patients with *acute* nonrespiratory acidosis or alkalosis are not mediated by central chemoreceptors, because CSF pH changes are in the wrong direction, and therefore must be attributed to chemosensitive mechanisms elsewhere, presumably the peripheral chemoreceptors.

CARBON DIOXIDE RESPONSE TESTS

Obviously, it would be desirable to be able to examine the responsiveness of the central chemoreceptors in patients who are suspected of having abnormalities in their control of breathing. An ideal test would measure the changes in ventilation that resulted from a given change in pH within the chemosensitive cells, but there are many theoretic and practical reasons why such a test cannot be designed. One approach to the problem has been through the use of CO_2 response curves; although these have proved useful, they have certain limitations. (1) The stimulus cannot be quantified precisely because it is impossible to measure pH in or even near the central receptors; (2) the peripheral chemoreceptors as well as the central chemoreceptors are stimulated by the pH effects of breathing CO_2; (3) there is a wide range of "normality"; and (4) the response is modified, and thus difficult to interpret, by changes in the mechanics of breathing.

A CO_2 response curve is obtained by measuring ventilation while the subject breathes increasing concentrations of CO_2 in O_2 (to remove any effect of changing P_{O_2} on ventilation). The CO_2 concentration of the inspired air is raised by rebreathing in a closed system or switching to mixtures with stepwise increases. Some representative CO_2 response curves are shown in Figure 9–11. The responsiveness to CO_2 is reflected in the increment in ventilation for a given change in PCO_2 or, in other words, the slope of the line. Figure 9–11 also demonstrates that a family of CO_2 response curves can be obtained by performing CO_2 tests at different values of inspired PO_2; at a given alveolar PCO_2, expired ventilation is greater when breathing a hypoxic gas mixture ($PO_2 = 40$ mm Hg) than when breathing an enriched gas mixture ($PO_2 > 600$ mm Hg). The family of lines usually (but not always) converges to a point (B) on the abscissa. The differences in the steepness of the three lines after acclimatization compared with that before acclimatization are accounted for, in part, by alterations in the buffering capacity of CSF.

CEREBROSPINAL FLUID

The ultimate response to the various afferent and direct stimuli that affect ventilation will be considered in the final section of this chapter. The central chemoreceptors play an important role in determining the net reaction and appear to respond to changes in pH in their immediate environment. Because CSF is a good mirror of brain extracellular fluid, it provides a convenient source of information about what is "going on" centrally. It is essential, therefore, to have some understanding about how CSF is formed, its chemical composition, and the effect of various systemic disturbances on CSF pH. Excellent reviews have been published about CSF and the regulation of respiration.[36,41]

It is generally agreed that CSF is formed mainly in the choroid plexus of the lateral cerebral ventricles. The

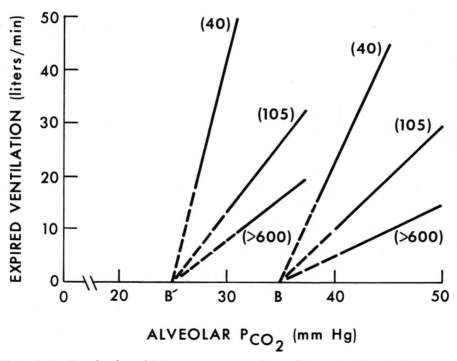

Figure 9–11 Two families of CO_2 response curves obtained at constant alveolar PO_2 values of 40, 105, and >600 mm Hg. Extrapolation of the three lines converge to point B in a subject studied at sea level and to point B' in the same subject after acclimatization at high altitude.

fluid flows through the ventricles and aqueduct into the subarachnoid space surrounding the brain and spinal cord. The CSF is absorbed into the venous bloodstream through arachnoid villi that protrude into cerebral venous sinuses.

Secretion of CSF is mainly determined by the activity of enzymes, chiefly carbonic anhydrase and adenosine triphosphatases, in the choroid plexus and brain tissue[41]; inhibition of these enzymes reduces the formation of both CSF and brain extracellular fluid. (Hence, the use of acetazolamide, a carbonic anhydrase inhibitor, in conditions associated with hydrocephalus and increased intercranial pressure.)

The fluid elaborated by the choroid plexus is not an ultrafiltrate of plasma, and the composition of CSF is modified as it flows through the cerebral ventricles.[41] These differences present a problem when trying to establish the exact composition of the CSF overlying the chemoreceptors. Furthermore, most studies (but not all) have revealed differences in P_{CO_2} and pH between cisternal CSF and lumbar fluid[42]; these differences tend to be increased during unsteady state conditions, so that lumbar CSF should not be relied upon as a source of valid information about central chemoreceptor stimulation when arterial P_{CO_2} is changing.

The concentrations of various substances in arterial blood and CSF (lumbar puncture) are given in Table 9–2. With the important exceptions of P_{CO_2}, HCO_3^-, and pH, the concentrations of the other components of CSF remain remarkably constant; even substantial variations in serum levels of electrolytes induce only small changes in CSF content.[41]

The pH of CSF is lower than that of arterial blood (Table 9–2). Because the $[HCO_3^-]$ values in CSF and blood are normally about the same, the lower pH in CSF can be accounted for mainly by the 7 to 9 mm Hg higher P_{CO_2} in CSF. Moreover, HCO_3^- is the only buffer of consequence in CSF, which means that CSF pH changes are completely governed by the relationship between CSF HCO_3^- and P_{CO_2} and can be expressed by the Henderson-Hasselbalch equation:

$$pH = pK + \log \frac{[HCO_3^-]}{[\alpha \cdot P_{CO_2}]}, \quad (1)$$

where α equals the solubility of CO_2 in CSF. This equation is exactly the same as Equation 14 in Chapter 8, but it should be pointed out that the pKs and solubilities differ between CSF and blood: those for CSF are 6.130 and 0.0312 and those for blood are 6.10 and 0.0301, respectively.

The chief role of CO_2 in deter-

Table 9–2   Normal Values (Mean ± SD) for the Composition of Cerebrospinal Fluid (CSF) and Arterial Blood

SUBSTANCE	CSF	ARTERIAL BLOOD
Na	141.2 ± 6.0 mEq/L	140.6 ± 7.2 mEq/L
K	2.96 ± 0.45 mEq/L	4.46 ± 0.45 mEq/L
Ca	2.43 ± 0.05 mEq/L	5.23 ± 0.27 mEq/L
Mg	2.40 ± 0.14 mEq/L	1.94 ± 0.15 mEq/L
Cl	127 ± 3 mEq/L	103 ± 3 mEq/L
HCO$_3$	21.5 ± 1.2 mEq/L	24.8 ± 1.4 mEq/L
Protein	15–45 mg/100 ml	6.6–8.6 gm/100 ml
Glucose	45–70 mg/100 ml	70–105 mg/100 ml
P$_{CO_2}$	50.2 ± 2.6 mm Hg	39.5 ± 1.2 mm Hg
pH	7.336 ± 0.012	7.409 ± 0.018

mining CSF pH, owing to the diffusibility of CO_2 across the blood-brain barrier, has already been emphasized. It can be shown that of the four variables that affect the amount of CO_2 in the brain and CSF (cerebral blood flow, CO_2 production, and the CO_2 contents of arterial and venous blood), the principal determinant of CSF P_{CO_2} in normal subjects and most patients is arterial CO_2 content. This is because brain metabolism is mainly aerobic and stable under varying conditions and because the cerebral arteriovenous difference is usually small so changes in blood flow have little effect on venous CO_2 content. Furthermore, because the CO_2 equilibrium curves are reasonably linear in the physiologic range, arterial CO_2 content is linearly related to arterial P_{CO_2}. The value of this relationship can be appreciated by recognizing that any deviations in arterial P_{CO_2} from normal levels promptly change CSF P_{CO_2} (and pH) in the direction that stimulates or depresses ventilation in an attempt to correct the abnormality in P_{CO_2}.

The discussion thus far has considered only the effects on CSF pH of *acute* changes in arterial P_{CO_2}. It is now well established that in patients with *chronic* acid-base disorders of both respiratory and nonrespiratory origin, CSF pH returns nearly to normal levels (7.34) regardless of the level of arterial P_{CO_2}. The only way that CSF pH can be restored in the face of sustained increases or decreases in CSF P_{CO_2} is through proportionate changes in CSF HCO_3^- that restore HCO_3^-:P_{CO_2} to a normal ratio.* Despite general agreement that this phenomenon occurs, and there is abundant clinical and experimental evidence that it does, there is considerable dispute concerning the mechanisms by which the changes in CSF HCO_3^-

---

*Reference to Equation 1 shows why reestablishing the ratio after P_{CO_2} changes is essential to restoring pH.

are brought about. All studies have indicated that changes in CSF HCO_3^- are independent of those that take place in plasma, but it is uncertain whether CSF HCO_3^- is controlled by an active transport process or responds passively to changes in the composition of the blood perfusing the brain.[41]

Once CSF HCO_3^- changes have occurred and pH is restored toward normal, the central chemoreceptors are reset to operate at the new level of ventilation. Moreover, ventilation tends to persist at the new level despite removal or correction of the stimulus that affected ventilation in the first place; the persistence of ventilation is also attributable to the slowness with which CSF HCO_3^- can change. Variations in CSF-buffering capacity modify the sensitivity to changes in P_{CO_2} and account for the differences in the slopes of the CO_2 response curves shown in Figure 9–11. When CSF HCO_3^- is low but pH is normal (e.g., in the acclimatized high altitude sojourner), any reduction in ventilation causes CO_2 retention, which in turn causes a greater reduction in CSF pH and stimulus to ventilation than would occur if CSF HCO_3^- were higher. Hence, the CO_2 response curve is steeper.

INTEGRATED RESPONSES

Breathing is regulated on a moment to moment basis, primarily in response to changing metabolic needs (see also Chapter 10 on Exercise). The regulatory systems also adjust breathing to minimize the effects of stresses that threaten the O_2, CO_2, and H^+ composition of blood and tissues such as breathing air with a low P_{O_2} and respiratory and nonrespiratory acid-base disturbances. The extent of adjustments in blood and CSF differs, depending upon whether the conditions are acute or chronic. The usual responses to acute and chronic hypoxia and acid-base abnormalities are shown in Table 9–3.

HYPOXIA

The usual response to acute hypoxia is an increase in the rate and depth of breathing. Acute hypoxic stimuli are not common in everyday life but are experienced by normal persons upon a change from low to high altitudes and can be produced in the laboratory by giving subjects low concentrations of O_2 to breathe. Patients with acute pulmonary disorders may suddenly become hypoxic, but in these conditions numerous afferent systems are stimulated and the ventilatory response is not due solely to hypoxia. (The multiplicity of receptors involved is demonstrated clinically by the failure of acutely hypoxic patients to breathe normally when their hypoxia is corrected by the administration of high concentrations of O_2.)

A reduction in arterial PO_2 is de-

Table 9–3 Relative Magnitude (0 to 3[+]) of the Changes in CSF and Arterial Blood pH in Acute and Chronic Acid-base Changes in Man

CONDITION	ARTERIAL pH	CSF pH
Nonrespiratory acidosis		
Acute	3+ Decrease	2+ Increase
Chronic	2+ Decrease	Normal
Nonrespiratory alkalosis		
Acute	3+ Increase	2+ Decrease
Chronic	2+ Increase	Normal
Respiratory acidosis		
Acute	3+ Decrease	3+ Decrease
Chronic	<2+ Decrease	1+ Decrease
Respiratory alkalosis		
Acute	3+ Increase	3+ Increase
Chronic	0-1+ Increase	Normal

tected by the peripheral chemoreceptors and, as indicated, primarily by the carotid bodies in man. Within a few seconds of exposure to low O_2, chemoreceptor activity results in an increase in ventilation; however, the resulting decrease in arterial PCO_2 quickly induces a decrease in CSF and brain extracellular PCO_2. Consequently, brain pH increases, which causes central inhibition of ventilation. Therefore, the acute ventilatory response to hypoxia, which is completed within minutes of exposure, represents a balance between the stimulating effects of hypoxia on the peripheral chemoreceptors and the inhibiting effects of hypocapnia on the central chemoreceptors.[25]

If the hypoxic stimulus is unremitting, additional mechanisms are activated that govern acclimatization. These are mainly adaptive because they improve arterial PO_2, enhance O_2 transport, and restore arterial pH toward normal. However, reductions in plasma volume and myocardial contractility also occur which are detrimental because they impair circulatory responses and maximal O_2 uptake during exercise.[43]

Ventilatory acclimatization is evident a few hours after exposure to sustained hypoxia and is complete within one to three days. Following the initial rapid reduction in CSF PCO_2 from peripheral chemoreceptor-induced hyperventilation, CSF $[HCO_3^-]$ begins to fall slowly. Accordingly, CSF pH also falls toward normal, which removes part of the central suppression of ventilation. Thus, a new balance between opposing chemoreceptor drives to ventilation is reached that permits an increase in ventilation. This adjustment is followed by a new series of incremental changes until finally the complete ventilatory response to chronic hypoxia is evident. Thereafter, the increased ventilation is maintained in part by continued peripheral chemoreceptor stimuli and in part because the changes in CSF HCO_3^- have reset the CO_2 chemosensitive cells to sustain the new level.

The differences between the acute and chronic adjustments to hypoxia can be demonstrated nicely by administering high concentrations of O_2, and thus removing the hypoxic stimulus, during the two conditions: in acute hypoxia, breathing is restored to normal rates, but in chronic hypoxia, it is only slightly reduced owing to the resetting of the CO_2-chemosensitive mechanism.

The magnitude of the ventilatory response to acute hypoxia varies widely in apparently normal persons. Besides those subjects who demonstrate what may be viewed as the low end of the continuum of normal responses to acute hypoxia, persons who were born at high altitude characteristically have an absent or blunted response.[44] On the basis of a similar lack of responsiveness to acute hypoxia in patients with surgically corrected cyanotic congenital heart disease,[45] although there is contradictory evidence about this group,[46] it was postulated that the defect is acquired, possibly within the first few years of life, and is not genetically determined.[44,45]

Despite failure to respond to acute hypoxia, persons born and living at high altitude hyperventilate during exposure to chronic hypoxia, though not quite as much as sojourners acclimatized to the same altitude; moreover, the CSF pHs in the high altitude natives are the same as in the sojourners. The sequence of changes in the CSF HCO_3^- must be different in the two groups because the response in sojourners is believed to be initiated by peripheral chemoreceptor-induced hyperventilation, which is obviously an impossibility in the high altitude natives in whom this capability is absent. It has been postulated, but not proved, that the fall in CSF HCO_3^- and stimulus to hyperventilation in those persons without an acute response depends upon the local production of lactate by the brain when it becomes hypoxic.[25]

Insensitivity to hypoxia has been proposed as the explanation for the failure of some patients with hypoxia from chronic bronchitis and obesity (Pickwickian syndrome) to ventilate appropriately. Failure to increase ventilation contributes to CO_2 retention, polycythemia, and cor pulmonale. It is not known whether the defect in the patients is acquired as part of their disease or whether their failure to hyperventilate is inherited and they belong to the low end of the normal frequency response curve.

RESPIRATORY ACIDOSIS

Although acute experiments have been performed using human subjects, the responses to pure long-standing CO_2 retention have not been examined in normal man. Data are available from studies in patients with ventilatory failure and experimental animals given CO_2 to breathe.[47,48] These conditions are not strictly comparable, but the results of the investigations provide a framework of understanding about the sequence of events in respiratory acidosis.

As expected, dogs breathing a gas mixture containing 12 per cent CO_2 developed an increase in arterial P_{CO_2} that was rapidly reflected by an increase in CSF P_{CO_2}. The resulting fall in pH in both fluid compartments caused brisk hyperventilation by stimulating peripheral and central chemoreceptors and also actuated mechanisms in the kidney and brain that regulate HCO_3^- in the blood and CSF. Figure 9-12 depicts the time course of the rises in $[HCO_3^-]$ in arterial blood plasma and cisternal CSF in dogs after exposure to 12 per cent CO_2.[48] The initial increase in CSF HCO_3^- is a little slower than in blood, but the maximum CSF response is achieved sooner—by 24 hours in the CSF com-

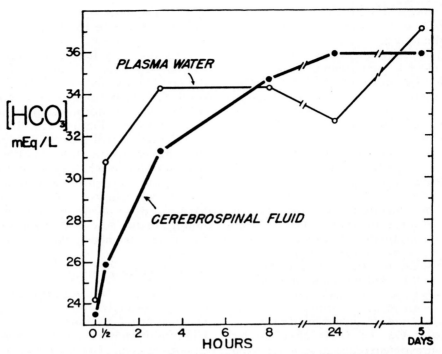

Figure 9-12 Time course of the changes in the concentration of bicarbonate in cerebrospinal fluid and in plasma water before (zero time) and during exposure to 12 per cent CO_2. (From Bleich, Berkman, and Schwartz.[48] Reprinted by permission from the authors and publisher.)

pared with three to five days in the blood (see also Figure 8–11). Despite the increase in CSF [HCO_3^-], CSF pH is not restored to normal but remains more acid than usual. This is true not only in experimental animals but also in patients.[47] The magnitude of the deviation of CSF pH from normality appears to depend upon the severity of the acidemia as reflected in arterial blood. Ordinarily, when the fall in arterial pH is less than 7.30, CSF pH remains stable, but when arterial pH falls below 7.30, CSF pH tends to become progressively lower than normal levels.[47] In patients with pulmonary diseases, an additional factor is the magnitude of any coexisting hypoxia that might affect ventilation independently.

The rise in CSF HCO_3^- that occurs, whether it restores CSF pH to normal or not, has two deleterious

consequences: it reduces central chemoreceptor drive to ventilation and it suppresses CO_2 responsiveness. The effect of the former is to allow arterial P_{CO_2} to rise even higher than it was at the outset, and the effect of the latter is to lower the sensitivity to any incremental increases in P_{CO_2}. These disadvantages are compounded because any rise in arterial P_{CO_2} is accompanied by a reciprocal fall in arterial P_{O_2}.

It is difficult to appreciate any "wisdom of the body" in these adjustments. Perhaps the respiratory control system evolved in order to defend the organism against the physiologic stresses of hypoxia and nonrespiratory acid-base disorders, which are much more common insults among animals than chronic CO_2 retention. The legacy inherited by patients with advanced chronic obstructive pulmonary disease can thus be viewed as the product, albeit an undesirable one, of the adaptive responses that usually serve to protect the biochemical environment of the body.

Assessment of the individual factors that contribute to respiratory regulation and CSF composition in patients with chronic CO_2 retention is complicated by the multiple effects of their underlying diseases. For example, the presence of hypoxia increases the total drive to ventilation, but increased work of breathing in patients with chronic bronchitis and emphysema decreases their capability of responding to the stimulus. Furthermore, there is considerable uncertainty about whether the impairment of ventilatory control that is evident in these patients is an acquired characteristic of their disorder or whether the patients are inherently "nonresponders."

The diminished CO_2 sensitivity that accompanies CO_2 retention removes the hyperventilatory response that ordinarily results from slight increases in PCO_2; as a result, the main stimulus to breathe in patients with hypercapnia from chronic pulmonary disease comes from their arterial hypoxia. This dependency is responsible for the clinical observation that elimination of the hypoxic drive to ventilate by the administration of high concentrations of O_2 depresses breathing and may cause CO_2 narcosis or even death. Part of the rationale of "low flow O_2," therapy for patients with chronic pulmonary diseases and respiratory failure is based on avoiding O_2-induced suppression of breathing.

RESPIRATORY ALKALOSIS

Acute hyperventilation lowers arterial PCO_2 and, secondarily, CSF PCO_2. Consequently, CSF pH rises and the central chemoreceptor drive diminishes in an effort to inhibit ventilation and restore PCO_2 to normal values in both blood and brain. If the initial hyperventilation is sustained, CSF HCO_3^- falls and CSF pH returns to normal levels; these changes occur faster than the comparable ones in blood.

Chronic hypocapnia is an adaptive response to hypoxia in normal persons living at high altitude. Sustained hyperventilation also occurs in patients with chronic infiltrative pulmonary diseases (presumably not from hypoxia but from afferent receptor drive), or with central nervous system or psychogenic disorders. Regardless of the cause, as already emphasized in a previous section (Hypoxia), once the compensatory adjustments are complete, CO_2 sensitivity is increased and ventilation tends to persist at the newly established level.

NONRESPIRATORY ACIDOSIS

Interpretation of data from studies of CSF composition in patients with nonrespiratory acidosis is complicated by uncertainties about the presence of a steady state at the time the specimens were obtained and by the lack of control measurements in the same subjects. Despite these shortcomings, there is general agreement that CSF pH is remarkably stable in patients with chronic nonrespiratory acidosis.[41] (This is not true for *acute* nonrespiratory acidosis, discussed later.) The constancy of CSF pH during prolonged acidemia means that CSF HCO_3^- must have changed proportionately to any reduction in CSF PCO_2. As emphasized previously, CSF HCO_3^- does not change nearly as fast as PCO_2, and the balance between the two variables that is encountered in nonrespiratory acidosis can be attributed to the timing of the sampling procedure and to the gradual rate of evolution of the underlying disorder that allows the mechanisms that regulate CSF HCO_3^- to keep pace with the slow reductions in CSF PCO_2 caused by peripheral chemoreceptor-induced hyperventilation.

Sudden acidemia is an uncommon clinical event but results occasionally from ingestion of certain poisons (methyl alcohol and propylene glycol) and from massive loss of base from the gastrointestinal tract (cholera); acute acidosis is easy to reproduce in the laboratory and has been studied extensively. The responses in both patients and experimental animals appear to be identical.

A rapid lowering of arterial pH stimulates peripheral chemoreceptors and causes hyperventilation. This results in a lowering of arterial and CSF PCO_2 and an inhibition of the central drive to respiration similar to that which occurs in acute hypoxia. Adaptation to chronic acidemia then proceeds in exactly the same manner as described for sustained hypoxia, i.e., by lowering of CSF HCO_3^- and pH, which allows a further increase in ventilation. Thus, the hyperventilation that develops in response to acute acidemia occurs in two phases: immediate and delayed. In contrast, the hyperventilation that accompanies prolonged, slow increases in blood $[H^+]$ is a more gradual and continuous (one phase) reaction.

Regardless of whether the nonrespiratory acidosis has an acute or a slow onset, once the blood pH is stable and the adjustments in CSF HCO_3^- are complete, ventilation tends to remain at the newly established increased level despite correction of the blood component of the acidemia. This response depends upon the heightened CO_2 sensitivity of the central chemoreceptors and is the same as that which perpetuates hyperpnea for a few days after an acclimatized subject descends from high altitude. This mechanism accounts for the persistent hyperventilation and respiratory alkalosis that have been observed after treatment of renal acidosis by dialysis[49] or diabetic acidosis by fluids and insulin.[50]

NONRESPIRATORY ALKALOSIS

There are only a few studies of CSF composition in patients or experimental subjects with nonrespiratory alkalemia, and in most of them the alkalemia was not severe. Moreover, it should be recalled (Chapter 8) that whether or not arterial PCO_2 changes at all appears to depend upon the cause of the condition. Alveolar hypoventilation developed in subjects made alkalotic by the administration of buffers and ethacrynic acid, but no change in arterial PCO_2 occurred in the same subjects when they were given thiazide diuretics or aldosterone.[51]

In general, CSF pH in patients with nonrespiratory alkalosis, as in those with respiratory acidosis, is within the normal range. This indicates that CSF HCO_3^- rises to offset any increase in CSF PCO_2 that may have occurred. The results of experiments in dogs agree with the observations in patients that CSF pH remains nearly normal during chronic nonrespiratory acidosis.[52] However, different conclusions have been reached about the changes that occur in nonrespiratory *alkalosis;* in contrast to a stable pH in man, slight but significant increases have been demonstrated in dogs. Figure 9–13 reproduces the results of experiments in dogs in which particular care was taken to ensure that a steady state was present[52]; the CSF pH was unchanged during acidosis, but rose during alkalosis. A change of this magnitude could easily have been overlooked in clinical alkalemia owing to the inherent difficulties in obtaining satisfactory studies in patients; the possibility also exists of a species variation in the responses to nonrespiratory alkalosis. In either case, it is clear that more data are needed for both blood and CSF composition in man under carefully controlled conditions to allow a more complete analysis of the factors that regulate CSF $[HCO_3^-]$.

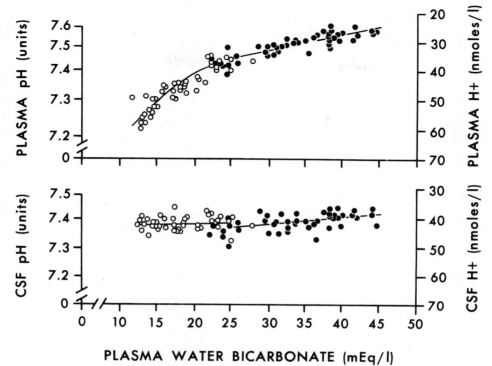

Figure 9–13 Cerebrospinal fluid (CSF) and plasma pH and H⁺ activity in nonrespiratory acidosis (O) and alkalosis (●) and their relation to plasma bicarbonate in dogs. (Replotted from Chazan, Appleton, London, and Schwartz.[52] Reprinted by permission from the authors and publisher.)

SUMMARY

Although much has been learned in recent years about the control of respiration, much more remains to be discovered. Important deficiencies remain in our understanding about regulatory processes in health and disease. For example, there are major uncertainties concerning the mechanisms that underlie the coupling of ventilation to the intensity of muscular exercise. Similarly, there are many mysteries enshrouding the various converging pathways that lead from disturbances of respiration, circulation, and neuromuscular and central nervous system functions to the symptom of *dyspnea*. The recent investigations of the role of abnormal afferent impulses in the pathogenesis of dyspnea are a useful beginning, but considerably more information is needed to clarify the mechanisms that lead from intrapulmonary receptor stimulation to the conscious perception of breathlessness.

REFERENCES

1. Pitts, R. F.: Organization of the respiratory center. Physiol. Rev., 26:609-630, 1946.
2. Batsel, H. L.: Localization of bulbar respiratory center by microelectrode sounding. Exp. Neurol., 9:410-426, 1964.
3. Wang, S. C., and Ngai, S. H.: General organization of central respiratory mechanisms. *In* Fenn, W. O., and Rahn, H. (eds.): Handbook of Physiology, Section 3. Respiration. Vol. I. Washington, D. C., American Physiological Society, 1964, pp. 487-505.
4. Baker, A. B., Matzke, H. A., and Brown, J. R.: Poliomyelitis. III. Bulbar poliomyelitis;

a study of medullary function. Arch. Neurol. Psychol., 63:257-281, 1950.

5. Batsel, H. L.: Some functional properties of bulbar respiratory units. Exp. Neurol., 11:341-366, 1965.

6. Campbell, E. J. M., Agostoni, E., and Newsom Davis, J.: The Respiratory Muscles. Mechanics and Neural Control. Philadelphia, W. B. Saunders Company, 1970, pp. 234-270.

7. Duffin, J.: The functional organization of respiratory neurones: a review. Canad. Anaesth. Soc. J., 19:1-7, 1972.

8. Kahn, N., and Wang, S. C.: Electrophysiologic basis for pontine apneustic center and its role in integration of the Hering-Breuer reflex. J. Neurophysiol., 30:301-318, 1967.

9. Magoun, H. W.: Caudal and cephalic influences of the brain stem reticular formation. Physiol. Rev., 30:459-474, 1950.

10. Hugelin, A., and Cohen, M. I.: The reticular activating system and respiratory regulation in the cat. Ann. N. Y. Acad. Sci., 109:586-603, 1963.

11. Guz, A., Noble, M. I. M., Widdicombe, J. G., Trenchard, D., Mushin, W. W., and Makey, A. R.: The role of vagal and glossopharyngeal afferent nerves in respiratory sensation, control of breathing and arterial pressure regulation in conscious man. Clin. Sci., 30:161-170, 1966.

12. Guz, A.: Clinical aspects of the nervous control of breathing. Acta Physiol. Pol., 22 (Suppl. 2):445-458, 1971.

13. Guz, A., Noble, M. I. M., Eisele, J. H., and Trenchard, D.: Experimental results of vagal block in cardiopulmonary disease. In Porter, R. (ed.): Ciba Foundation Symposium: Breathing: Hering-Breuer Centenary Symposium. London, J. & A. Churchill, 1970, pp. 315-329.

14. Trenchard, D., Gardner, D., and Guz, A.: Role of pulmonary vagal afferent nerve fibres in the development of rapid shallow breathing in lung inflammation. Clin. Sci., 42:251-263, 1972.

15. Jain, S. K., Trenchard, D., Reynolds, F., Noble, M. I. M., and Guz, A.: The effect of local anaesthesia of the airway on respiratory reflexes in the rabbit. Clin. Sci., 44:519-538, 1973.

16. Plum, F.: Neurological integration of behavioural and metabolic control of breathing. In Porter, R. (ed.): Ciba Foundation Symposium: Breathing: Hering-Breuer Centenary Symposium. London, J. & A. Churchill, 1970, pp. 159-175.

17. Heymans, C, Bouckaert, J. J., and Dautrebande, L.: Sinus carotidien et réflexes respiratoires. II. Influences respiratoires réflexes de l'acidose, de l' alcalose, de l'anhydride carbonique, de l'ion hydrogène et de l'anoxémie. Sinus carotidien

et échanges respiratoires dans les poumons et au dela des poumons. Arch. Int. Pharmacodyn. Ther. 39:400-450, 1930.

18. Comroe, J. H., Jr.: The location and function of the chemoreceptors of the aorta. Am. J. Physiol., 127:176-191, 1939.

19. McDonald, D. M. and Mitchell, R. A.: The innervation of glomus cells, ganglion cells, and blood vessels in the rat carotid body: a quantitative ultrastructural analysis. J. Neurocytol, 4:1-77, 1975.

20. Comroe, J. H., Jr.: Peripheral chemoreceptors. In Fenn, W. O., and Rahn, H. (eds.): Handbook of Physiology, Section 3. Respiration. Vol. I. Washington, D. C., American Physiological Society, 1964, pp. 557-583.

21. Coleridge, H. M., Coleridge, J. C. G., and Howe, A.: Thoracic chemoreceptors in the dog. A histological and electrophysiological study of the location, innervation and blood supply of the aortic bodies. Circ. Res., 26:235-247, 1970.

22. Hornbein, T. F., and Roos, A.: Specificity of H ion concentration as a carotid chemoreceptor stimulus. J. Appl. Physiol., 18:580-584, 1963.

23. Comroe, J. H., Jr., and Mortimer, L.: The respiratory and cardiovascular responses of temporally separated aortic and carotid bodies to cyanide, nicotine, phenyldiguanide and serotonin. J. Pharmacol. Exp. Ther., 146:33-41, 1964.

24. Lugliani, R., Whipp, B. J., Seard, C., and Wasserman, K.: Effect of bilateral carotidbody resection on ventilatory control at rest and during exercise in man. New Eng. J. Med., 285:1105-1114, 1971.

25. Sorensen, S. C.: The chemical control of ventilation. Acta Physiol. Scand., 361 (Suppl.):1-72, 1971.

26. Weil, J. V., Byrne-Quinn, E., Sodal, I. E., Friesen, W. O., Underhill, B., Filley, G. F., and Grover, R. F.: Hypoxic ventilatory drive in normal man. J. Clin. Invest., 49:1061-1072, 1970.

27. Landgren, S., and Neil, E.: Chemoreceptor impulse activity following haemorrhage. Acta Physiol. Scand., 23:158-167, 1951.

28. Eyzaguirre, C., and Lewin, J.: The effect of sympathetic stimulation on carotid nerve activity. J. Physiol. (Lond.), 159:251–267, 1961.

29. Biscoe, T. J.: Carotid body: structure and function. Physiol. Rev., 51:437-495, 1971.

30. Mitchell, R. A., Sinha, A. K., and McDonald, D. M.: Chemoreceptive properties of regenerated endings of the carotid sinus nerve. Brain Res., 43:681-685, 1972.

31. Liljestrand, A.: Respiratory reactions elicited from medulla oblongata of the cat. Acta Physiol. Scand., 29(Suppl. 106):321-393, 1953.

32. Leusen, I. R.: Chemosensitivity of the re-

spiratory center. Influence of CO_2 in the cerebral ventricles on respiration. Am. J. Physiol., *176*:39-44, 1954.

33. Leusen, I. R.: Chemosensitivity of the respiratory center. Influence of changes in the H^+ and total buffer concentrations in the cerebral ventricles on respiration. Am. J. Physiol., *176*:45-51, 1954.

34. Mitchell, R. A., Loeschcke, H. H., Massion, W. H., and Severinghaus, J. W.: Respiratory responses mediated through superficial chemosensitive areas on the medulla. J. Appl. Physiol., *18*:523-533, 1963.

35. Schlaefke, M. E., See, W. R., and Loeschcke, H. H.: Ventilatory response to alterations of H^+ ion concentration in small areas of the ventral medullary surface. Resp. Physiol., *10*:198-212, 1970.

36. Mitchell, R. A.: Cerebrospinal fluid and the regulation of respiration. *In* Caro, C. G. (ed.): Advances in Respiratory Physiology. London, Edward Arnold Ltd., 1966, pp. 1-47.

37. Pappenheimer, J. R.: Ion transport between blood, cerebrospinal fluid and brain. *In* Brooks, McC., Kao, F. F., and Lloyd, B. B. (eds.): Cerebrospinal Fluid and the Regulation of Respiration. Philadelphia, F. A. Davis Company, 1964, pp. 43-54.

38. Gesell, R., and Hertzman, A. B.: The regulation of respiration. IV. Tissue acidity, blood acidity and pulmonary ventilation; effects of semipermeability of membranes and the buffering action of tissues with the continuous method of recording changes in acidity. Am. J. Physiol., *78*:610-629, 1926.

39. Jacobs, M. H.: To what extent are the physiological effects of carbon dioxide due to hydrogen ions? Am. J. Physiol., *51*:321-331, 1920.

40. Jacobs, M. H.: The production of intracellular acidity by neutral and alkaline solutions containing carbon dioxide. Am. J. Physiol., *53*:457-463, 1920.

41. Leusen, I.: Regulation of cerebrospinal fluid composition with reference to breathing. Physiol. Rev., *52*:1-56, 1972.

42. Plum, F., and Price, R. W.: Acid-base balance of cisternal and lumbar cerebrospinal fluid on hospital patients. New Eng. J. Med., *289*:1346-1351, 1973.

43. Alexander, J. K., Hartley, L. H., Modelski, M., and Grover, R. F.: Reduction of stroke volume during exercise in man following ascent to 3,100 m altitude. J. Appl. Physiol., *23*:849-858, 1967.

44. Sorensen, S. C., and Severinghaus, J. W.: Irreversible respiratory insensitivity to acute hypoxia in man born at high altitude. J. Appl. Physiol., *25*:217-220, 1968.

45. Sorensen, S. C., and Severinghaus, J. W.: Respiratory insensitivity to acute hypoxia persisting after correction of tetralogy of Fallot. J. Appl. Physiol., *25*:221-223, 1968.

46. Edelman, N. H., Lahiri, S., Braudo, L., Cherniack, N. S., and Fishman, A. P.: The blunted ventilation response to hypoxia in cyanotic congenital heart disease. New Eng. J. Med., *282*:405-411, 1970.

47. Huang, C. T., and Lyons, H. A.: The maintenance of acid-base balance between cerebrospinal fluid and arterial blood in patients with chronic respiratory disorders. Clin. Sci., *31*:273-284, 1966.

48. Bleich, H. L., Berkman, P. M., and Schwartz, W. B.: The response of cerebrospinal fluid composition to sustained hypercapnia. J. Clin. Invest., *43*:11-16, 1964.

49. Cowie, J., Lambie, A. T., and Robson, J. S.: The influence of extracorporeal dialysis on the acid-base composition of blood and cerebrospinal fluid. Clin. Sci., *23*:397-404, 1962.

50. Kety, S. S., Polis, B. D., Nadler, C. S., and Schmidt, C. F.: The blood flow and oxygen consumption of the human brain in diabetic acidosis and coma. J. Clin. Invest., *7*:500-510, 1948.

51. Goldring, R. M., Cannon, P. J., Heinemann, H. O., and Fishman, A. P.: Respiratory adjustment to chronic metabolic alkalosis in man. J. Clin. Invest., *47*:188-202, 1968.

52. Chazan, J. A., Appleton, F. M., London, A. M., and Schwartz, W. B.: Effects of chronic metabolic acid-base disturbances on the composition of cerebrospinal fluid in the dog. Clin. Sci., *36*:345-358, 1969.

Chapter Ten

EXERCISE

INTRODUCTION

Most chest physicians and pulmonary physiologists are not as concerned or informed about muscular exercise as they should be. There are several important reasons for examining both healthy subjects and patients with cardiopulmonary disorders during exercise as well as during rest. (1) Movement from one place to another (locomotion) is a characteristic of the entire animal kingdom, and the ability to run, to swim, to climb trees, and to

253

perform a variety of physical activities is required for the pursuit of food and the escape from predators; in other words, movement is essential for survival. Thus, study of the responses of normal persons to exercise and of the factors that limit the maximum amount of exercise that can be carried out provides information about adjustments to what is undoubtedly the most common and important physiologic stress that man must endure. (2) Almost all diseases, not only those of the cardiorespiratory systems, either reduce the maximum amount of exercise that can be accomplished or modify the usual physiologic responses to muscular work. Dyspnea, weakness, excessive fatigue, cramps, angina, and syncope, to mention only a few, are all symptoms of exertion that testify to the interaction among contracting skeletal muscles and the circulatory, respiratory, neural, and erythropoietic systems of the body. However, only limited knowledge is available about the mechanisms that impair exercise capacity in disease states, especially the pathways by which the abnormal physiologic factors are translated into symptoms such as dyspnea. (3) Despite their obvious importance, there are remarkably few data concerning how purposeful physical conditioning, or the lack of it, protects or modifies the responses of growing children and of young or old adults to the influences of diseases, accidents, or degenerative changes.[1] A detailed understanding about muscular exercise, therefore, is useful not only for the knowledge it provides about an important physiologic phenomenon but also because of the potential for prevention and treatment of a variety of common diseases.

Exercise can be differentiated clearly from the resting state by the simple fact that in exercise various skeletal muscles are actively contracting under the influence of neurogenic stimuli; in complete rest, on the other hand, with the exception of those muscles engaged in quiet breathing,

skeletal muscles are relaxed.[1] Under normal conditions, man's ability to perform exercise depends upon the capacity of the circulatory and respiratory systems to increase the transport of O_2 to the participating muscles and upon the status of local factors that determine whether the increased quantity of O_2 reaches the cell interior where it is utilized to provide energy for muscle fiber contraction. This chapter will consider chiefly the respiratory and circulatory mechanisms that augment O_2 transport during exercise; excellent reviews are available that provide additional information about the physiologic and metabolic responses to exercise and training.[2-4]

CIRCULATION

CARDIAC OUTPUT

Contracting muscles require additional O_2, and it is generally recognized that the increase in O_2 consumption that occurs during exercise is the best available measurement of the total muscular effort expended (Figure 10–1).[5] Increased O_2 demands can be satisfied either by an increase in O_2 transport or by an increase in O_2 extraction; in muscular exercise, the additional O_2 requirements are met by increases in *both* transport to and extraction by the working muscles.

Systemic O_2 transport, as defined and discussed in Chapter 7, depends upon the total blood flow to the tissues of the body (the cardiac output) and the content of O_2 in arterial blood (which is determined by arterial P_{O_2}, the amount of hemoglobin available, and the affinity of hemoglobin for O_2). In normal subjects, the elevated O_2 transport during exercise is achieved almost entirely by an increase in cardiac output, and a well-defined relationship has been established between cardiac output and O_2 consumption or O_2 uptake (the variable that is actually measured) during exercise. This rela-

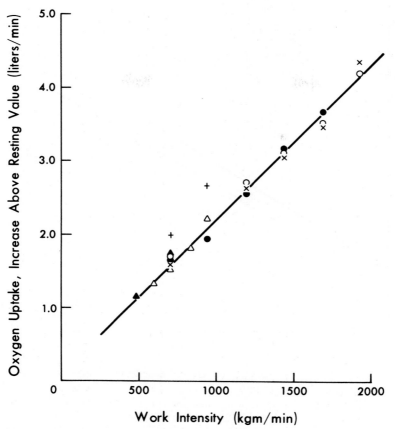

Figure 10–1 Relationship between O_2 uptake in excess of resting uptake and work intensity. Data from six healthy subjects studied on a bicycle ergometer by Christensen.[5]

tionship is linear at progressively greater intensities of exercise, but ultimately a plateau is reached that is called maximal O_2 uptake.[6] When studies are properly conducted, this level is a stable and reproducible physiologic characteristic of the subject being tested.

The magnitude of the increase in cardiac output as work load is steadily increased is shown in Figure 10–2; increasing muscular effort in this and subsequent figures is reflected by the increasing O_2 uptake on the abscissa. Figure 10–2 indicates that cardiac output at a given level of exercise will be 1 to 2 L/min higher if the exercise is performed while the subject is supine compared with the value while he is in the upright position.[7] The influence of posture is primarily due to the effects of gravity on venous return to the heart; cardiac filling and, consequently, right and left ventricular volumes and stroke volume are all greater when the subject is supine than when he is upright.

Another important determinant of the cardiac output response to exercise is the age of the subject. Older persons have lower cardiac outputs at a given work load than younger persons in both the supine and upright positions.[7] Exactly why the heart "wears out" with advancing years is not known, but the effect of aging is reflected in a

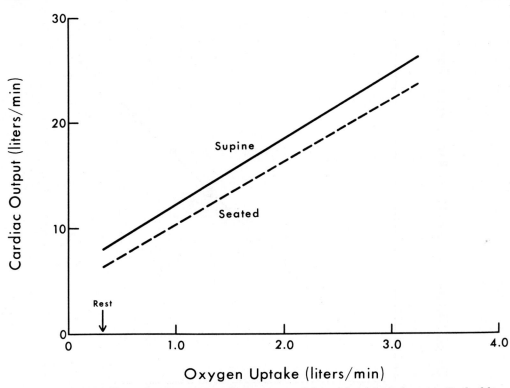

Figure 10-2 Relationship between cardiac output and O_2 uptake during exercise. Dashed line represents normal subjects in seated position, and solid line represents the same subjects supine. (Adapted from Ekelund and Holmgren.[7] Reprinted by permission from the authors and publisher.)

reduction in heart rate and usually stroke volume at any O_2 uptake.

Cardiac output is apportioned differently during exercise compared with rest; redistribution is achieved by vasodilation in the working muscles and skin and vasoconstriction in the viscera and nonworking muscles. These variations in regional blood flow are produced by a complex interplay of local and general vasodilator and vasoconstrictor mechanisms. Vasoconstriction in the splanchnic and renal vascular beds causes a redistribution of 70 to 80 per cent of resting blood flow (or about 2.2 L/min) from these organs to exercising muscles.[6] The increase in cardiac output above the resting value during strenuous exercise is distributed mainly (80 to 90 per cent) to the working muscles, but blood flow to the skin also increases, owing to the elevation in body temperature and the requirements for heat dissipation. Because the vasoconstriction in some organs is more than offset by vasodilation in others, peripheral vascular resistance decreases and becomes an important mechanism that governs the magnitude of the cardiac output response during exercise.

HEART RATE AND STROKE VOLUME

An increase in cardiac output can result from an increase in either heart rate or stroke volume, or both. Normally, most of the increase in cardiac output during exercise is caused by an increase in heart rate, and the changes in stroke volume are proportionately smaller. Although the rate of cardiac contractions increases linearly with O_2 consumption during muscular work (Figure 10–3), the magnitude of the change in rate (i.e., the slope of the line) is determined by the size of the stroke volume: the smaller the stroke volume, the greater the increase in heart rate. Stroke volume may vary under different circumstances and depends upon the physical condition of the subject, the mass of muscles that are performing the work, and the distribution of blood flow.[2] Each of these affects the ventricular volumes and/or the filling and emptying conditions of the heart. These factors also account for the variations in stroke volume encountered in patients with various diseases and for the fact that stroke volume is usually smaller when the patient is in the upright than in the supine position at a given cardiac output.

MYOCARDIAL RESPONSES

Muscle contractility is an elusive but important physiologic phenomenon that can be defined as "an increase in the force developed during isometric contraction at constant muscle length and stimulus." Myocardial contractility, according to this definition, can only be measured with precision under highly artificial laboratory conditions, and its assessment in man presents formidable problems. There are, however, several indexes related to contractility* that can be derived from measurable variables in normal subjects at rest and during exercise. Regardless of which index is

---

*Indexes of contractility can be divided into two categories: the rate of change of pressure with respect to time during isovolumic contraction (e.g., dP/dT/IT, where IT equals developed pressure at dP/dT minus end-diastolic pressure), and derivatives of contractile element shortening velocity (e.g., circumferential shortening rate at a given developed pressure).

used, there is abundant evidence that myocardial contractility increases during exercise.[9,10] Presumably, two separate components interact to augment myocardial contractility during exercise: (1) an increase in heart rate (the treppe effect) that is independent of adrenergic influences and is believed to result from an increase in the rate of interaction of specific sites in the contractile elements; and (2) heightened activity of the sympathetic nervous system. The contributions of these two mechanisms have been separated by the use of β-adrenergic blocking drugs and cardiac pacing.[10]

It is not widely appreciated that under *resting* conditions, cardiac output remains relatively constant despite large changes in heart rate (e.g., induced by artificial pacing) because stroke volume goes down as frequency goes up and vice versa. The experimental data plotted in Figure 10–4 reveal that cardiac output remained within ± 20 per cent of control levels because stroke volume changed opposite to heart rate when heart rate was varied from less than 50 to greater than 200 per cent of control values.[11] This means that during *exercise*, because stroke volume is always higher than it would be at the same heart rate under resting conditions, other mechanisms are actuated that maintain or even increase stroke volume. One of these is the Frank-Starling mechanism through which the extra stretch imparted to the muscle fibers of the ventricles consequent to the increased filling of the heart causes stroke volume to increase; thus, at any given heart rate, end-diastolic volume (i.e., initial myocardial fiber length) and stroke volume are both larger during exercise than at rest. Normally, the increase in contractility and the Frank-Starling effect are complementary and interact during exercise to raise cardiac output, but when one of the mechanisms cannot be utilized, as may result from disease, drugs, or experimental intervention, the heart makes great-

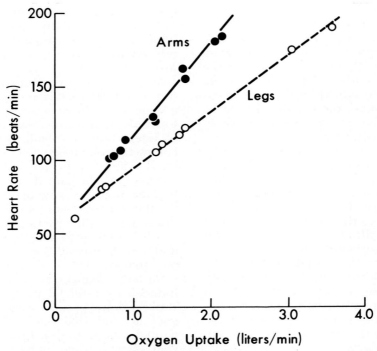

Figure 10–3 Relationship between heart rate and O₂ uptake in the same subject during work with the arms and with the legs. (Adapted from Asmussen and Hemmingsen.[8] Reprinted by permission from the authors and publisher.)

er use of the other to increase blood flow. A good example of the heart taking advantage of its available resources for increasing cardiac output is shown by experiments in trained greyhounds that had their adrenergic-mediated contractility mechanisms eliminated by surgical cardiac denervation.[12] The total cardiac output response to racing after denervation was the same as before because those animals that could not reflexly increase their myocardial performance during exercise simply relied more heavily on the Frank-Starling mechanism than they had before denervation.

BLOOD VOLUME AND HEMATOCRIT

The changes in blood volume and hematocrit that accompany exercise are variable and depend upon the severity and duration of the work load and the physical condition of the subject. Maximal exercise usually causes a reduction in plasma volume and an increase in hematocrit ratio (8 per cent).[13] However, the magnitude of any change that may develop in hemoglobin concentration or blood volume during submaximal exercise is sufficiently small that O₂ transport is not greatly affected by this mechanism.

Extremely hard exercise, particularly in a hot environment, may be associated with minor amounts of hemolysis. In contrast, severe exercise in well-trained athletes or workers accustomed to it did not produce detectable changes in either blood volume or hemoglobin concentration[14]; the constancy of blood volume may reflect the effects of conditioning, because it is well established that highly trained persons have larger total amounts of hemoglobin and greater circulating

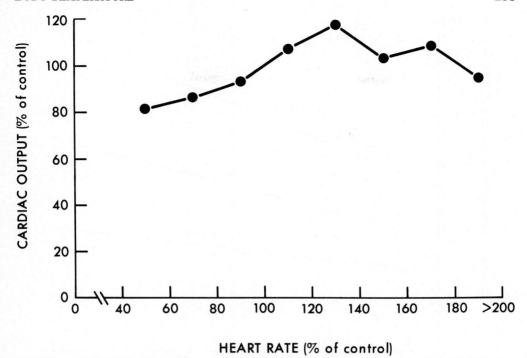

Figure 10–4 Effect of experimentally induced changes in heart rate on cardiac output. Mean values of multiple observations from 11 dogs. (From data of Bristow, Ferguson, Mintz, and Rapaport.[11])

blood volumes and heart volumes than unconditioned persons of similar body build.[4]

VASCULAR PRESSURES

Systolic, diastolic, and mean systemic arterial blood pressures increase gradually during exercise and in the steady state bear a relationship to the intensity of the work performed (Figure 10–5).[7] At very heavy work loads, especially in untrained subjects, systolic pressures above 200 mm Hg are common. Systolic, diastolic, mean pulmonary arterial, and wedge pressures also increase linearly with increasing levels of exercise (Figure 10–6).[7]

Because systolic pressures in both pulmonary and systemic arterial systems increase during exercise, there must be corresponding changes in right and left ventricular systolic pressures. However, the diastolic pressure responses differ in the two ventricular cavities: right ventricular end-diastolic pressure decreases, but left ventricular end-diastolic pressure increases (as indicated by the elevated pulmonary arterial wedge pressure). These responses must reflect differences in the distensibilities of right and left ventricular myocardiums.

BODY TEMPERATURE

The exercising body resembles a machine in the sense that only a fraction of the total energy produced by the consumption of fuel is transformed into useful work. The work:energy ratio is a measure of the *efficiency* of the human "machine" and has been shown to vary depending upon the kind and severity of work, the fre-

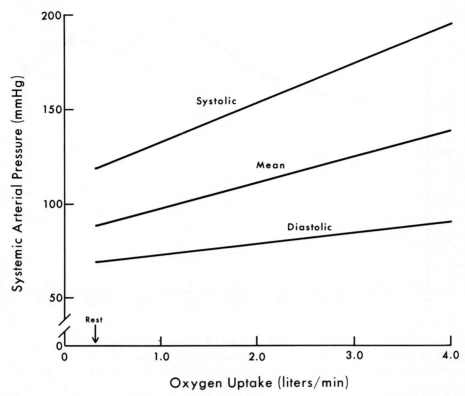

Figure 10–5 Relationship between systolic, diastolic, and mean systemic arterial pressures and O_2 uptake during exercise in the supine position. (From data of Ekelund and Holmgren.[7])

quency of movements, the skill of the performer, and the diet of the subject. Under ordinary conditions of stair climbing, for example, the net efficiency of normal persons varies between 19 and 25 per cent.

The quantity of energy that is not converted into mechanical work (i.e., the remaining 75 to 81 per cent in stair climbing) degenerates into heat. The heat production of an exercising subject has a particular value for a given work intensity and during strenuous exercise may reach values 15 to 20 times the value at rest. Some of the extra heat is stored in the body and raises its temperature (Figure 10–7), and the remainder is dissipated.[15] Once the body temperature is elevated to the steady state value that corresponds to the amount of work being performed,

all the heat produced by the muscles must be eliminated. In man, heat dissipation occurs mainly through the skin, and this requires a considerable increase in blood flow to the body surface. In hot and humid environments where heat loss is impaired, an unusually large amount of blood flow may be diverted to the skin at the expense of blood flow to exercising muscles and other parts of the body; this may limit exercise and produce symptoms such as exercise fatigue, unsteadiness, and even syncope. Heat exhaustion is caused by dehydration from excessive sweating during exercise, and heat cramps appear to result from severe loss of NaCl in sweat; cramps are especially likely to occur in this setting if only water losses are replaced.

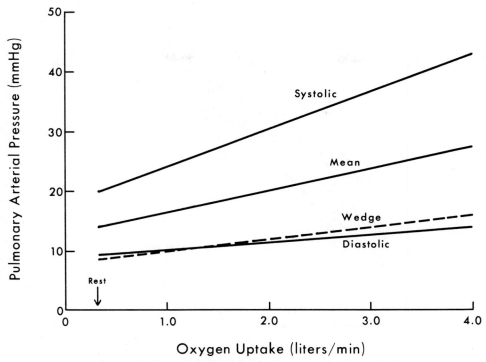

Figure 10-6 Relationship between systolic, diastolic, mean, and "wedge" pulmonary arterial pressures and O_2 uptake during exercise in the supine position. (From data of Ekelund and Holmgren.[7])

GAS EXCHANGE

VENTILATION

The demands of exercise for increased O_2 uptake and CO_2 elimination require that ventilation be closely coupled with the intensity of the work load. As shown in Figure 10–8, minute volume increases almost immediately upon initiating muscular exercise and reaches a plateau within a few minutes during mild to moderate exercise; however, minute volume increases progressively during severe exercise.[16]

The increased minute volume during exercise is achieved mainly by an increase in tidal volume during light work, and respiratory frequency increases only as the work performed becomes heavier. With strenuous exercise, the tidal volume is usually about 50 per cent of a normal subject's vital

capacity, and the respiratory frequency is 40 to 50 breaths/min.[2]

From rest to moderate levels of exercise, the increase in ventilatory volume is linearly related to the increase in O_2 uptake. But beginning with moderate work loads, the increase in ventilation becomes progressively greater than the increase in O_2 consumption (Figure 10–9). The additional "drive" to ventilation reflects mainly the progressive accumulation of lactic acid in the bloodstream. The contribution of anaerobic metabolism and lactate production was demonstrated by experiments using supplemental O_2[17]; breathing air mixtures enriched with O_2 lowered ventilation during heavy work but had no effect in the same subjects at rest or during light work (Figure 10–9). It has also been suggested that stimulation of J receptors (see Chapter 3) by intersti-

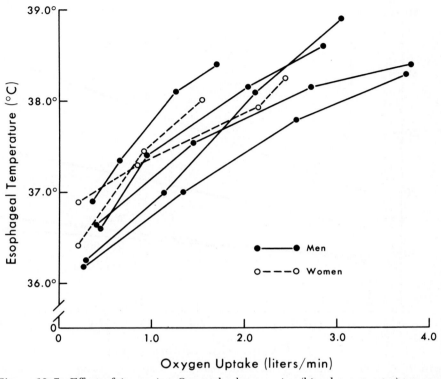

Figure 10-7 Effect of increasing O_2 uptake by exercise (bicycle ergometer) on esophageal temperature. Individual measurements in seven healthy subjects. (Adapted from Saltin and Hermansen.[15] Reprinted by permission from the authors and publisher.)

tial congestion during very strenuous exercise may cause dyspnea and a reflex increase in ventilation; however, studies of pulmonary extravascular water volume in normal subjects after one hour of heavy exercise failed to provide evidence in support of this theory.[18]

ALVEOLAR VENTILATION AND WASTED VENTILATION

The volume of anatomic dead space usually increases slightly during exercise owing to the distension of airways that accompanies deep breathing (Figure 7–9); in contrast, the volume of alveolar dead space normally present at rest decreases. Thus, because the two components of (total) wasted ventilation change in opposite direc-

tions, the absolute values of wasted ventilation are nearly constant during exercise (Figure 10–10). However, because tidal volume increases considerably in response to increasing work loads, the wasted ventilation: tidal volume ratio decreases from 30 per cent (rest) to 10 to 15 per cent (exercise). By this mechanism, alveolar ventilation increases from about 70 per cent of minute volume at rest to about 85 to 90 per cent of minute volume during heavy exercise.[20]

DIFFUSING CAPACITY

The changes in intravascular pressures within the pulmonary artery and left atrium during exercise serve both to recruit previously closed pulmonary capillaries and to distend capillar-

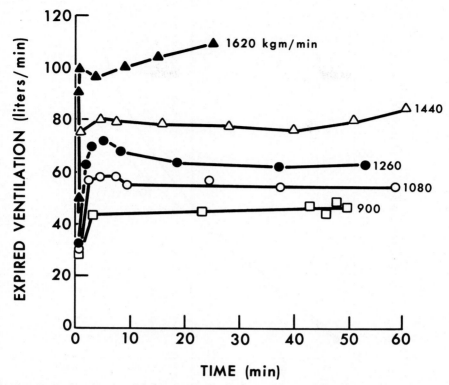

Figure 10–8 Time course of changes in expired ventilation at different work intensities. (Data from Nielsen.[16] Adapted from Asmussen.[2] Reprinted by permission from the author and publisher.)

ies that had been perfused but were not maximally dilated. The consequences of these phenomena are (1) a better matching of ventilation and perfusion, with resulting improvement of gas exchange, and (2) an increase in pulmonary capillary blood volume and membrane-diffusing capacity.[21]

In most but not all studies, pulmonary diffusing capacity for CO has been found to increase linearly and continuously as O_2 uptake increases to maximal values. In contrast, it has been shown that pulmonary diffusing capacity for O_2 reaches its maximal level at submaximal work loads.[22] Whether or not diffusing capacity reaches a plateau during exercise is an important question that needs to be investigated further.

As stressed in Chapter 6, pulmo-

nary diffusion does not limit exchange of O_2 and CO_2 in healthy resting subjects; in fact, there is considerable utilizable reserve in this function so that large reductions in diffusing capacity must occur before differences become apparent between the Po_2 of alveolar gas and of red blood cells at the end of their passage through pulmonary capillaries. The increase in diffusing capacity during exercise serves to promote O_2 uptake and ensure that alveolar-capillary Po_2 differences remain negligible. If a maximal limit to diffusing capacity is reached at submaximal work loads, exercise at higher intensities would be associated with an increase in alveolar-arterial Po_2 difference (see next section); whether or not this occurs has not been settled. Therefore, during exercise at sea level,

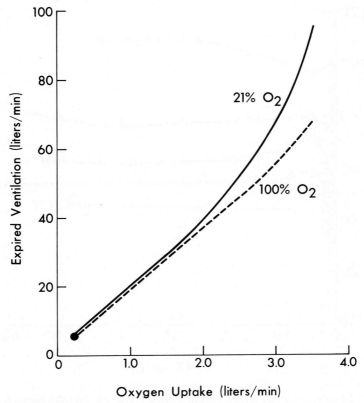

Figure 10–9 Effect of increasing O_2 uptake by exercise (bicycle ergometer) on expired ventilation while breathing room air (21 per cent O_2) and 100 per cent O_2. (Adapted from Asmussen and Nielsen.[17] Reprinted by permission from the authors and publisher.)

pulmonary diffusing capacity is adequate to maintain equilibrium at the completion of gas exchange across the air-blood barrier except possibly during maximal or near-maximal work loads. In normal persons living at high altitudes, however, owing to the low Po_2 in the inspired air, the total amount of O_2 that can diffuse into the blood per unit time is reduced despite the presence of a perfectly normal alveolar-capillary membrane and normal or increased pulmonary capillary blood volume. The reduction in diffusion of O_2 is of little consequence at rest but does reduce maximal O_2 uptake and thereby maximal attainable work loads. Similarly, the presence of pulmonary abnormalities that impair diffusion is seldom important when patients are resting, but imposes serious limitations on gas transfer, evidenced by a reduction in maximal O_2 uptake and exercise capacity.

ALVEOLAR-ARTERIAL OXYGEN TENSION

Despite the considerable increases in O_2 consumption, minute volume of ventilation, and cardiac output during exercise, alveolar and arterial Po_2 compositions remain remarkably constant. Figure 10–11 depicts the mean alveolar and arterial values of both O_2 and CO_2 at rest and during progressively increasing work loads in the upright position (bicycling); the alveolar-arterial Po_2 difference during exercise initially decreases slightly from the resting value and then increases at very high work loads.[23]

The resting alveolar-arterial P_{O_2} difference of 8 mm Hg, as discussed in Chapter 7, results from a mismatching of ventilation and perfusion and from a small right-to-left shunt. The ventilation-perfusion imbalance is mainly due to the effects of gravity on the distribution of pulmonary blood flow. At rest in the upright position, blood flow is about ten times greater to the base than to the apex, but during exercise, the increase in pulmonary artery pressure causes blood flow to become more uniformly distributed throughout the lungs[24]; this improves the matching of ventilation and blood flow and, consequently, reduces the alveolar-arterial P_{O_2} difference. (This phenomenon is reflected in the decreased height of the vertical dashed lines in Figure 10–11.) At very high levels of work, the alveolar-arterial P_{O_2} difference increases to a value greater than the resting value (Figure 10–11). The mechanism of the increase is not known, but there are two possibilities: (1) an increased right-to-left shunt (either an increase in the quantity or a decrease in the mixed venous P_{O_2} of the shunted blood) or

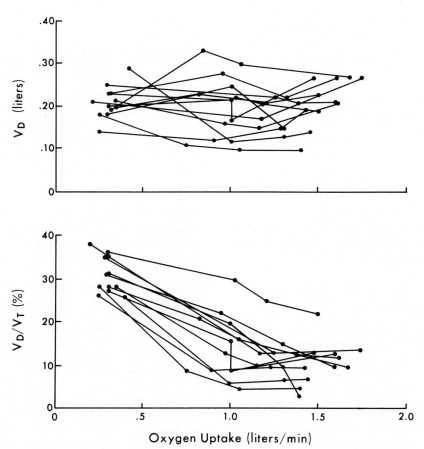

Figure 10–10 Effect of increasing O_2 uptake by exercise (bicycle ergometer) on wasted ventilation (V_D) and wasted ventilation:tidal volume ratio (V_D/V_T). (From data of Glazier and Murray.[19])

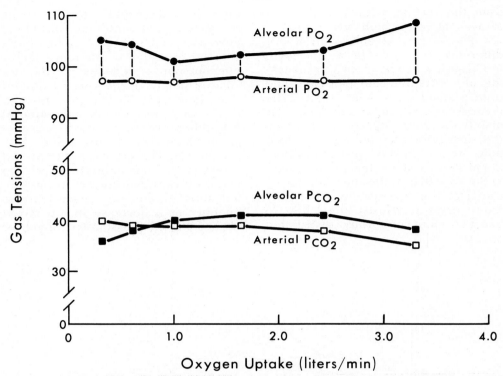

Figure 10–11 Effect of increasing O_2 uptake by exercise (bicycle ergometer) on alveolar and arterial P_{O_2} and P_{CO_2}. Mean values from studies in five healthy subjects. The vertical dashed line represents the alveolar-arterial P_{O_2} difference. (From data of Whipp and Wasserman.[23])

(2) a limitation of diffusion so that complete equilibration of O_2 between alveolar gas and pulmonary capillary blood does not occur.

ALVEOLAR-ARTERIAL CARBON DIOXIDE TENSION

Figure 10–11 shows the relationship between mean alveolar and arterial P_{CO_2} values at rest and during exercise. The fact that alveolar P_{CO_2} is lower than arterial P_{CO_2} at rest may at first seem surprising, but it is also accounted for by the poor perfusion of the upper regions of the lungs that results from the gravitational distribution of blood flow. Mean alveolar P_{CO_2} reflects gas composition in those air spaces in which CO_2 uptake has oc-

curred as well as in the apices that are ventilated but poorly perfused. This so-called alveolar dead space effect disappears during exercise, owing to the improved perfusion of the upper regions of the lungs, and thus alveolar P_{CO_2} becomes equal to or slightly higher than arterial P_{CO_2}. The latter discrepancy reflects increased CO_2 delivery to the lungs and oscillation of alveolar and arterial values around slightly different mean levels.[25]

During heavy exercise, both alveolar and arterial P_{CO_2} values begin to fall, owing to the hyperventilation that occurs in response to the lactic acid that begins to accumulate at these work intensities (Figure 10–9); the fall in alveolar P_{CO_2} is associated with the rise in alveolar P_{O_2}, as shown in Figure 10–11. In exhaustive work, alveolar P_{CO_2} may decrease to about 30 mm Hg.[17]

REGULATION OF VENTILATION

Arterial P_{O_2} and P_{CO_2} are almost exactly the same during mild and moderate exercise as at rest. Simply maintaining arterial blood gases at their resting levels may not sound like much of an adjustment, yet this constancy can only be achieved by a remarkable correspondence between the intensity of work on the one hand and the amount of ventilation on the other. Despite extensive investigation, the mechanisms that couple alveolar ventilation to increases in O_2 consumption and CO_2 production are poorly understood. The prevailing theory holds that no single factor controls breathing during exercise and that those processes responsible can be separated into two categories, depending on their time of onset: a fast component that is probably reflex in origin and a slow component that is probably humoral in origin.[26]

ROLE OF CARBON DIOXIDE

Since Haldane and Priestley[27] studied the problem in the early 1900s, much attention has been directed toward the role that CO_2 plays in the regulation of ventilation during exercise. Carbon dioxide has always been a logical choice as a regulator because its production parallels the severity of muscular work and because the medullary chemoreceptors are able to respond quickly to new levels of CO_2 in the brain and CSF. Although the CO_2 theory has been found deficient in part, it is a convenient place to begin an examination of the factors involved in the control of breathing during exercise.

As discussed in Chapter 7, arterial P_{CO_2} varies directly with CO_2 production and inversely with alveolar ventilation (see Equation 7–2); accordingly, at any constant CO_2 production, the relationship between alveolar ventilation, or the more commonly measured total expired ventilation, and arterial P_{CO_2} is expressed by a hyperbolic curve similar to those shown in Figure 10–12: the lower curve defines possible values for arterial P_{CO_2} and expired ventilation at resting CO_2 production, and the upper curve depicts the same variables during mild exercise when CO_2 production is quadrupled. Normal values for resting arterial P_{CO_2} and expired ventilation are 40 mm Hg and 8 L/min, respectively (point A, Figure 10–12); however, if ventilation is either suppressed (e.g., by sedative drugs) or stimulated (e.g., by apprehension or anxiety), the resulting values of arterial P_{CO_2} and expired ventilation will be *on the curve*, but to the right or left (respectively) of point A. Similarly, if ventilation is abnormally high or low while exercising, the resulting arterial P_{CO_2} will differ from the normal value of 40 mm Hg and will lie to the right or left of point B on the upper curve.

If the change in ventilation during exercise were due solely to the ventilatory drive from newly produced CO_2 that is beginning to accumulate in the bloodstream, the response would be determined by the subject's sensitivity to CO_2.* Normal CO_2 responsiveness is shown by the dashed line moving up and to the right from point A in Figure 10–12 (see Chapter 9 for discussion of CO_2 response lines). The CO_2 response line intersects the exercise CO_2 production curve at point C and thereby defines the arterial P_{CO_2} and expired ventilation values that would

---

*Evidence supporting the assumption that the response to metabolically produced CO_2 is the same as that to inhaled CO_2 has been obtained in man[28]; furthermore, the slight increase in CO_2 sensitivity found in exercising dogs is insufficient to account for the ventilatory response during exercise.[29]

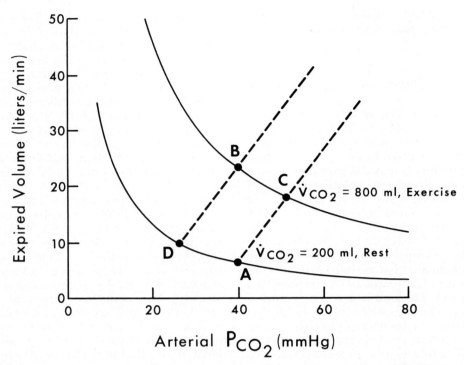

Figure 10–12   Relationship between expired ventilation and arterial P_{CO_2} when CO_2 output is 200 ml (rest) and 800 ml (exercise). The dashed lines represent "normal" CO_2 response curves. (For details, see text.)

occur during exercise if the patient's sensitivity to CO_2 were the *only* mechanism controlling breathing. Although the differences between the arterial P_{CO_2} and minute ventilation values represented by points B and C are small, they are readily detectable. Thus, because the effect of CO_2 sets conditions at point C rather than point B, other stimuli must be present to account for the observed increment in ventilation during exercise.

NONMETABOLIC FACTORS

One way of reaching point B is to move along the exercise CO_2 production curve from C to B. Another way is to move along the resting CO_2 production curve from A to D and then up a CO_2 response line of normal sensitivity from D to B. Although it is controversial, some investigators believe that

the latter process (A to D to B) is what actually happens during exercise[28, 29] and that at least two distinct regulatory mechanisms are involved.[30]

1. The first (fast) factor is presumably nonmetabolic (i.e., unrelated to CO_2) and occurs almost immediately after exercise is begun. The rapid effect of this stimulus suggests strongly that it is reflex in origin. The nonmetabolic factor causes ventilation to increase and because CO_2 production has not had time to rise, the values of arterial P_{CO_2} and expired ventilation change from those at point A to those at point D (Figure 10–12).

2. The second (slow) factor is presumably metabolic in origin and requires seconds to minutes to exert its complete effect on ventilation. The time sequence suggests that this factor is humorally mediated, and metabolically produced CO_2 provides a

straightforward explanation for the shift from point D to point B. The hyperventilation that occurs during strenuous work has been related to lactic acid (or other products of anaerobic metabolism) acting on carotid chemoreceptors.

ROLE OF REFLEXES

An extensive search has been made to identify the nonmetabolic stimulus to ventilation. The evidence available at present favors a reflex mechanism that originates from the exercising muscles and limbs. Experiments have demonstrated (1) that passive movements of the limbs of man or experimental animals cause ventilation to increase, (2) that the increase in ventilation is almost instantaneous and is not affected by occluding the blood supply to the limb, and (3) that the ventilatory response disappears after section of the peripheral nerve or dorsal root subserving the muscle and during spinal anesthesia. These observations, although controversial, support the contention that mechanoreceptors of some type are situated in skeletal muscles. However, a major deficiency in the reflex theory of control of breathing during exercise is the lack of convincing evidence concerning the morphology and location of the presumed receptors. Muscle spindles, once candidates for the role, have been shown not to be involved.[31]

Recent experiments demonstrated that ventilation increased in unanesthetized dogs in the breath following an isoproterenol-induced increase in cardiac output.[32] These results illustrate that ventilation rapidly adjusts to changes in cardiac output or one of its derivatives. Furthermore, the response was shown not to be mediated by the carotid or aortic bodies and to be linked closely to the level of alveolar, and hence arterial, CO_2. Thus it is possible that rapidly responding CO_2 receptors are responsible for the prompt increase in ventilation at the onset of exercise and that other sources of reflex stimulation are relatively unimportant.

OTHER FACTORS

The main stimulus to ventilation during exercise results from the interaction of presumed chemical and neurogenic influences. However, other factors, especially those related to temperature regulation and conditioned responses, are known to be important.

Ventilation is closely linked to temperature regulation in animals in which the chief mechanism of excess heat elimination is panting. The extent to which this highly complex system, presumably involving hypothalamic and medullary interconnections, is present in man has not been fully established. The data that are available from hypothermia experiments suggest that normal subjects do not rely on their respiratory systems to regulate body temperature during short episodes of mild exercise.[33] It is likely, however, that the effects of temperature on ventilation would be more discernible during prolonged and/or heavy exercise, owing to the increases caused by an elevated body temperature in CO_2 production and CO_2 sensitivity, both of which should increase ventilation.

Psychogenic influences, particularly conditioned responses, may profoundly affect ventilation before and during exercise; for example, it is well known that dogs trained to run on a treadmill anticipate the stress of exercise and change their breathing pattern before the treadmill is even turned on. Undoubtedly, similar influences are actuated in man under certain conditions. Furthermore, breathing is often modified to suit the rhythmic pattern of the exercise being undertaken; thus, the swimmer and the cross-country runner, at the same work intensity, demonstrate different combinations of tidal volumes and breathing frequencies.

TRAINING

The effects of training are remarkably complex and have been the subject of countless investigations. However, it should be emphasized at the outset of a discussion about the topic that it is virtually impossible to design suitable experiments that will answer some of the important and unsolved questions about the effects of training. For example, five Olympic cross-country skiers had an average maximal O_2 uptake of 5.6 L/min and two champions had values above 6.0 L/min; in contrast, sedentary men had maximal O_2 uptakes of about 3.0 L/min.[34] Clearly, there is a remarkable difference in maximal O_2 uptake, transport, and utilization between top athletes and untrained men. Some of these differences are due to the fact that outstanding athletes have large hearts, increased blood volumes and red blood cell masses, and greater than "normal" pulmonary diffusing capacity measurements. What is *not* known is whether these attributes are inherited and champions are genetically endowed with superior ability or whether these so-called "dimensional" characteristics of athletic prowess are acquired through years of rigorous exercise. On the one hand, training has been shown to affect several circulatory and respiratory physiologic variables; on the other hand, an influence of training on several of the critical physical dimensions that enhance maximal O_2 uptake and delivery during exercise has not been demonstrated.

The chief difficulty in designing experiments lies in the selection of appropriate subjects. Not only is the person who is willing to be a test subject in a strenuous physical conditioning program highly motivated but also his interest in athletics is likely

to be manifested in a certain degree of physical conditioning at the outset. In contrast, the unfit person has already demonstrated his lack of interest in athletic activities; accordingly, it is difficult to enroll him in a serious physical training program and to maintain his enthusiastic participation throughout. Furthermore, some of the variables that are being measured, especially the dimensional characteristics, may require years to change, or may be changeable only during growth of the subject, and experiments of sufficient duration with suitable control subjects are obviously difficult to carry out.

Despite the experimental problems of design and interpretation, it is widely recognized that it is possible to increase the maximum amount of muscular exercise that a subject can perform by a period of physical training. Improvement is demonstrated by an increased O_2 uptake and an increased maximal work intensity. The physiologic variables that have been examined to determine whether they contribute to the increased work capacity that follows training are summarized in Table 10–1. It should be emphasized that not all of those that *may* change actually *do* change in a given person. There appears to be considerable individual variation in the response to exercise training that depends, in part, upon the subject's physical fitness at the time training is begun.

CARDIAC FACTORS

Some studies have documented that training leads to an increase in maximal cardiac output,[35] but this change is by no means an invariable one.[36] A more universal response is that at the same submaximal work load, cardiac output is lower in the trained than in the untrained subject. Maximal heart rate does not change with exercise training but, like car-

Table 10–1   Summary of the Effects of Training on Circulatory and Respiratory
Function During Physical Exercise

VARIABLE	RESPONSE
Maximal O_2 uptake	Increased
Work output	Increased
Mechanical efficiency	Unchanged
Cardiac output	Increased
Maximal heart rate	Unchanged
Heart rate at submaximal loads	Decreased
Stroke volume	Increased
Arteriovenous O_2 difference	Increased
Hemoglobin, hematocrit	Unchanged
Blood lactate level at maximal loads	Increased
Blood lactate level at submaximal loads	Decreased
Blood flow per unit muscle	Decreased
Maximal ventilation	Unchanged
Ventilation at submaximal loads	Decreased
Pulmonary diffusing capacity	Unchanged
Capillary density in muscles*	Increased
Oxidative enzymes in muscles	Increased

*Not demonstrated in man.

diac output, it is lower at a given work load in the trained than in the untrained person. The changes in stroke volume with training are small and inconstant, although in those studies in which maximal cardiac output increased, the changes were achieved mainly by an increase in stroke volume.[35]

PERIPHERAL FACTORS

Knowledge about the effects of training on the mechanisms that contribute to improved delivery and uptake of O_2 by exercising muscles is incomplete. From a theoretic point of view, peripheral mechanisms may adapt to training and these responses may be at least as important as those that regulate either cardiac output or gas exchange.

Muscle Blood Flow. The effects of training on blood flow to exercising muscles have not been studied systematically. It is known that trained athletes have a lower blood flow *per unit of muscle* than untrained subjects performing the same work load.[37] This observation is not as surprising as it

appears at first glance and may be accounted for by two interrelated factors: first, athletes usually have large muscle masses, so the *total* blood flow to their working muscles may be increased compared with nonathletes, even though the flow per unit of muscle is less; second, the muscles of a trained person are able to extract more O_2 than those of an untrained subject, so that muscle O_2 requirements are satisfied by a lower blood flow.

At maximal work loads, blood flow per unit of exercising muscle was the same in trained as in untrained subjects.[37] Thus, the effects of training on muscle blood flow in these subjects appear to be similar to the effects on other physiologic variables in which the maximal attainable value does not change but the work accomplished at a given submaximal value increases. It is possible that champion athletes may have superior muscle blood flow, but this has not been examined. There is general agreement that sympathetic vasoconstrictor activity is increased to nonworking organs in proportion to the severity of exercise, and it appears from the evidence that has recently been reviewed that training may affect the redistribution of cardiac output that occurs with exercise.[6] However, the problem has not been systematically studied, and the conclusion is by no means definite.

It has been demonstrated that repetitive exercise has an important effect on the density of muscle capillaries in experimental animals. In guinea pigs made to run on a treadmill, the number of capillaries increased in muscles whose work output increased (heart and gastrocnemius) compared with those muscles that were not exercised (masseter).[38] An increased density of capillaries would have the obvious advantage of improving the diffusion of O_2 and other metabolic substrates by effectively shortening the distance for transfer between the capillary lumens and the mitochondria and other sites of utilization within the contracting fibers. In contrast to the results in experimental animals, no changes could be documented in young men studied before and after physical conditioning.[3] Furthermore, capillary density was the same in specimens of the quadriceps muscles of untrained and highly trained young men[39]; although it was also demonstrated that both the average size of muscle cells and the number of capillaries surrounding each cell were higher in the trained than in the untrained subjects, there was no difference in calculated diffusion distance between adjacent capillaries.[39] Nevertheless, it is possible that increases in local myoglobin concentration may facilitate diffusion of O_2 in trained athletes.

Oxygen Extraction. The amount of O_2 extracted from the blood perfusing contracting muscles, reflected by the arteriovenous O_2 difference "across" the muscles, is increased by physical training. Most of the increased extraction is attributable to the local effects of decreased pH and increased temperature on oxyhemo-

globin dissociation. Another factor that may decrease hemoglobin-O_2 affinity, so that more O_2 is released from the bloodstream at the prevailing P_{O_2}, is an increase in erythrocyte DPG (see Chapter 7). This possibility has been examined, and although in one study an increase in the concentration of erythrocyte DPG was observed, there was no change in P_{50}; the decreased O_2 affinity that should have occurred from the increased DPG was offset by a concomitant decrease in mean corpuscular hemoglobin concentration, which increased O_2 affinity.[40] In any case, the physiologic benefits are likely to be small, and other factors are more important in determining the arteriovenous O_2 difference.[41]

Oxygen Utilization. Exercise training programs can be designed specifically to increase either aerobic or anaerobic work capacity. However, in most physical conditioning programs both capacities increase to some degree and are reflected by changes in the blood level of lactate and the muscle cell biochemical composition. After training, the level of lactate in the blood is lower at a given submaximal load but higher at the maximal load than it was before; the reduced blood levels at submaximal exercise after training are caused by lower muscle lactate concentrations in the exercising muscles.[42] These changes are probably caused by an increase in the amount of energy produced aerobically, because training has been shown to increase oxidative capacity.[43] Long-term exercise induces muscle mitochondrial proliferation, increases the concentration of oxidative enzymes, and increases the synthesis of glycogen and triglyceride, which are important intracellular energy sources.[44] Although it is possible that the observed increase in mitochondria and enzymes could allow the muscle to function at a lower P_{O_2}, this explanation for the increased O_2 extraction after training is purely speculative.

RESPIRATORY FACTORS

Maximal ventilation in some normal subjects is unchanged by physical training.[36] In some subjects, however, ventilation increases after training corresponding to the increase in maximal O_2 uptake that occurs.[34] At submaximal exercise loads, ventilation is always less after training than before.

The pulmonary diffusing capacity of competitive athletes, especially swimmers, is higher than that of non-athletes.[45] Although this difference is caused by a higher pulmonary capillary blood volume in the athletes, the basic explanation for its occurrence is unknown. Most studies of the effect of training on pulmonary diffusing capacity have failed to demonstrate any changes attributable to short-term exercise programs.[46] These investigators, however, did not rule out the possibility that training of longer duration — for example, beginning in childhood — could lead to improvements in diffusing capacity; such an increase, if it did

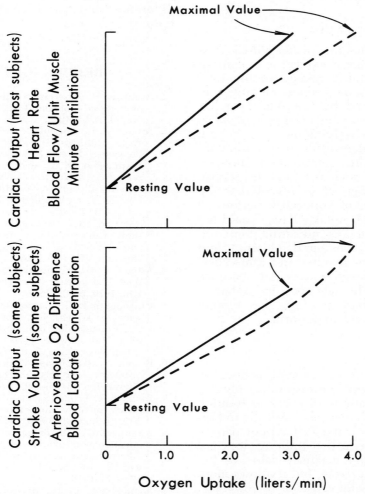

Figure 10–13 Schematic representation of the before (solid lines) and after (dashed lines) effects of training on physiologic variables.

develop, might be related to the large total blood volumes, especially red blood cell masses, that athletes characteristically have.[47] The other explanation is, of course, that athletes are endowed by heredity and then selected on the basis of their superior physical attributes.

Recent studies of ventilatory control in athletes revealed a marked depression of hypoxic and hypercapnic responses at rest.[48] These results suggested diminished peripheral chemoreceptor function, but whether or not this behavior is acquired as a result of training is unknown.

WORK EFFICIENCY

The efficiency of *individual* muscle fibers (measured as the amount of work performed related to the total energy consumed) does not appear to by influenced by training. This has been demonstrated for simple physical acts such as walking on level ground. However, the results of training involving more complicated physical maneuvers, such as treadmill exercise and bicycling, often reveal that the same amount of work can be performed at a lower O_2 uptake. This should not be interpreted as indicating increased muscle efficiency but that learning and practice have resulted in a more coordinated relaxed movement; because fewer muscles (agonists and antagonists) are participating, the motion requires less O_2 to perform.

SUMMARY

There are two general patterns to the circulatory and respiratory physiologic adaptations to exercise training which are shown schematically in Figure 10–13. In the first (upper panel), it can be seen that training does not influence the maximal value of the particular variable, but it allows more work to be achieved at any given value, up to and including the maximal one.

Physiologic functions that are affected by training according to this sequence are cardiac output (in most subjects), heart rate, blood flow per unit of muscle, and minute ventilation. In the second general pattern (lower panel), the maximal value is increased by the effects of training, but owing to a shift in the relationships between the variables and O_2 uptake, submaximal work loads are attained at lower values after training than before. Functions that are affected by training according to this sequence are cardiac output (in some subjects), stroke volume (in some subjects), arteriovenous O_2 difference, and blood lactate concentration.

REFERENCES

1. Asmussen, E.: Exercise: General statement of unsolved problems. Circ. Res., *20 & 21* (Suppl. 1):2-5, 1967.
2. Asmussen, E.: Muscular exercise. *In* Fenn, W. O., and Rahn, H. (eds.): Handbook of Physiology, Section 3. Respiration. Vol. II. Washington, D. C., American Physiological Society, 1965, pp. 939-978.
3. Saltin, B., Blomqvist, G., Mitchell, J. H., Johnson, R. L., Wildenthal, K., and Chapman, C. B.: Response to exercise after bed rest and after training. A longitudinal study of adaptive changes in oxygen transport and body composition. Circulation, 38(Suppl. VII):1-78, 1968.
4. Åstrand, P.-O., and Rodahl, K.: Textbook of Work Physiology. New York, McGraw-Hill, 1970, pp. 1–669.
5. Christensen, E. H.: Beiträge zur Physiologie schwerer körperlicher Arbeit; der Stoffwechsel und die respiratorischen Funktionen bei schwerer körperlicher Arbeit. Arbeitsphysiologie, 5:463–478, 1932.
6. Rowell, L. B.: Human cardiovascular adjustments to exercise and thermal stress. Physiol. Rev., *54*:75-159, 1974.
7. Ekelund, L. G., and Holmgren, A.: Central hemodynamics during exercise. Circ. Res., *20 & 21*(Suppl. 1):33-43, 1967.
8. Asmussen, E., and Hemmingsen, I.: Determination of maximum working capacity at different ages in work with the legs or with the arms. Scand. J. Clin. Lab. Invest., *10*:67-71, 1958.
9. Sonnenblick, E. H., Braunwald, E., Williams, J. F., Jr., and Glick, G.: Effects of

exercise on myocardial force-velocity relations in intact unanesthetized man: relative roles of changes in heart rate, sympathetic activity, and ventricular dimensions. J. Clin. Invest., 44:2051-2062, 1965.

10. Braunwald, E., Sonnenblick, E. H., Ross, J., Jr., Glick, G., and Epstein, S. E.: An analysis of the cardiac response to exercise. Circ. Res., 20 & 21(Suppl. 1):44-58, 1967.

11. Bristow, J. D., Ferguson, R. E., Mintz, F., and Rapaport, E.: The influence of heart rate on left ventricular volume in dogs. J. Clin. Invest., 42:649-655, 1963.

12. Donald, D. E., and Shepherd, J. T.: Response to exercise in dogs with cardiac denervation. Am. J. Physiol., 205:393-400, 1963.

13. Van Beaumont, W., Greenleaf, J. E., and Juhos, L: Disproportional changes in hematocrit, plasma volume, and proteins during exercise and bed rest. J. Appl. Physiol., 33:55-61, 1972.

14. Åstrand, P.-O., and Saltin, B.: Plasma and red cell volume after prolonged severe exercise. J. Appl. Physiol., 19:829-832, 1964.

15. Saltin, B., and Hermansen, L.: Esophageal, rectal, and muscle temperature during exercise. J. Appl. Physiol., 21:1757-1762, 1966.

16. Nielsen, M.: Untersuchungen über die Atemregulation beim Menschen. Skand. Arch. Physiol., 74(Suppl. 10):83-208, 1936.

17. Asmussen, E., and Nielsen, M.: Studies on the regulation of respiration in heavy work. Acta Physiol. Scand., 12:171-188, 1946.

18. Vaughan, T. R., DeMarino, E. M., and Staub, N. C.: Extravascular lung water in prolonged heavy exercise. Circulation, 50 (Suppl. III):24, 1974.

19. Glazier, J. B., and Murray, J. F.: Unpublished observations, 1974.

20. Jones, N. L., McHardy, G. J. R., Naimark A., and Campbell, E. J. M.: Physiological dead space and alveolar-arterial gas pressure differences during exercise. Clin. Sci., 31:19-29, 1966.

21. Johnson, R. L., Jr., Spicer, W. S., Bishop, J. M., and Forster, R. E.: Pulmonary capillary blood volume, flow and diffusing capacity during exercise. J. Appl. Physiol., 15:893-902, 1960.

22. Shepard, R. H., Varnauskas, E., Martin, H. B., White, H. A., Permutt, S., Cotes, J. E., and Riley, R. L.: Relationship between cardiac output and apparent diffusing capacity of the lung in normal man during treadmill exercise. J. Appl. Physiol., 13:205-210, 1958.

23. Whipp, B. J., and Wasserman, K.: Alveolar-arterial gas tension differences during graded exercise. J. Appl. Physiol., 27:361-365, 1969.

24. West, J. B.: Distribution of gas and blood in the normal lungs. Brit. Med. Bull., 19:53-58, 1963.

25. Staub, N. C.: Alveolar-arterial oxygen tension gradient due to diffusion. J. Appl. Physiol., 18:673-680, 1963.

26. Dejours, P.: Control of respiration in muscular exercise. In Fenn, W. O., and Rahn, H. (eds.): Handbook of Physiology, Section 3. Respiration. Vol. I. Washington, D. C., American Physiological Society, 1965, pp. 631-648.

27. Haldane, J. S., and Priestley, J. G.: The regulation of the lung-ventilation. J. Physiol. (Lond.), 32:225–266, 1905.

28. D'Angelo, E., and Torelli, G.: Neural stimuli increasing respiration during different types of exercise. J. Appl. Physiol., 30:116-121, 1971.

29. Bainton, C. R.: Effect of speed vs. grade and shivering on ventilation during active exercise. J. Appl. Physiol., 33:778-787, 1972.

30. Kao, F. F.: An experimental study of the pathways involved in exercise hyperpnoea employing cross-circulation techniques. In Cunningham, D. J. C., and Lloyd, B. B. (eds.): The regulation of Human Respiration. Philadelphia, F. A. Davis Company, 1963, pp. 461-502.

31. Horbein, T. F., Sørensen, S. C., and Parks, C. R.: Role of muscle spindles in lower extremities in breathing during bicycle exercise. J. Appl. Physiol., 27:476-479, 1969.

32. Wasserman, K., Whipp, B. J., and Castagna, J.: Cardiodynamic hyperpnea: hyperpnea secondary to cardiac output increase. J. Appl. Physiol. 36:457–464, 1974.

33. Whipp, B. J., and Wasserman, K.: Effect of body temperature on the ventilatory response to exercise. Resp. Physiol., 8:354–360, 1970.

34. Saltin, G., and Åstrand, P.-O.: Maximal oxygen uptake in athletes. J. Appl. Physiol., 23:353-358, 1967.

35. Ekblom, B., Åstrand, P.-O., Saltin, B., Stenberg, J., and Wallström, B.: Effect of training on circulatory response to exercise, J. Appl. Physiol., 24:518-528, 1968.

36. Douglas, F. G. V., and Becklake, M. R.: Effect of seasonal training on maximal cardiac output. J. Appl. Physiol., 25:600-605, 1968.

37. Grimby, G., Häggendal, E., and Saltin, B.: Local xenon 133 clearance from the quadriceps muscle during exercise in man. J. Appl. Physiol., 22:305-310, 1967.

38. Petrén, T., Sjöstrand, T., and Sylvén, B.: Der Einfluss des Trainings auf die Häufigkeit der Capillaren in Herz und Skeletmuskulatur. Arbeitsphysiologie, 9: 376–386, 1936.

39. Hermansen, L., and Wachtlova, M.: Capillary density of skeletal muscle in well-

trained and untrained men. J. Appl. Physiol., *30*:860-863, 1971.

40. Shappel. S. D., Murray, J. A., Bellingham, A. J., Woodson, R. D., Detter, J. C., and Lenfant, C.: Adaptation to exercise: role of hemoglobin affinity for oxygen and 2,3-diphosphoglycerate. J. Appl. Physiol., *30*:827-832, 1971.

41. Rand, P. W., Norton, J. M., Barker, N., and Lovell. M.: Influence of athletic training on hemoglobin-oxygen affinity. Am. J. Physiol., *224*:1334-1337, 1973.

42. Karlsson, J., Nordesjö, L.-O., Jorfeldt, L., and Saltin, B.: Muscle lactate, ATP, and CP levels during exercise after physical training in man. J. Appl. Physiol., *33*:199-203, 1972.

43. Gollnick, P. O., Armstrong, B., Sanbert, C. W., Piehl, K., and Saltin, B.: Effect of training on enzyme activity and fiber composition of human skeletal muscle. J. Appl. Physiol., *34*:107-111, 1973.

44. Morgan, T. E., Cobb, L. A., Short, F. A., Ross, R., and Gunn, D. R.: Effects of long-term exercise on human muscle mitochondria. *In* Pernow, B. and Saltin, B. (eds.): Muscle Metabolism During Exercise. New York, Plenum Press, 1971, pp. 87-95.

45. Mostyn, E. M., Helle, S., Gee, J. B. L., Bentivoglio, L. G., and Bates, D. V.: Pulmonary diffusing capacity of athletes. J. Appl. Physiol., *18*:687-695, 1963.

46. Anderson, T. W., and Shephard, R. J.: Physical training and exercise diffusing capacity. Int. Z. Angew. Physiol., *25*:198-209, 1968.

47. Bevegård, S., Holmgren, A., and Jonsson, B.: Circulatory studies in well trained athletes at rest and during heavy exercise, with special reference to stroke volume and the influence of body position. Acta Physiol. Scand., *57*:26-50, 1963.

48. Byrne-Quinn, E. Weil, J. V., Sodal, I. E., Filley, G. F., and Grover, R. F.: Ventilatory control in the athlete. J. Appl. Physiol., *30*:91-98, 1971.

Chapter Eleven

DEFENSE MECHANISMS

INTRODUCTION

The body is in direct contact with its external environment through the air inhaled during breathing. Each day the tracheobronchial tree and terminal respiratory units are exposed to more than 10,000 L of ambient air that may contain infectious microorganisms and hazardous dusts or chemicals. Tuberculosis, a classic example of a communicable disease acquired by inhalation, was once the scourge of the entire world, including the United States and Europe, and still is a major cause of illness and death in underdeveloped countries. In many communities, as pulmonary tuberculosis and its complications have declined, they have been replaced by the effects of inhaled toxic substances, particularly cigarette smoke and occasionally other chemical pollutants, as the major cause of disabling pulmonary disease. In the United States, cancer of the lung is the most common cause of death from malignancies in men, and chronic obstructive pulmonary disease has been among the most rapidly increasing serious medical disorders during the last two decades. The medical and socioeconomic importance of inhalation pulmonary diseases has resulted in a large amount of research on how the lung defends itself against the continuous onslaught of the various noxious substances it may encounter during normal breathing. A large amount of valuable information has resulted from these investigations, and it is now possible to piece together the various elements that contribute to pulmonary defenses and to understand, in part, how the lung resists development of disease from infectious agents, chemicals, physical injury, immunologic phenomena, and neoplasia.

The separate roles of the numerous components of the system of defenses that interact to protect the lung and the rest of the body against injury and disease are too complex (and often poorly understood) to review in detail here. This chapter will consider briefly the main determinants that affect the outcome of the battle between a beleaguered host, who is constantly challenging himself in the process of breathing, and an endless array of potentially harmful parasites and chemical substances. Thus, it is necessary to examine how certain particles and vapors are removed from the airstream within the normal respiratory tract, and once deposited, how some substances are handled by nonspecific (i.e., nonimmunologic) defense mechanisms of the respiratory tract and others are handled by cell-mediated and antibody-mediated immunologic responses. The components of the nonspecific and immunologic defense mechanisms that will be considered successively in this chapter are outlined in Table 11–1.

A distinction should be made between use of the general term *"immunity"* and the specific term *"immunologic."* Immunity means a condition of being exempt from injury or harmful influences (disease, taxes, military conscription), and immunologic denotes highly specific biologic phenomena characterized by recall or memory and the capability of mounting an anamnestic reaction.

DEPOSITION OF PARTICLES AND VAPORS

AEROSOLS

The term aerosol is used to describe any system of liquid droplets or solid particles dispersed in air (or some other gas) that remains airborne for a reasonable length of time.[1] The essential requirements of an aerosol are for the particles to be so small that they settle slowly and for the aerial suspension to be a stable one. Because large particles tend to settle

Table 11-1 Mechanisms that Contribute to the Defense of the Respiratory Tract

Nonspecific defense mechanisms
  Clearance
    Nasal clearance
    Tracheobronchial clearance
    Alveolar clearance
  Secretions
    Tracheobronchial lining (mucus)
    Alveolar lining (surfactant)
    Lysozyme
    Interferon
    Complement
  Cellular defenses
    Nonphagocytic
      Airway epithelium
      Terminal respiratory epithelium
  Phagocytic
    Blood phagocytes (polymorphonuclear
      neutrophilic leukocytes, monocytes)
    Tissue phagocytes (alveolar macrophages)
Specific defense (immunologic) mechanisms
  Antibody-mediated (B lymphocyte–dependent) immunologic
    responses
    Serum immunoglobulins
    Secretory immunoglobulins
  Cell-mediated (T lymphocyte–dependent) immunologic responses
    Lymphokine-mediated
    Direct cellular cytotoxicity

rapidly, clinically important aerosols, whether industrial, natural, or therapeutic, are composed for the most part of particles less than 10 μm in diameter.

Particles are removed from the airstream the instant they contact any portion of the lining of the respiratory tract. Furthermore, once a particle has touched the epithelial surface, it cannot be resuspended in the airstream and must be cleared from the body by some other means. Three different physical forces govern the deposition of particles within the respiratory system: inertia, sedimentation, and diffusion.

Inertia. During inhalation, particles are forced to change their directions repeatedly as they travel through the numerous curves and branches in the nasopharynx and tracheobronchial tree. However, once in motion, a particle tends to move in the same direction owing to inertial forces. This means that if a particle continues in its original direction when it should turn, it will touch and hence be deposited upon the epithelial surface. Because inertial forces increase with air velocity, inertial deposition of particles is greater in the upper than in the lower airways and is enhanced by increased frequency of breathing.

Sedimentation. Although an aerosol is a reasonably stable suspension, the particles are under the influence of gravity and will settle if given enough time. The speed at which a particle settles is determined by the density of the particle and the square of its diameter; accordingly a silica particle settles faster than a grain of pollen the same size. Deposition by sedimentation occurs more readily in relatively still air and thus is greater toward the terminal respiratory units than in the conducting airways. For similar reasons, at a given minute volume, sedimentation is augmented by breathing slowly and deeply.[2]

Diffusion. Aerosol particles may

demonstrate random (brownian) motion if the particles are small enough to be influenced by the continuous bombardment of the surrounding gas molecules. Consequently, deposition by diffusion is negligible for particles larger than 0.5 μm and is important only in the terminal respiratory units where the mass movement of air is trivial. It will be recalled (Chapter 6) that the mixing of newly inspired fresh air with air remaining from the previous breath takes place in the distal units by diffusion of gas molecules rather than by bulk flow; however, owing to differences in size, the diffusion of gas molecules is orders of magnitude faster than the diffusion of particles.

Whether or not a particle is deposited in the respiratory tract depends upon the airflow at different levels within the system and the size, density, and shape of the particle. It is obviously desirable to know both the distribution and deposition of particles in order to understand the pathogenesis of various pneumoconioses and the mode of action of therapeutic aerosols. It is possible to calculate air-

flow velocity at a given tidal volume and respiratory frequency from the dimensions of the airways and terminal respiratory units; from these data, the behavior of varying-sized spherical particles of unit density can be approximated. An example of the deposition of different-sized particles during normal quiet breathing (tidal volume 750 ml, 15 breaths/min) through the nose is shown in Figure 11–1. Although the distribution of aerosols is difficult to examine precisely in man, the results of most studies support the calculations diagramed in Figure 11–1.[3]

The following conclusions are warranted about the differing characteristics of particle trapping at various levels within the respiratory system.[2]

1. Almost all particles larger than 10 μm are deposited in the nasal passages and hence do not penetrate as far as the tracheobronchial tree. Conversely, the efficiency of nasopharyngeal filtering decreases as particle size decreases and becomes negligible at about 1 μm.

2. Accordingly, the percentage of

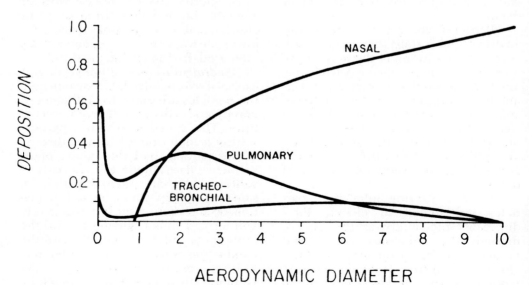

Figure 11–1 Nasal, tracheobronchial, and pulmonary deposition as a function of particle size; breathing pattern, 15 breaths/min, 750 ml tidal volume. (From Task Group on Lung Dynamics.[3] Reprinted by permission from the author and publisher.)

particles that penetrate into the terminal respiratory units rises from essentially zero with particles 10 μm and above to a maximum with particles 1 μm and below.

3. On a scale of graded particle sizes (Figure 11–1) those about 2 μm in aerodynamic diameter demonstrate a peak of deposition within terminal respiratory units; larger particles are trapped in the airways, and smaller particle retention decreases because impaction in alveoli decreases down to a particle size of about 0.5 μm.

4. Particles smaller than 0.5 μm are also retained in considerable numbers owing to a relative increase in the force of impaction by diffusion with decreasing particle size.

It should be emphasized that these statements apply only to "idealized" aerosols that contain spherical particles of unit density. When considering the distribution and retention behavior of irregularly shaped materials of varying densities, appropriate corrections must be introduced. Moreover, particles may change size as they move through the upper respiratory passages if they are sensitive to moisture (hygroscopic), and thus gain or lose water.

GASES (VAPORS)

According to toxicologic nomenclature, gases are classified into three main groups[4]: therapeutic, inert, and toxic. Therapeutic gases include O_2 and inhalation anesthetics and occasionally CO_2. Inert gases are normally of no physiologic consequence, but they are frequently used under controlled conditions in the laboratory to study various aspects of respiratory function. Toxic gases produce an undesirable physiologic effect that is usually accompanied by a pathologic response. Sometimes gases must be classified in more than one category; for example, a therapeutic gas may also be toxic (O_2 in high concentrations),

and an inert gas may be therapeutic (He). Because this chapter is concerned with the defenses of the lung, only the deposition and fate of noxious gases will be considered. The respiratory handling of O_2 and CO_2 has already been discussed (Chapter 5), and excellent reviews are available on the behavior of inert gases.[5, 6]

The penetration into and retention within the respiratory tract of toxic gases is exceedingly variable and depends upon the physical properties of the gas, its concentration in the inspired air, and the rate and depth of ventilation. Inhalation of a noxious gas usually has an immediate and profound effect on the pattern of breathing. Reflexes are triggered by chemical stimulation of receptors located in the nose (sneezing, laryngeal closure[7]), larynx (coughing, laryngeal closure, slowing of breathing[7,8]), airways (coughing, laryngeal narrowing, hyperpnea, bronchoconstriction[9,10]), and lung parenchyma (rapid shallow breathing[8]). When the entire system is activated, breathing consists of a variable mixture of sneezes, coughs, wheezes, gasps, grunts, and pants.

As indicated earlier, a force is required to impact a particle on the respiratory surfaces. In contrast, part of the airstream containing an inhaled toxic gas is always in contact with the moist epithelial lining of the nasopharynx, conducting airways, and distal airspaces. Therefore, some of the foreign gas is absorbed as the mixed inspirate flows through the upper air passages, and the amount removed varies according to the solubility of the gas. Highly water-soluble gases like SO_2 are completely extracted by the nose of healthy subjects during brief exposures[11]; in contrast, insoluble gases like phosgene and Cl_2 are removed much less completely and hence penetrate deeper into the respiratory tract. The amount of water-soluble gas that can be contained in tissues is limited, and saturation occurs quickly unless the amount already dissolved is removed by blood flow or chemical degradation. This means that if a highly soluble gas is present in high concentration, the absorptive capacity of the nasal passages becomes overwhelmed and the gas penetrates deep into the tracheobronchial tree. Less soluble gases that are poorly extracted in the conducting airways reach and mix with the air contained in distal respiratory units, and a fraction of the foreign gas is absorbed immediately. The amount taken up is proportional not only to the solubility and alveolar concentration of the foreign gas but also to the volume of tissue to which the gas is exposed. Because the alveolar surface is so extensive, large amounts of a toxic gas may be extracted by the lung even though the solubility of the gas is relatively low.

TEMPERATURE AND HUMIDITY

It is generally believed that inspired air is quickly brought to body temperature (37° C) and fully saturated with water vapor (PH$_2$O 47 mm Hg), regardless of the temperature and humidity of the ambient air. Both processes take place in the nasopharynx and under conditions of quiet nasal breathing are completed before the airstream reaches the larynx and upper trachea.[12] The nasopharyngeal mucosa serves as a heat source when cool air is breathed and as a heat absorber when excessively hot air is inhaled. Similarly, the epithelial lining is the source of the water vapor necessary for complete humidification. A rich blood supply and extensive surface area endow the nasal turbinates with these functional capabilities.

Changing from nasal breathing to mouth breathing also shifts the chief site of temperature control and humidification from the nose to the pharynx and larynx; bypassing the upper airway with an endotracheal tube or tracheostomy cannula moves the site

farther peripherally into the trachea and bronchi. Obviously, it is also possible to overburden the efficiency of the upper airway mechanisms, enabling air of unusual characteristics to penetrate into the tracheobronchial tree. This mechanism accounts for thermal injuries of the larynx and trachea, but in such cases superficial burns of the face and nose are apt to be particularly severe and indicate the difference in the intensity of heat that contacts the surface of the body and that which reaches the airways.

NONSPECIFIC DEFENSE MECHANISMS

The filtering system of the respiratory tract is not perfect, and a certain amount of potentially harmful material is deposited within the airways or airspaces during ordinary daily activities. To guard itself and the rest of the body, the respiratory system is normally furnished with several different nonspecific defense mechanisms, including clearance pathways, secretions with antimicrobial properties, and cells that impose barriers and actively phagocytize particles. The processes are nonspecific because they are effective against a variety of substances, not just specific ones (for comparison see subsequent section on immunologic mechanisms). Moreover, all nonspecific defenses are present from birth, and because they are not acquired by exposure, they are sometimes referred to as innate responses.

CLEARANCE

Highly water-soluble gases and liquid particles are absorbed at the sites of contact with the epithelial lining of the respiratory tract. Less soluble substances may be either eliminated or absorbed, depending upon the balance between the effectiveness of the clearance mechanisms and the rate of solution of the substance. The physiologic and pathologic consequences of absorption are determined by how much cellular damage and malfunction result from the biochemical reactions produced by the toxic substance and may vary from mild to lethal.

The fate of solid (insoluble) particles is considerably different. Coarse particles are filtered in the nose; finer ones are trapped in the nasopharynx and along the airways. Only very small particles (Fig. 11–1) penetrate to the terminal respiratory units, where some are deposited and the remainder are exhaled. Almost all of the solid particles that impact in the airways and lung parenchyma are ultimately eliminated from the body, but the mechanisms involved and the time required for complete removal vary greatly, depending upon the chemical properties of the particles and how far into the respiratory tract they penetrate before impacting. There are two interdigitating clearance systems that serve to remove particles deposited in different locations: clearance from the nasopharynx and tracheobronchial tree is achieved by *mucociliary transport*, and clearance from terminal respiratory units by *macrophage transport*. The efficiency of these processes can be appreciated by recognizing that residents of most cities inhale several hundred grams of solid particles over their lifetimes, yet analysis of their lungs after death reveals only a few grams of mineral ash.[2] The efficiency of clearance is also believed to be crucial to the pathogenesis of the slowly developing pneumoconioses because the severity of these diseases depends not only upon the quantity of dust initially deposited but also upon its subsequent removal.[2]

Nasal Clearance. The nose is structured anatomically so that most of the particulate matter that is inhaled through it impacts near the front on nonciliated epithelium where the passages are narrow and tortuous and where hairs are located; deposition of particles anteriorly facilitates their removal by nose blowing and sneez-ing.[13] Particles deposited more posteriorly are swept backward over the mucus-lined, ciliated epithelium to the nasopharynx where they are swallowed. It has been estimated that the mucous layer of the main nasal passages is normally cleared every 10 to 15 min, and that the rate of movement of particles placed on the mucosal surface is 4.8 mm/min.[13]

Tracheobronchial Clearance. As with the posterior nasopharynx, removal of particles from the entire system of conducting airways is carried out by mucociliary clearance: a film of mucus is continuously impelled proximally by the beating motion of cilia that cover most of the surface of the tracheobronchial epithelium. Any particles that deposit on the film of mucus are carried along with it to the oropharynx where they are swallowed or expectorated.

The number of cilia on the surface of each ciliated cell varies from one species to another; human ciliated cells have 200.[14] A characteristic of ciliated cells, as shown in Figure 11–2, is their numerous mitochondria, which cluster beneath the basal bodies of the cilia and are presumably the chief sources of energy for ciliary activity. A cilium is a complex structure that contains several pairs of separate filaments, each surrounded by a membrane. The cilia of a single cell and those of contiguous cells, though not anatomically connected, appear to be coordinated so that a wave of effective surface motion spreads in a proximal direction. Cilia beat rapidly with a characteristic biphasic stroke—a fast forward flick followed by a slow backward movement.

The mucous lining throughout most of the airways is composed of a double (sol-gel) layer on the surface of the bronchial epithelium, depicted in Figure 11–3. The inner layer, in which the cilia beat, is the liquid or sol phase of the transport medium, and the outer layer is the viscous or gel phase.[15] The viscous layer is nonabsorbent to water and presumably

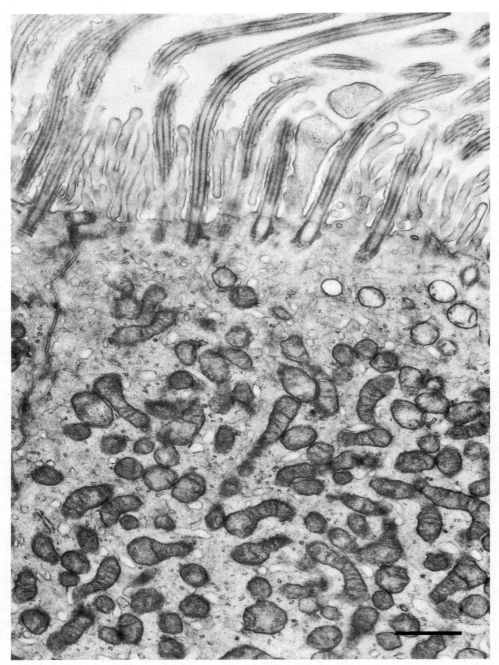

Figure 11–2 Electron photomicrograph of the luminal portion of a ciliated epithelial cell. Numerous mitochondria cluster beneath the basal bodies of the cilia. Horizontal bar = 1 μm. ($\times$ 12,500. Courtesy of Dr. Donald McKay.)

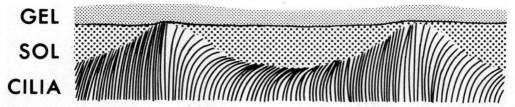

Figure 11–3 Schematic representation of cilia beating with a wave-like motion within the sol layer of the mucous lining; the tips of the cilia strike the inner surface of the gel layer. (Adapted from Hilding.[15] Reprinted by permission from the author and publisher.)

serves to protect the sol phase from desiccation; moreover, the tips of the beating cilia just strike the innermost portion of the gel covering them, thus facilitating proximal movement of the layer.

Because of the obvious difficulty in conducting suitable *in vivo* studies of mucociliary function in man, most of the available information has been derived from experimental animals. In the rat, for example, cilia have been observed to beat at a frequency of 1300 beats/min and to move the overlying mucous film at an average rate of about 13.5 mm/min.[16] Judging from studies in man, employing direct observations of small plastic disks through a cine-bronchofiberscope, the speed of tracheobronchial clearance is almost twice as fast (21.5 mm/min)[17]; however, clearance is distinctly slower in the peripheral divisions of the conducting airways than in the more central bronchi, owing to the necessity for the rate to increase progressively as the mucous streams converge. Mucociliary clearance varies widely, even in normal healthy subjects; in 14 nonsmokers, the mean 90 per cent clearance time of a radio-labeled aerosol was 494 min but the standard deviation was 130 min.[18]

Alveolar Clearance. The fate of solid particles that settle on the alveolar surface differs from that of particles deposited on the airway surface. The majority of the particulate load reaches the gastrointestinal tract via the mucociliary escalator and by swallowing, some is sequestered within the lung parenchyma, some reaches intrapulmonary, hilar, or other lymph nodes, and some enters the bloodstream and may circulate to any organ in the body[19]; which of these pathways is utilized depends upon the quantity and physicochemical properties of the substances deposited and the capabilities of the host's removal mechanisms.

Particles may traverse these routes in either the naked state or, more commonly, within phagocytes. Thus, considerable variation is possible in the means of removing substances from the alveolar surface, and this is reflected in the enormous range of alveolar clearance half-times (<1 day to >1400 days).[3]

1. Under normal conditions in which the aggregate dust load is light, almost all of the particles are phagocytosed by alveolar macrophages (Figure 11–4) which then eliminate the particle either by digesting it or by carrying it along the alveolar surface to the beginning of the mucociliary transport system.[20] From there, both the macrophage and its particulate contents are propelled centrally to the oropharynx where they are swallowed.

2. The second pathway of alveolar clearance also depends upon macrophages for phagocytosis and transport. In this instance, instead of moving along the alveolar surface the particle-laden macrophage moves through the interstitial space of the interalveolar septum until it reenters the lumen of the airspaces, often at the site of or ac-

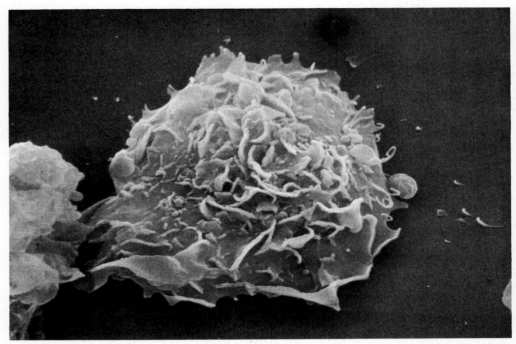

Figure 11-4 Scanning electron photomicrograph of a rat macrophage. Characteristic ruffles (lamellipodia) facilitate enfolding of particles during phagocytosis. (× 7400. Courtesy of Marguerite M. Kay, National Institute of Aging.)

tually through the lymphatic aggregates at the junctions of respiratory and terminal bronchioles.[21] Septal transport represents a "shortcut" from alveolus to respiratory bronchiole compared with surface transport but takes longer to traverse.

3. Some of the particles that reach the interstitial space enter lymphatic capillaries instead of reentering bronchioles. Once inside the lymphatic system, the particle has access to more centrally located lymph channels and lymph nodes. If the particle successfully navigates these sites of possible retention, it reaches the bloodstream and may circulate anywhere in the body.

It is generally agreed that unless the particle load is heavy and macrophage transport via surface and septal pathways is overwhelmed, little, if any, of the inhaled material reaches the hilar lymph nodes or bloodstream. However, with increasing exposure and saturation of phagocytic capacity, more and more particles can be found in regional lymph nodes and elsewhere in the body.

4. Some of the particles originally deposited in alveoli may be sequestered in the lung parenchyma by a tissue reaction. This reaction is complex, and many details about the mechanisms involved are lacking. The pathogenesis of the response clearly relates to the cytotoxicity of the inhaled substance. For example, silica (SiO_2) particles are usually lethal to the macrophages that engulf them; the dead cells (or their products) may give rise to a tissue reaction that prevents further ingestion or the silica particles may be recycled from one macrophage to another.

SECRETIONS

The respiratory tract distal to the larynx is normally sterile. The absence of culturable microorganisms depends not only upon the swift and efficient mucociliary and alveolar clearance mechanisms but also upon the constituents of the secretions that overlie the respiratory epithelium. Thus, defense against penetration into the lung's interior is imposed by the physical and chemical barriers of the surface film and the epithelial lining and is enhanced by the presence in the secretions that cover the epithelium of several antimicrobial substances, such as lysozyme, lactoferrin, and interferon, that serve to destroy or inhibit many bacteria and viruses.

Tracheobronchial Lining. The surface layer of liquid that normally lines the entire tracheobronchial tree is not a simple substance but a mixture of secretions derived from several sources: the liquid film that lines the surfaces of the terminal respiratory units, the secretions from goblet cells, and the secretions from mucous glands. Normally, mucous glands are found only in cartilaginous airways, whereas goblet cells are located in cartilaginous and membranous airways but not in terminal bronchioles. This means that unless there is retrograde movement of goblet cell secretions, the surface film in terminal bronchioles should be composed of secretions from Clara cells (and possibly other sources) and of surfactant that has been extruded or massaged from respiratory bronchioles into nonrespiratory bronchioles.*

The composition and physical properties of the lining layer are known to change dramatically in various bronchopulmonary and cardiac diseases. Inflammatory processes, allergic reactions, cystic fibrosis, circulatory failure, and respiratory tract neoplasms all usually increase the volume and change the character of the secretions from those normally produced. Furthermore, a striking increase or decrease in mucus viscosity affects mucociliary clearance,[23] and this is probably one reason why patients with these diseases have such a high incidence of pulmonary infections.

Alveolar Lining. Studies in experimental animals have revealed marked variations in the rate at which different species of bacteria are killed after inhalation (Figure 11–5). Part of the variation may be attributed to the capacity of some bacteria to multiply within the respiratory tract[25] and another part to varying bactericidal activity of alveolar macrophages.[24] Recent unconfirmed experiments suggest that the presence of alveolar lining material may enhance bactericidal activity *in vivo* by coating bacteria with lipids that undergo peroxidation to bactericidal aldehydes after phagocytosis.[26]

Lysozyme. The enzyme lysozyme is one of the most well-characterized antimicrobial substances found in respiratory tract secretions and other tissues and fluids of man. Lysozyme attacks muramic acid, a constituent of all bacterial cell walls. When the antimicrobial activity of lysozyme is studied in the absence of other factors normally present in respiratory secretions, it is found to be more effective against gram-positive than against gram-negative bacteria; the decreased susceptibility of gram-negative organisms is owing to the outer mainly lipoprotein layers of their cell walls, which protect the inner muramic acid–containing portion.[27] The activity of lysozyme against gram-negative bacteria is enhanced in the presence of antibody and activated complement. The combined action of antibody and complement on the outer wall of the bacterium exposes the inner layers to the enzymatic action of lysozyme.

---

*It has been speculated that if surfactant still retains its surface tension–lowering properties, it provides stability to the small airways in which it is normally present.[22] Accordingly, the increased distribution of goblet cells to within terminal bronchioles in patients with chronic bronchitis is probably accompanied by an alteration in the type of secretions in the airways that, in turn, may impair their stability and contribute to airways obstruction.

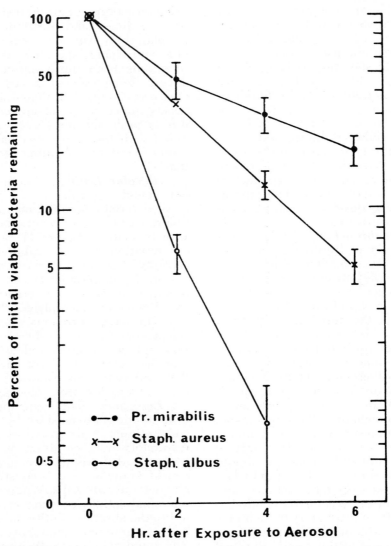

Figure 11–5 Clearance of *Proteus mirabilis, Staphylococcus aureus,* and *Staphylococcus albus* by normal mouse lung. (From Green and Kass.[24] Reprinted by permission from the authors and publisher.)

Lysozyme is also one of the important hydrolytic enzymes contained in lysosomes, the membrane-bound intracellular structures that participate in the killing of bacteria after phagocytosis. For example, lysozyme has been demonstrated in large quantities within alveolar macrophages from patients with tuberculosis and probably represents an important adaptive host response in the defense against spread of the infection.

Interferon. In 1957, Isaacs and Lindenmann[28] reported the discovery of a potent antiviral substance that they called *interferon*. Since then, interferons have been the subject of intensive investigations that have progressed to the threshold of development of methods for the prevention and treatment of important clinical diseases. It is now known that in addition to their antiviral activity, interferons confer protection against experimental infections of cell cultures with other intracellular parasites such as bacteria and protozoa; however, the clinical analogues of these *in vitro* phenomena have not been established. Of considerable interest and possible importance is the knowledge that interferons have an effect on the behavior of both viral- and nonviral-induced neoplasms.[29]

Interferons are a family of related proteins rather than single homogeneous molecules and constitute part of the natural defense system of vertebrate species from the teleost fishes up to and including man. In general, there is limited cross reactivity among interferons from different species, and interferons are most effective in the cells of the same animal species that produced them. The chief natural stimulus for *in vivo* interferon production appears to be viral infections; however, a variety of biologic and synthetic materials can also provoke cells to synthesize large amounts of interferon. These substances have proved extremely valuable in laboratory analysis of the interferon system, and their clinical usefulness is being examined.

The exact sequence of intracellular biochemical events that culminate in increased resistance to viral infection is not known but appears to incorporate two separate processes. The first step entails the synthesis and release of interferon by infected cells, and the second step involves the stimulation by interferon of an intracellular antiviral polypeptide that protects uninfected cells. The second step is necessary because interferon has no antiviral activity per se and can only act in the cells that it contacts by enhancing the production of antiviral substances.

Although cells from man, in general, are not as efficient synthesizers of interferons as cells from other vertebrates, interferon has been found in secretions from the respiratory tract and is known to be produced by alveolar macrophages.[30] Interferon is also one of the biologically active factors released by sensitized lymphocytes during cell-mediated immunologic reactions; it is of interest that macrophages, one of the chief effectors of cell-mediated immunity, are able to transfer the information for interferon production to lymphocytes.[31]

The precise role of interferon in defending against viral respiratory infections is uncertain, but there is every reason to believe that it is extremely important. Furthermore, interferon has a broad spectrum of antiviral activity, and only a few kinds of viruses have been found to be resistant. There is some doubt, at least at present, about the therapeutic value of interferon or its inducers in the treatment or prevention of common virus infections in normal subjects who are capable of synthesizing their own supply. However, the observation that 13 otherwise healthy patients with benign varicella or herpes zoster had high titers of interferon in their vesicular fluid, whereas three patients with neoplasms had disseminated herpes zoster and much less interferon, suggests a possible therapeutic benefit from interferon in the compromised host.[32] The use of interferon or interferon-inducers in the therapy of life-threatening virus infections and even of neoplasms has remarkable possibilities that need to be defined.

Complement. The activity of complement was once believed to be limited mainly to its role as an essential cofactor that allowed certain antigen-antibody sequences to reach completion. Now, complement is known to participate in various aspects of the inflammatory response such as enhancement of vascular permeability and chemotaxis of polymorphonuclear leukocytes; moreover, it also possesses clot-promoting activity. These multiple properties have recently been reviewed extensively.[33]

The complement system is composed of nine component proteins that participate in a sequential, or "cascading," reaction that results in active products that are both cell-bound and in the liquid phase. The cell-bound complexes contribute to cell lysis and death, and the liquid phase ingredients contribute to the humorally mediated portion of the inflammatory response.

Complement may be activated, as shown in Figure 11–6, by antigen-antibody complexes, plasmin, and certain insoluble polysaccharides, such as those contained in bacteria (e.g., pneumococcal) capsules. Two principal sequences are involved: the "classic" pathway including both early (C1, C2, C4) and late (C3, C5-9) components and the "alternate," or *properdin*, pathway incorporating only late components. The early components of the complement reaction sequence have been shown to participate in the neutralization of certain viruses[34]; the late components, especially C3, serve to enhance phagocytosis.[33] Late products also contribute to chemotaxis and cytolysis (Figure 11–6). It is important to emphasize that the alternate pathway can be activated in the absence of specific antibody and thus may play an important role in nonspecific defenses at the onset of primary infections before specific antibodies have been generated. This concept is supported by the increased frequency of bacterial infections, particularly pneumococcal, in patients with sickle cell anemia in whom the alternate pathway is deficient.[35]

CELLULAR DEFENSES

In addition to the antimicrobial substances that are naturally present in the secretions lining the respiratory tract, both nonphagocytic and phagocytic cell populations also contribute

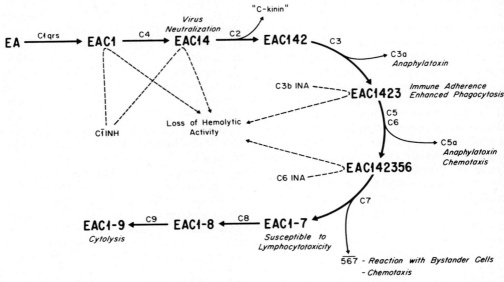

Figure 11–6 Classic complement-reaction sequence leading to the lysis of erythrocytes (E) treated with antibody (A) and the biologic activities of the various components (C1 to C9). (From Ruddy, Gigli, and Austen.[33] Reprinted by permission from the authors and publisher.)

to the defense of the lung and the rest of the body.

Nonphagocytic Cells. The surface epithelium and basement membrane of the airways and terminal respiratory units impose a physical barrier that guards the interior of the lung, and hence its lymphatic channels and blood vessels, from penetration by infectious agents and toxic substances. Furthermore, even if harmful materials reach the interior of the epithelial cells, the cells are probably capable of some inactivation by intracellular neutralization or digestion. The efficacy of this physical defense system is demonstrated by the frequency with which respiratory tract infections develop after injury to the epithelium (e.g., following viral infections of the tracheobronchial tree, especially influenza, and chemical damage from aspiration or inhalation of corrosive chemicals).

Phagocyctic Cells. Nearly a century ago, Metchnikoff[36] argued that phagocytosis is an important defense mechanism against the constant assault on the body by pyogenic microorganisms. The logic of Metchnikoff's deductions has been amply confirmed and his conclusions extended. Now, much is known about the cell types involved and the factors that regulate their production, how phagocytes recognize infection and "home in" on parasites, and how phagocytes engulf and kill microorganisms.[37] There are three types of "professional scavengers" that are constantly on duty in a state of functional readiness in the bloodstream (polymorphonuclear neutrophilic leukocytes and monocytes) and tissues throughout the body (tissue macrophages, including alveolar macrophages).

Blood Phagocytes. Polymorphonuclear neutrophilic leukocytes and monocytes are the two types of circulating phagocytes. In addition to their presence in the bloodstream, small numbers of both cell types are normally encountered in tissue spaces throughout the body; furthermore, a dramatic increase in the concentration of either polymorphonuclear neutrophilic leukocytes or monocytes in tissues constitutes one of the histologic hallmarks of differing kinds and durations of inflammatory processes. Both kinds of circulating phagocytes are derived from precursor cells in the bone marrow. Maturation in the marrow of polymorphonuclear neutrophilic leukocytes is slow, but once released into the circulation, they have a short half-time of survival of only six to seven hours; in contrast, monocytes mature faster in the marrow and spend more time in the circulation.[37] Also, as mentioned earlier in the case of alveolar macrophages (Chapter 2), some circulating monocytes enter interstitial tissues of the lung where they differentiate into alveolar macrophages and may replicate.

Early in the evolution of an inflammatory response, circulating granulocytes and monocytes stick to the endothelium of small blood vessels at the site of injury. If the damage is of sufficient intensity, both cell types migrate into the interstitial space surrounding the vessels. Extravascular emigration occurs by ameboid motion through the intercellular clefts in response to chemotaxis. The chemotactic factors involved have not been fully identified, but in addition to bacterial products, many appear to be closely related to components and products of the complement reaction sequence.

Polymorphonuclear neutrophilic leukocytes emigrate more quickly and in greater numbers than monocytes and so are the principal cell type early in the genesis of an inflammatory response. Although the emigration of mononuclear cells is delayed, it persists for a much longer period than that of granulocytes; therefore, mononuclear cells gradually become the predominant cell type as most inflammatory processes evolve. But the time course and extent of participation by the two species of cells vary greatly with different damaging stimuli.[38] Ordinarily, polymorphonuclear neutrophilic leukocytes degrade substances more effectively than monocytes, and this may be one reason why granulocytes are mobilized first.

It has already been pointed out that the defense mechanisms on the surface of the respiratory tract deal more effectively with relatively insoluble particles than with highly soluble substances. The same disparity exists for materials that penetrate the surface barriers: particulate matter, such as microorganisms, is phagocytosed and detoxified more readily than soluble chemicals. Both types of phagocytes, and other cells as well, take up soluble materials that have not caused a direct chemical injury (such as soluble antigens) by the mechanism of pinocytosis, after which the substances may be detoxified.

The cellular component of the inflammatory response appears to facilitate the isolation and detoxification of the offending agent through phagocytosis and digestion. These activities often cause the death of the participating cells, which results in the release of their proteolytic enzymes and further tissue necrosis. Usually, however, the process is a limited one, and the debris is removed by the ultimate scavengers, the monocytes.

Tissue Macrophages. The resident tissue macrophage in the lung, as discussed earlier, is the alveolar macrophage. These cells are sparse in the interstitium of the lung and common within the liquid film lining the

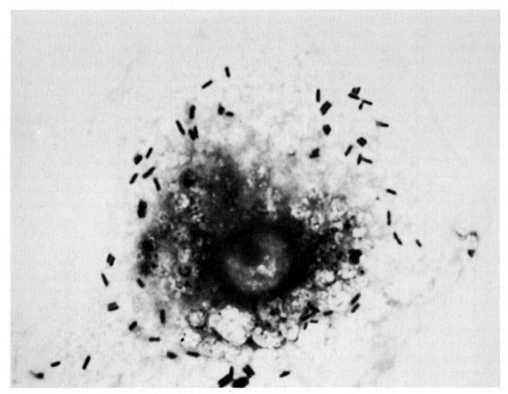

Figure 11-7 Photomicrograph of cultured human alveolar macrophage, obtained by lung lavage, showing phagocytosed *Listeria monocytogenes*. (× 7000. Courtesy of Dr. Allen B. Cohen.)

alveolar surface. Alveolar macrophages are avid phagocytes (Figure 11–7) and are able to dispose of a wide variety of microorganisms[39]; thus, they must be regarded as the chief guardians of the extensive surface of the terminal respiratory units.

However, once a microorganism or other particle impacts on the alveolar surface, no one knows how a macrophage locates it. Presumably, most particles do not exhibit tropism that would attract phagocytes, and macrophages move slowly in random fashion as they scavenge. Although the statistical likelihood of encountering a particle is small, the chance of contact is probably considerably enhanced by the rapid movement of the particles themselves, due to a combination of brownian forces in the alveolus and slipperiness of the surfactant lining.

It is also unknown how macrophages, and occasional unengulfed particles, find their way in such a purposeful manner out of the labyrinthine terminal respiratory unit to the mucociliary escalator. A minor pulling force may be imparted to the peripheral surface film by the activity of the more centrally located cilia, and gradients in surface tension have been described. However, the most important force for movement toward the hilum of alveolar secretions, cells, and debris appears to be derived from respiratory movements. Clinical and experimental data clearly demonstrate an impairment of dust clearance with appropriate pathologic sequelae (depending upon the dust) when movement of the lung is impaired,[2] but how respiratory movements are transmitted to cells and particles on the alveolar surface is unknown.

SPECIFIC DEFENSE (IMMUNOLOGIC) MECHANISMS

Nonspecific resistance of the respiratory tract depends upon normally functioning clearance mechanisms, antimicrobial substances, anatomic barriers, and circulating and tissue phagocytes. Each of these defenses is present at birth and demonstrates nonselectivity by operating against a wide variety of noxious intruders. In contrast, specific defense mechanisms are latent until actuated by natural exposure to foreign antigenic materials or by artificial induction (vaccination). Thus, specific defenses are acquired (in contrast to innate defenses) and are considered synonymous with immunologic defenses because they involve highly specific stimuli that cause equally specific responses. There are several pathways through which immunologic resistance may be acquired (Table 11–2), but this discussion will consider primarily the mechanisms of development of naturally acquired immunity.

Acquired immunity is mainly mediated by the capability of *specific antibodies* or *sensitized cells* to recognize and to react with individual *antigens* possessed by the offending agent. An antigen is defined by its capacity to induce specific antibodies or sensitized cells against it. Whether or not a substance is antigenic depends upon its molecular weight, physical shape, and chemical constituents; antigenicity also depends upon the capacity of the host to react to the given substance, a response which may vary considerably from one animal species to another. A *hapten* is a substance that pos-

Table 11–2   Pathways by Which Immunologic Defenses May be Acquired: Classification and Clinical Examples

---

Acquired naturally
   Active; e.g., following a bout of measles
   Passive; e.g., from placental transfer of immunity to mumps in the newborn

Acquired artificially
   Active; e.g., following immunization with diphtheria toxoid
   Passive; e.g., from injection of tetanus antitoxin

---

sesses antigenic capabilities, but this potential only becomes expressed after the hapten has complexed with an appropriate "carrier" molecule. Transformation of haptens into antigens is an important process because it provides a mechanism by which small and/or simple substances, which by themselves are not antigens, become antigenic following spontaneous *in vivo* combinations. This process allows the body to mount a defense against virtually any chemical substance that enters it and is of clinical significance in the formation of antibodies against toxins and other bacterial products.

The specialized ability to form antibodies is found only in vertebrates but is present in all that have been studied, including the most primitive one, the hagfish.[40] Among vertebrates, increasing complexity of immunologic responsiveness correlates with the evolutionary development of lymphoid tissue. It is not yet fully understood why it was essential to develop a system of specific immunity in addition to nonspecific defenses, but undoubtedly part of the explanation lies in the inherent flexibility of the antibody-manufacturing and cell-sensitizing systems. These mechanisms endow vertebrates with the capability of responding to the diverse antigens, such as infectious agents and cellular mutations, that are likely to be encountered during a lifetime. Certainly, the penalties of multiple infections and a high incidence of neoplasia in immunosuppressed patients are vivid testimony to the importance of acquired immunologic defenses (although it must be appreciated that immunosuppression usually impairs nonspecific defenses as well).

The human fetus produces only small amounts of antibodies, and the newborn depends mainly upon passively transferred maternal antibodies for protection during the first few weeks of extrauterine life. The meager production of antibodies by the fetus probably reflects the lack of sufficient antigenic challenge in the sheltered uterine environment to provoke an antibody response but may also be due to incomplete maturation of the lymphoid system and its control mechanisms. Antibody synthesis increases in the newborn infant a few weeks after delivery and accelerates even further during the first few years of life. The serum concentration of immunoglobulins reaches a plateau about 15 to 25 years of age and thereafter increases slowly (see Chapter 12 for further details about age-related changes).

This chapter will not consider the complexities and uncertainties concerning the interactions among antigens, lymphoid cells, and the immune response; these subjects are being investigated extensively and have been reviewed recently.[41,42] It will suffice to indicate that immunologic phenomena depend upon two major subpopulations of cells of the lymphocyte series[43]: (1) one population of cells differentiates under the control of the thymus, and accordingly, the cells are designated thymus-derived lymphocytes or T cells; (2) a second population of cells differentiates independently of the thymus but under the control of the bursa of Fabricius in birds, and although the analogue of the bursa in man is unknown, the cells are called bursa-derived lymphocytes or B cells. As will be emphasized subsequently in this chapter, the two populations of immunocompetent cells participate in two distinct immunologic reactions: B cells are the precursors of immunoglobulin-synthesizing plasma cells and thus are the effectors of antibody-mediated immunologic responses; T cells release lymphokines or may be directly cytotoxic and thus are the effectors of cell-mediated immunologic responses.

It is now possible to identify T and B cells by testing for specific surface markers. The commonly used marker for B cells is surface immunoglobulin and for T cells is their ability to participate in rosette formation (Figure 11–8). Using these methods, it has been shown that about 70 per cent of peripheral lymphocytes are T cells and the remainder are B cells.[45]

The morphologic and functional distinctions between T and B cells have led to the traditional view that there are two separate and independent components of the specific defense system. However, recent reviews emphasize that collaboration between both arms of the system is necessary to allow full expression of immunologic responsiveness.[46,47]

Most antigens that are introduced into the body are either "captured" by macrophages within lymphoid tissues or transported by macrophages to lymphoid tissue. Much of the new antigen is rapidly degraded, but a sufficiently large pool is retained to serve as an initial source of long-term antigenic stimulation. Arrival of a new antigen in the lymphoid system causes stimulation of those lymphoid cells predetermined to recognize the antigen. A wave of cellular proliferation ensues that is followed by differentiation into plasma cells or specifically sensitized T cells. Although most sensitization is believed to occur within lymphoid aggregates, in the case of allograft rejection circulating lymphocytes may become sensitized as they perfuse the foreign tissue. Depending upon the characteristics of the newly encountered antigen, the previously uncommitted cells that become stimulated belong to either the B or T cell series. However, the precise mechanisms of

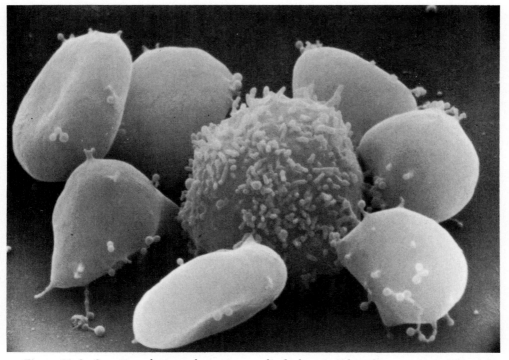

Figure 11–8 Scanning electron photomicrograph of a human T lymphocyte rosette. The ability of human lymphocytes to bind sheep red blood cells in the absence of antibody and complement has been shown to be a marker for T (thymus-derived) cells; T cells usually have greater than 300 microvilli per cell. (× 9400. From Kay, Belohradsky, Yee, Vogel, Butcher, Wybran, and Fudenberg.[44] Reprinted by permission from the authors and publisher.)

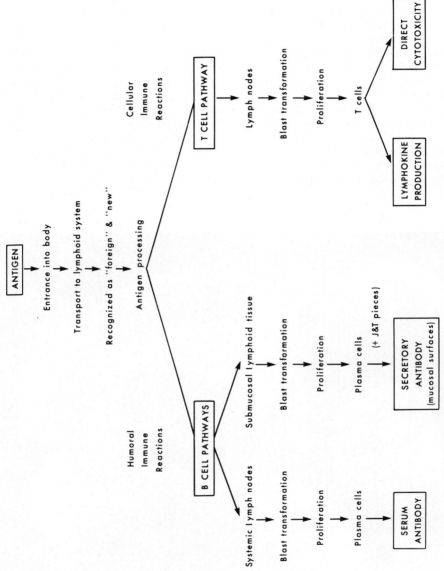

Figure 11-9 Schematic representation of the pathways by which antigens actuate B cell or T cell pathways and the resulting effector substances or mechanism of activity.

antigenic induction of either antibody-producing plasma cells or sensitized lymphocytes, or both, is not known but is an important problem that is being investigated extensively. Most antigens stimulate both B and T cell responses, but usually one or the other is greater in magnitude. Which one predominates depends upon the physicochemical properties of the antigen and its mode of presentation (e.g., with or without adjuvant). The different pathways of immunologic responsiveness that will be discussed subsequently are shown schematically in Figure 11–9.

Antibody-Mediated (B Lymphocyte-Dependent) Immune Responses

Induction of B lymphoid cells into antibody producers after antigenic challenge appears to be rapid: morphologic changes in target cells are apparent within six hours of exposure, and newly synthesized antibodies can be detected as early as 24 hours after exposure. After formation, antibodies are apparently released into the liquid environment surrounding the plasma cells. Additional factors, discussed later, lead to important differences be-

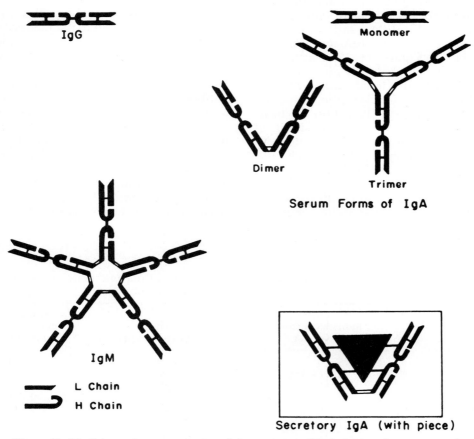

Figure 11–10 Schematic representation of the structure of IgG, IgM, and secretory and serum forms of IgA immunoglobulins. (From Weiser, Myrvik, and Pearsall.[27] Adapted from Tomasi, T. B., Hospital Practice 2:26, 1967. Reprinted by permission from the authors and publisher.)

tween the antibody constituents of internal secretions (including serum and pleural fluid) and external secretions (including tracheobronchial mucus). Most antibodies in the bloodstream are uncombined (or "free"), whereas others are cytophilic and become attached to cells.

Antibodies are known collectively as immunoglobulins and constitute the major fraction of serum gamma globulin. Immunochemical techniques have subdivided the immunoglobulins into at least five distinct classes: IgG, IgA, IgM, IgD, and IgE. All immunoglobulins consist basically of two long or heavy (H) chains and two short or light (L) chains; they differ in the amino acid constituents of the H and L chains and how the molecules are complexed. A schematic representation of IgG, IgM, and serum and secretory forms of IgA antibodies is shown in Figure 11–10. Further refinements of chemical analysis have permitted additional differentiation of the five chief classes of immunoglobulins into subclasses on the basis of variation in the composition of their H chains. In this context, it should be emphasized that each antibody-producing cell is highly specialized and produces a homogeneous protein that is uniform with respect to its electrophoretic mobility, antigen-

combining specificity, and immunoglobulin class and subclass.[48]

The designation, chemical characteristics, and normal concentrations of the major classes of serum and secretory immunoglobulins are presented in Table 11–3. Different classes of antibodies are now known to participate in antigen-antibody reactions with different physiologic and pathologic consequences (e.g., virus neutralization or anaphylaxis), and several clinical disorders have been linked to abnormalities of certain classes of immunoglobulins.

Serum Immunoglobulins. Circulating antibodies may function in several different ways to provide protection against microorganisms or their toxins. The "classic" reactions between antigens and antibodies that have been delineated in the laboratory are precipitation, agglutination, opsonization, cytolysis through complement activation, and neutralization.[27] It is widely accepted that a given antigen-antibody combination can be made to demonstrate many or all of these reactions by controlling the conditions under which it is studied and that a given reaction might be produced by several subclasses of antibody. Thus, examination of antigen-antibody reactions under rigorously controlled experimental circumstances *in vitro* is a

Table 11–3 Classification, Characteristics, and Normal Concentrations of Serum and Secretory Levels of Human Immunoglobulins*

CLASS	SEDIMENTATION CONSTANT	APPROXIMATE MOLECULAR WEIGHT	NORMAL SERUM LEVEL, MG/100 ML
IgG	7S	160,000	800-1680
IgA (serum)	7S, 11S, 18S	170,000	140-420
IgA (secretions)	11S	390,000	
IgM	19S	900,000	50-190
IgD	7S	160,000	0.3-40
IgE	8S	160,000	~0.003

*Data in part from Weiser et al.[27] and Cohen and Milstein.[48]

useful means of detecting and quantifying their presence in the body, and undoubtedly there are important biologic counterparts to the laboratory reactions that have clinical significance.

Precipitation occurs as a result of the combination of antibodies with soluble antigens in multiple proportions depending upon the amount of each reactant that is available. The number of antibodies that will react with a given molecule of antigen is determined by the number of antigen sites on the molecule; large molecules, therefore, have more sites for combination than small molecules. After the rapid initial combination between antigens and their specific antibodies is completed, secondary cross-links form among adjacent complexes and precipitation occurs. Precipitation is believed to be an important mechanism *in vivo* for converting soluble antigens into insoluble particles that are then subject to phagocytosis.

Agglutination is similar to precipitation except that the sizes of the cells involved in agglutination (e.g., bacteria or even red blood cells) are orders of magnitude greater than the sizes of the molecules of soluble antigens involved in precipitation. Antibodies cause agglutination by serving as bridges that link antigens on the surface of one cell with those on adjacent cells. This explains why IgM antibodies, which are large and have five reaction sites radially dispersed, are more likely to cause agglutination than IgG antibodies, which are much smaller and have only two reaction sites. For similar reasons, agglutination is markedly affected by the number and topographic distribution of the antigen-determinant sites on the cell surface. Agglutination *in vivo* probably assists in phagocytosis of particles by macrophages and histiocytes.

Cytolysis results from the reaction of specific antibody with antigens located on the cell surface in the presence of activated complement. Addi-

tion of complement to the antigen-antibody combination produces a complex that leads to injury of the outer cell wall and is lytic to susceptible cells. This system is highly bactericidal for gram-negative bacteria *in vitro* and is believed to be an important *in vivo* defense. The greater effectiveness of antibody-activated complement complexes against gram-negative bacteria compared with gram-positive bacteria is explained by differences in the composition of the outer cell wall; those with lipoprotein surfaces provide suitable substrates for the reaction that is presumably enzyme-mediated. (This also explains why red blood cells and other human cells, which have similar lipoprotein membranes, may also be lysed by the action of antibodies and activated complement.)

Some bacteria and other particulate materials possess the capacity to resist phagocytosis that may be overcome by *opsonization*. A coating of antibodies (opsonins) considerably enhances the ability of phagocytic cells to engulf particles and may augment the capacity of the cells to degrade the material. It appears likely that some nonspecific opsonins are normally present in serum and contribute to innate resistance, but most opsonins are IgG and IgM antibodies and represent an acquired response to antigenic challenge. Antibodies of IgA and IgE do not appear to be able to activate the complement reaction sequence and hence do not contribute to cellular lysis or complement-mediated opsonization.

Some of the most important consequences of certain infectious diseases are caused by toxins elaborated by the causative microorganisms. The value of antibody *neutralization* against these toxins is obvious and provides the basis for the acquired immunity, usually artificial by immunization, against diphtheria and tetanus. Some of the toxins that are neutralized by antibodies are known to be enzymes (e.g., lecithinase produced in gas gangrene), and there is a similarity in the reactions between antibodies and both toxins and enzymes.*

Viral neutralization by specific antibodies of the IgG, IgM, and IgA classes is more complex than toxin neutralization and appears to vary from one virus species to another. Different mechanisms may involve retention of virus within the phagocytic cells and inhibition of cellular penetration, but serum antibodies appear primarily to prevent hematogenous dissemination from the portal of entry to distant organs.[49]

Secretory Immunoglobulins. The long-standing suspicion that a local or regional immune system exists that is independent of the circulating antibody system has recently been confirmed. The evidence rests primarily upon the finding that the immunoglobulin content of external secretions is clearly different from that of serum (Table 11–3). In contrast, internal secretions, such as pleural and peritoneal fluids, CSF, amniotic fluid, and aqueous humor, contain immunoglobulins in nearly the same proportions as in serum, the exception being IgM, which, owing to its large size and limited diffusibility, is present in lower proportions in internal fluids than in serum. Furthermore, additional evidence supports the concepts of independent regulation of the antibody concentrations in external secretions on the one hand and the bloodstream on the other and, consequently, of a dissociation between systemic and local mucous membrane immunity.[50]

The chief immunoglobulin component of all external secretions is IgA, which, as indicated in Table 11–3, is physicochemically different from IgA in serum. Although the data are limited, it appears that the IgG, IgE,

and most of the IgM present in secretions are virtually identical with their circulating counterparts. Secretory IgA, designated SIgA, differs from serum IgA in that SIgA is a dimer of two IgA molecules linked by a secretory component (SC) and a joining chain (J chain) (Figure 11–10).

Monomeric 7S IgA is synthesized by plasma cells situated within or near mucous membranes and their glandular constituents. Some of the locally produced 7S IgA ultimately reaches the bloodstream, but the contribution from this source to the total circulating pool of IgA has not been established in man. Most of the IgA produced within the mucosa appears to combine with SC and J chain into an 11S complex and reaches the neighboring epithelial surface. The SC is synthesized by the epithelial cells and is believed to facilitate the transport of SIgA into external secretions by protecting the molecules from intracellular degradation during their passage through the cytoplasm of epithelial cells. The J chain is probably also produced locally in the mucosa by the same plasma cells that synthesize immunoglobulins. Whereas SC is found only in external secretions, J chain is present in immunoglobulin complexes of both internal and external secretions and appears to characterize the formation of polymers.[50]

The exact biologic role of SIgA is not completely documented. There is no doubt that it has neutralizing activity against viruses, and the levels of SIgA in various secretions correlate better than the serum levels with immunity, acquired either by spontaneous infection or by immunization, against certain viral infections. Moreover, adequate levels of SIgA may be necessary to eliminate the carrier state for viruses that have become established within various epithelial barriers (e.g., poliovirus in the intestine). On this basis, it has been inferred that the presence of SIgA in tracheobronchial and nasopharyngeal secretions pro-

---

*In both cases, antibodies are believed to be beneficial because they *indirectly* affect the chemical properties of the molecules by reacting with antigen-determinant sites near the toxin sites or enzyme-active sites.

vides an important defense against many viruses with a predilection for the respiratory tract, notably respiratory syncytial, influenza, parainfluenza, and rhino viruses.

The role of SIgA against bacterial infections is not clear, but it may enhance phagocytosis. Moreover, the recent discovery of antiragweed SIgA antibodies in respiratory tract secretions suggests that these antibodies may act locally and thus block, or prevent, allergic reactions that might otherwise occur. If this hypothesis proves to be correct, desensitization may be enhanced if expressed at the mucosal rather than the systemic level.[50]

CELL-MEDIATED (T LYMPHOCYTE-DEPENDENT) IMMUNE RESPONSES

The functional significance of acquired cellular immunity is not as immediately obvious as that of humoral immunity. However, cellular defenses are essential to combat infectious agents once they have reached an intracellular environment where they are protected from circulating antibodies.[51] In addition, cell-mediated immunity provides the mechanisms for surveillance and rejection of foreign and neoplastic cells. Although rejection creates special clinical problems related to the transplantation of tissues and organs, its physiologic role appears to protect the host against danger from cellular mutations and neoplastic transformations.[52] Similarly, cell-mediated immunity underlies tuberculin-type delayed hypersensitivity and contact hypersensitivity. All cell-mediated immune reactions have a common basis through involvement of T cells but are carried out by two basically different effector mechanisms[46]: (1) sensitized T cells in the presence of appropriate antigen elaborate and release a variety of biologically active factors known as *lymphokines* that, in turn, cause the tissue response to become fully developed; and (2) sensi-

tized T cells in the presence of suitable membrane antigen are directly *cytotoxic* against cells carrying the antigen. Whether these cytolytically active T cells are the same or are distinct from lymphokine-producing T cells is unknown at present.

The delayed hypersensitivity skin tests (e.g., with tuberculin or other antigens) has been the traditional means of demonstrating cell-mediated immunity. These tests, although clinically valuable, suffer from shortcomings as quantitative methods and in their failure to detect the presence of regional (e.g., respiratory) cell-mediated immunity in the absence of systemic involvement. Useful new tests are available such as allograph rejection and *in vitro* production of lymphokines, especially macrophage migration inhibition factor.[53]

Lymphokine-Mediated Cellular Immunity. As mentioned earlier, the essential mediator of specific cellular defenses is the immunologically committed, small, thymus-derived lymphocyte. After inoculation with intracellular parasites or certain antigens that provoke cell-mediated responses, there is an intense proliferative response in the lymphoid tissue (blast transformation and differentiation) that results in an expanded population of a specifically sensitized clone of lymphocytes. However, the direct attack against the given antigen is carried out not by the lymphocytes themselves but by chemical mediators, macrophages, polymorphonuclear neutrophilic leukocytes, and eosinophils. Lymphocytes "find" the antigen by their specific recognition capabilities and then, by releasing lymphokines, mobilize and activate nonsensitized cells that isolate, phagocytose, and attempt to destroy the foreign material.[54] This accounts for the usual finding of a few small lymphocytes in areas of delayed hypersensitivity inflammation. Thus, the essential characteristics of cellular defenses are collaboration between committed lymphocytes and uncommitted cells, especially macrophages; this relationship is beneficial because it amplifies considerably the magnitude of the cellular response. On the basis of *in vitro* experiments, it has been shown that only a few sensitized lymphocytes produce enough lymphokines to activate large numbers of normal cells.[55]

More than a dozen biologic activities have been attributed to factors elaborated by committed lymphocytes sensitized by specific antigen (Table 11–4). It appears likely that at least some and perhaps many of the properties listed in the table represent activities of similar substances tested under varying experimental conditions. However, the physiologic utility of these responses, assuming there are *in vivo* counterparts to the *in vitro* activities, is obvious. The factors serve to attract, to localize, and to stimulate macrophages and other effector cells. Accordingly, committed lymphocytes are endowed with the capacity to release chemicals with potent and varied biologic properties that serve to bring the cellular reaction to maturity.

Lymphokines have also been isolated from nonsensitized lymphocytes that have been "tricked" into behaving like committed cells after stimulation with certain mitogenic agents such as phytohemagglutinin or concanavalin. Although there appears to be no physiologic counterpart to this response, it is a useful method of studying lymphocyte behavior.

Cooperation among the cell types that participate in cellular defenses also takes advantage of the fact that lymphocytes are not equipped to function as phagocytes and degraders of foreign material whereas macrophages and polymorphonuclear leukocytes are. Furthermore, once macrophages are activated, their intracellular metabolism is greatly increased, which confers upon them an augmented capacity to migrate, phagocytose, and dispose of ingested material unrelated to the original activating antigen. In other words, immunologically committed lymphocytes induced in the defense against tuberculosis will react only to the presence of tubercle bacilli; however, the macrophages activated in the process will demonstrate increased effectiveness against not only tubercle bacilli but also other microorganisms.[56]

Although most lymphokines arm effector cells, *transfer factor* appears to induce noncommitted T cells to form T cells of the same antigen-specific clone as the original cells.[57] The physiologic usefulness of transfer factor in normal subjects may be by providing a

Table 11–4   Biologic Activities of Factors Elaborated by Committed Lymphocytes
Stimulated by Specific Antigen*

Transfer factor
Migration inhibitory factor
Chemotactic factor for macrophages
Chemotactic factor for neutrophilic polymorphonuclear
    leukocytes
Macrophage-activating factor
Cytotoxic factor
Growth-inhibiting factor
Cloning inhibition factor
Factor preventing DNA synthesis
Mitogenic factor
Skin-reactive factor
Macrophage aggregation factor

*Data in part from David.[54]

mechanism for both perpetuating antigenic memory and amplifying the response to specific antigen by stimulating the formation of additional numbers of committed T cells. Transfer factor also may be a powerful therapeutic substance in the treatment of patients who have genetic or acquired diseases associated with loss of cell-mediated immunity, and this is currently the subject of numerous clinical trials. The efficacy of transfer factor and the indications for its use are not yet established.

Direct Cellular Cytotoxicity. It is now evident from *in vitro* studies that at least three separate mechanisms involving several different cell types participate in cell-mediated cytotoxicity.[58] The first involves a cell-cell interaction between sensitized T cells and membrane-bound antigens carried by foreign tissues; serum antibodies are not required and if present may inhibit the cytotoxicity of the T cells. The second involves the reaction of IgG antibody with target cells and linkage with receptor sites on effector cells; the type(s) of effector cells is unknown, but they are present in unsensitized persons and are not T cells. The third involves macrophages that are equipped with either cytophilic antibodies or lymphokines elaborated by sensitized T cells.

Thus, a fully expressed graft rejection *in vivo* is an extremely complex process involving antibody-mediated immune responses as well as cell-mediated phenomena (including direct cytotoxicity and release of lymphokines). T cells presumably initiate the reaction by ferreting out the incompatible antigens and then after blast transformation and proliferation invade the graft and react with the tissues. Thus, T cells constitute both the afferent, or sensitizing, limb and the efferent, or effector, limb of this pathway.

T cell cytotoxicity is probably an important mechanism that contributes to immune surveillance against neoplasms. However, the means by which T cells kill other cells is unknown despite many attempts to identify a cytotoxic substance from *in vitro* experiments. Clearly, much more needs to be learned about cellular cytotoxicity.

IMMUNOLOGIC REACTIONS IN THE LUNG

Recent experimental evidence indicates that both antibody- and cell-mediated immunologic responses occur in the lung and, of considerable importance, that these responses can be expressed independently of changes in systemic immune factors. Thus, the concept of the lung having its own "local" immune system is gaining strength. However, the issue is by no means settled.

Several pieces of evidence support the presence of a local antibody-producing system in the lung: (1) it is known (Chapter 3) that the human lung contains submucosal aggregates of lymphoid tissue along conducting airways and respiratory bronchioles; (2) fluorescent-staining methods have revealed IgA in intercellular spaces of the epithelium and basement membrane area and in scattered plasma cells in the lamina propria of bronchial mucosa of normal subjects[59]; (3) B cells can be detected in lung washings from man[60] and dogs[61]; (4) B cells from the lower respiratory tract of dogs are capable of responding to antigen with a specific antibody-mediated response[62]; and (5) secretory IgA has been identified in respiratory tract secretions.[50] Thus, it is clear that "local" B cell-mediated responses do occur.

Evidence in favor of the existence of local T cell-mediated immunity is not as completely convincing as that of local B cell responses. Even though morphologically and functionally intact T cells were found in lung washings from normal subjects,[60] it is possible that the cells originated in the pulmonary circulation and not from local lymphoid aggregates. Furthermore, it was not possible to identify

T cells in lung washings from normal dogs until they were challenged with intra-alveolar instillations of antigenic material[61]; in these experiments, it was uncertain whether the T cells were recruited from the bloodstream or from local lymphoid tissue. Similarly, the large numbers of presumed T cells that accumulated in the bronchial lamina propria of experimental animals may have been derived from the circulation and not local precursors.[63]

More convincing evidence in support of the existence of local pulmonary cell-mediated immunity is provided by the results of experiments in which the effects of different routes of immunization were compared. It was possible to differentiate local from systemic T cell-mediated responses by inoculating guinea pigs either subcutaneously or by nose drops.[64] Furthermore, the general conclusions from these studies have been supported by recent experiments using subcutaneous and aerosol inoculations of influenza virus in human subjects.[65] The evidence from both these studies must be considered inconclusive because it is not known exactly where the drops or aerosol were distributed, how much was absorbed systemically, and what was the origin of the lymphocytes that participated in the response.

Another unsettled problem in the genesis of local pulmonary cell-mediated immune responses concerns the role of alveolar macrophages as effector cells in lymphokine-dependent reactions. It would seem to be to the host's advantage for local rather than circulating macrophages to participate in locally mediated responses. Yet, the limited data available from immunization and bacterial challenge experiments indicate that alveolar macrophages are not as effective as hepatocytes in clearing bacteria and that most of the macrophages recovered in the lung that phagocytosed and killed the bacteria came from the circulation.[66]

To summarize, local antibody-mediated immunity has been demonstrated in the lung.[67] However, it is still uncertain whether or not the lung can mount local cell-mediated immunity. As a corollary, the role of the lymphocytes in the airway mucosa as precursors of T cells and the contribution of alveolar macrophages to the tissue response need to be clarified.

REFERENCES

1. Muir, D. C. F.: Deposition and clearance of inhaled particles. In Muir, D. C. F. (ed.): Clinical Aspects of Inhaled Particles. London, Heinemann, 1972, pp. 1–20.
2. Hatch, T. F., and Gross, P.: Pulmonary Deposition and Retention of Inhaled Aerosols. New York, Academic Press, 1964, pp. 67-85.
3. Task Group on Lung Dynamics: Deposition and retention models for internal dosimetry of the human respiratory tract. Health Phys., 12:173-207, 1966.
4. Oberst, F. W.: Factors affecting inhalation and retention of toxic vapours. In Davies, C. N. (ed.): Inhaled Particles and Vapours. New York, Pergamon Press, 1961, pp. 249-266.
5. Forster, R. E.: Diffusion of gases. In Fenn, W. O., and Rahn, H. (eds.): Handbook of Physiology, Section 3. Respiration. Vol. I. Washington, D. C., American Physiology Society, 1964, pp. 839-872.
6. Farhi, L. E.: Elimination of inert gas by the lung. Resp. Physiol., 3:1-11, 1967.
7. Szereda-Przestaszewska, M., and Widdicombe, J. G.: Reflex effects of chemical irritation of the upper airways on the laryngeal lumen in cats. Resp. Physiol., 18:107-115, 1973.
8. Widdicombe, J. G., and Sterling, G. M.: The autonomic nervous system and breathing. Arch. Intern. Med., 126:311-329, 1970.
9. Mills, J. E., Sellick, H., and Widdicombe, J. G.: Activity of lung irritant receptors in pulmonary microembolism, anaphylaxis and drug-induced bronchoconstrictions. J. Physiol. (Lond.), 203:337-357, 1969.
10. Nadel, J. A., Salem, H., Tamplin, B., and Tokiwa, Y.: Mechanism of bronchoconstriction during inhalation of sulfur dioxide. J. Appl. Physiol., 20:164-167, 1965.
11. Speizer, F. E., and Frank, N. R.: A comparison of changes in pulmonary flow resistance in healthy volunteers acutely exposed to SO_2 by mouth and by nose. Brit. J. Industr. Med., 23:75-79, 1966.
12. Ingelstedt, S.: Studies on the conditioning

of air in the respiratory tract. Acta Otolaryngol. (Suppl.), *131*:1-80, 1956.

13. Proctor, D. F., Andersen, I., and Lundqvist, G.: Clearance of inhaled particles from the human nose. Arch. Intern. Med., *131*: 132-139, 1973.

14. Rhodin, J. A. G.: Ultrastructure and function of the human tracheal mucosa. Am. Rev. Resp. Dis., *93* (Suppl.):1-15, 1966.

15. Hilding, A. C.: Experimental studies on some little understood aspects of the physiology of the respiratory tract and their clinical importance. Trans. Am. Acad. Ophthal. Otolaryngol., *65*:475-495, 1961.

16. Dalhamn, T.: Mucus flow and ciliary activity in the trachea of healthy rats and rats exposed to respiratory irritant gases (SO_2, H_3N, HCHO); functional and morphologic (light microscopic and electron microscopic) study, with special reference to technique. Acta. Physiol. Scand. *36* (Suppl. 123):1-161, 1956.

17. Santa Cruz, R., Landa, J., Hirsch, J., and Sackner, M. A.: Tracheal mucous velocity in normal man and patients with obstructive lung disease; effects of terbutaline. Am. Rev. Resp. Dis., *109*:458-463, 1974.

18. Albert, R. E., Lippmann, M., Peterson, H. T., Jr., Berger, J., Sanborn, K. and Bohning, D.: Bronchial deposition and clearance of aerosols. Arch. Intern. Med., *131*:115-127, 1973.

19. Green, G. M.: Lung defense mechanisms. Med. Clin. N. America, *57*:547-562, 1973.

20. La Belle, C. W. and Brieger, H.: The fate of inhaled particles in the early postexposure period. Arch. Environ. Health *1*:432-437, 1960.

21. Green, G. M.: Alveolobronchiolar transport mechanisms. Arch. Intern. Med., *131*:109-114, 1973.

22. Macklem, P. T., Proctor, D. F., and Hogg, J. C.: The stability of peripheral airways. Resp. Physiol., *8*:191-203, 1970.

23. Barton, A. D., and Lourenco, R. V.: Bronchial secretions and mucociliary clearance. Arch. Intern. Med., *131*:140-144, 1973.

24. Green, G. M., and Kass, E. H.: The influence of bacterial species on pulmonary resistance to infection in mice subjected to hypoxia, cold stress, and ethanolic intoxication. Brit. J. Exp. Pathol., *46*:360-366, 1965.

25. Johanson, W. G., Jr., Jay, S. J., and Pierce, A. K.: Bacterial growth in vivo. An important determinant of the pulmonary clearance of *Diplococcus pneumoniae* in rats. J. Clin. Invest., *53*:1320-1325, 1974.

26. LaForce, F. M., Kelly, W. J., and Huber, G. L.: Inactivation of staphylococci by alveolar macrophages with preliminary observations on the importance of alveolar lining material. Am. Rev. Resp. Dis., *108*:784-790, 1973.

27. Weiser, R. S., Myrvik, Q. N., and Pearsall, N. N.: Fundamentals of Immunology for Students of Medicine and Related Sciences. Philadelphia, Lea & Febiger, 1969, p. 363.

28. Isaacs, A., and Lindenmann, J.: Virus interference: I. The interferon. Proc. Roy. Soc. Lond. (Biol) Series B, *147*:258-267, 1957.

29. Grossberg, S. E.: The interferons and their inducers: molecular and therapeutic considerations. New Eng. J. Med., *287*:13-19, 79-85, 122-128, 1972.

30. Acton, J. D., and Myrvik, Q. N.: Production of interferon by alveolar macrophages. J. Bacteriol., *91*:2300-2304, 1966.

31. Epstein, L. B., Cline, M. J., and Merigan, T. C.: The interaction of human macrophages and lymphocytes in the phytohemagglutinin-stimulated production of interferon. J. Clin. Invest., *50*:744-753, 1971.

32. Armstrong, R. W., Gurwith, M. J., Waddell, D., and Merigan, T. C.: Cutaneous interferon production in patients with Hodgkin's disease and other cancers infected with varicella or vaccinia. New Eng. J. Med., *283*:1182-1187, 1970.

33. Ruddy, S., Gigli, I., and Austin, K. F.: The complement system of man. New Eng. J. Med., *287*:489–495, 545–549, 592–596, 642-646, 1972.

34. Daniels, C. A., Borsos, T., Rapp, H. J., Snyderman, R., and Notkins, A. L.: Neutralization of sensitized virus by purified components of complement. Proc. Nat. Acad. Sci. USA, *65*:528-535, 1970.

35. Johnston, R. B., Jr., Newman, S. L., and Struth, A. G.: An abnormality of the alternate pathway of complement activation in sickle-cell disease. New Eng. J. Med., *288*:803-808, 1973.

36. Metchnikoff, E.: Immunity in Infective Diseases. London, Cambridge University Press, 1905, p. 591.

37. Stossel, T. P.: Phagocytosis. New Eng. J. Med., *290*:717–723, 774–780, 833–839, 1974.

38. Hurley, J. V., Ryan, G. B., and Friedman, A.: The mononuclear response to intrapleural injection in the rat. J. Pathol. Bacteriol., *91*:575-587, 1966.

39. Green, G. M., and Kass, E. H.: The role of the alveolar macrophage in the clearance of bacteria from the lung. J. Exp. Med., *119*:167-176, 1964.

40. Grey, H. M.: Phylogeny of immunoglobulins. Adv. Immunol., *10*:51-104, 1969.

41. Good, R. A., and Fisher, D. W.: *Immunobiology*. Stamford, Conn., Sinauer Associates, Inc., 1971, pp. 1-305.

42. Eisen, H. N.: Immunology. An introduction to molecular and cellular principles of the immune response. Hagerstown, Harper and Row, 1974, pp. 352-624.

43. Craddock, C. G., Longmire, R., and McMillan, R.: Lymphocytes and the immune response. New Eng. J. Med., 285:324-331, 378-384, 1971.
44. Kay, M. M., Belohradsky, B., Yee, K., Vogel, J., Butcher, D., Wybran, J., and Fudenberg, H. H.: Cellular interactions: scanning electron microscopy of human thymus-derived rosette-forming lymphocytes. Clin. Immunol. Immunopathol., 2:301-309, 1974.
45. Jondal, M., Holm, G., and Wigzell, H.: Surface markers on human T and B lymphocytes. I. A large population of lymphocytes forming nonimmune rosettes with sheep red blood cells. J. Exp. Med., 136:207-215, 1972.
46. Bloom, B. R.: In vitro approaches to the mechanism of cell-mediated immune reactions. Adv. Immunol., 13:101-208, 1971.
47. Katz, D. H., and Benacerraf, B: The regulatory influence of activated T cells on B cell response to antigen. Adv. Immunol., 15:1-94, 1972.
48. Cohen, S., and Milstein, C.: Structure and biological properties of immunoglobulins. Adv. Immunol., 7:1-89, 1967.
49. Merigan, T. C.: Host defenses against viral disease. New Eng. J. Med., 290:323-329, 1974.
50. Tomasi, T. B., Jr.: Secretory immunoglobulins. New Eng. J. Med., 287:500-506, 1972.
51. Mackaness, G. B.: The J. Burns Amberson Lecture—the induction and expression of cell-mediated hypersensitivity in the lung. Am. Rev. Resp. Dis., 104:813-828, 1971.
52. Burnet, F. M.: Implications of cancer immunity. Aust. New Zeal. J. Med., 3:71-77, 1973.
53. Rocklin, R. E., Rosen, F. S., and David, J. R.: In vitro lymphocyte response of patients with immunologic deficiency diseases: correlation of production of macrophage inhibitory factor with delayed hypersensitivity. New Eng. J. Med., 282:1340-1343, 1970.
54. David, J. R.: Lymphocyte mediators and cellular hypersensitivity. New Eng. J. Med., 288:143-149, 1973.
55. David, J. R., Lawrence, H. S., and Thomas, L.: Delayed hypersensitivity in vitro. II. Effect of sensitive cells on normal cells in the presence of antigen. J. Immunol., 93:274-278, 1964.
56. Mackaness, G. B.: The immunological basis of acquired cellular resistance. J. Exp. Med., 120:105-120, 1964.

57. Lawrence, H. S.: Transfer factor. Adv. Immunol., 11:195-266, 1969.
58. Cerottini, J-C., and Brunner, K. T.: Cell-mediated cytotoxicity, allograft rejection, and tumor immunity. Adv. Immunol., 18:67-132, 1974.
59. Tourville, D. R., Adler, R. H., Bienenstock, J., and Tomasi, T. B., Jr.: The human secretory immunoglobulin system: immunohistological localization of γA, secretory "piece," and lactoferrin in normal human tissues. J. Exp. Med., 129:411-429, 1969.
60. Daniele, R. P., Altose, M. D., Salisbury, B. G., and Rowlands, D. T.: Characterization of lymphocyte subpopulations in normal human lungs. In Proceedings of the 17th Aspen Lung Conference. Chest 67 (Suppl.):52S–53S, 1975.
61. Kaltreider, H. B., and Salmon, S. E.: Immunology of the lower respiratory tract. Functional properties of bronchoalveolar lymphocytes obtained from the normal canine lung. J. Clin. Invest., 52:2211-2217, 1973.
62. Kaltreider, H. B., Kyselka, L., and Salmon, S. E.: Immunology of the lower respiratory tract. II. The plaque-forming response of canine lymphoid tissues to sheep erythrocytes after intrapulmonary or intravenous immunization. J. Clin. Invest., 54:263-270, 1974.
63. Fernald, G. W., Clyde, W. A., Jr., and Bienenstock, J.: Immunoglobulin-containing cells in lungs of hamsters infected with Mycoplasma pneumoniae. J. Immunol., 108:1400-1408, 1972.
64. Waldman, R. H., and Henney, C. S.: Cell-mediated immunity and antibody responses in the respiratory tract after local and systemic immunization. J. Exp. Med., 134:482-494, 1971.
65. Jurgensen, P. F., Olsen, G. N., Johnson, J. E., III, Swenson, E. W., Ayoub, E. M., Henney, C. S., and Waldman, R. H.: Immune response of the human respiratory tract. II. Cell-mediated immunity in the lower respiratory tract to tuberculin and mumps and influenza viruses. J. Infect. Dis., 128:730-735, 1973.
66. Truitt, G. L., and Mackaness, G. B.: Cell-mediated resistance to aerogenic infection of the lung. Am. Rev. Resp. Dis., 104:829-843, 1971.
67. Tomasi, T. B., Jr., and DeCoteau, E.: Mucosal antibodies in respiratory and gastrointestinal disease. Adv. Intern. Med., 16:401-425, 1970.

Chapter Twelve

AGING

INTRODUCTION

Most people recognize that improvements in socioeconomic conditions and in health care during the last several decades have extended the *average* life span of human beings by many years, but it is not so well known that the *maximum* duration of life in modern times is nearly the same as it was in antiquity.[1] Thus, every person is mortal, and contrary to popular belief, there is no foreseeable practical way of extending maximum life span. Elimination of cardiovascular diseases and cancer, today's two biggest killers in the western world, would increase life expectancy from birth only nine years by allowing persons to approach more closely their biologically determined maximums.[2]

Development from fertilization to complete maturation is clearly a time-dependent process and thus related to aging. These processes differ, however, because growth is characterized by the elaboration of cells, tissues, and organs with new structures or functions, whereas senescence is associated with loss of adaptation and in-

307

creased vulnerability to disease.[3] Embryogenesis and postnatal development of the lungs' structure are considered in Chapters 1 and 2. This chapter will discuss mainly the effects of aging on respiration during both growth and senescence; the structural basis for these changes will be included when information is available.

The mechanisms responsible for the cellular effects of aging are unknown, but most theories involve alterations, either genetically programmed or acquired, in genetic machinery.[2,3] Some organs (e.g., thymus, ovaries) involute and cease to function long before death usually occurs. However, the lungs appear to be relatively durable and, even though important alterations in their structure and function develop with age, are capable of maintaining adequate gas exchange for the maximum life span of otherwise normal persons.

It is important to document the effects of growth and senescence on pulmonary function in order to establish the limits of "normal" development and aging; this is obviously necessary before functional impairment from pulmonary diseases can be identified. In children, there are abundant data to document the effects of growth between about 5 and 15 years of age on pulmonary function variables, and some data are available from the newborn period. But little is known about changes during the early infancy-preschool period and the puberty-young adulthood period.[4] It should also be pointed out that differences in the rate of growth and age of maturation lead to differences between male and female persons in the age-related changes of many pulmonary function variables. Similarly, the effects of senescence on respiratory function tests are usually less marked in women than in men. The boundary between normality and disease is often ill-defined and presents a problem of definition that is especially troublesome in the aged. Therefore, some of the data from which conclusions about the effects of senescence on respiration have been reached must be accepted with reservations owing to uncertainties about smoking habits, environmental exposure, and physical activity.

STATIC PROPERTIES

COMPLIANCE

As discussed in Chapter 4, the determinants of static lung volumes are the elastic properties of the lungs and chest wall and the forces that can be generated by the muscles of respiration to inflate and deflate the respiratory system. Although there is some increase during growth followed by progressive weakening in old age of maximal inspiratory and expiratory muscle strength,[5] the chief physiologic effects of aging on pulmonary function are attributable to changes in the compliance of both the lungs and the chest wall. Recent studies have supplied much needed information about the compliance of human lungs in relation to age,[6,7] and knowledge about existing gaps in the continuum of information can be inferred with reasonable confidence. In contrast, studies about the age-related behavior of the chest wall are extremely limited, especially in infants and children; these data are needed because they are necessary to allow examination of the entire respiratory system and because they may explain the serious clinical consequences of lower respiratory infections in infants. For example, it was mentioned in Chapter 4 that children younger than five years of age may be at a disadvantage compared with adults because their small airways are disproportionately smaller; however, changes in the functional capabilities of the chest wall could either compound or minimize the effects of differences in airway caliber.

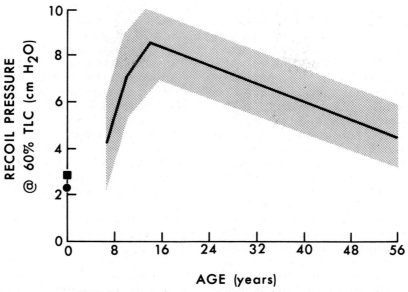

Figure 12–1 Static elastic recoil at 60 per cent total lung capacity (TLC) as a function of age. (Data of Turner, Mead, and Wohl[7] and Zapletal, Misur, and Samanek.[8]) Shaded area represents ± one standard deviation of mean values. Mean values in newborn period (■ ●) from Gribetz, Frank, and Avery[9] and Nelson.[10] (Adapted from Mansell, Bryan, and Levison.[6] Reprinted by permission from the authors and publisher.)

Figure 12–1 summarizes the relationship between static elastic recoil at 60 per cent of TLC and age based on separate studies of different age groups.[6-10] Static elastic recoil increases from birth until growth ceases and then gradually diminishes. These changes, in turn, offer a convenient explanation about the cause of age-related changes in lung volumes, expiratory flow rates, and arterial blood gases.

In the final analysis, the elastic properties of the lung can be separated into two components: surface and tissue forces. There is no evidence that the surface-active lining of terminal respiratory units alters its basic mechanical behavior with age. Thus, changes in surface forces do not appear to contribute to age-related changes with the exception that variations in elastic recoil from surface forces may occur secondary to the influence of tissue forces on alveolar dimen-

sions.[7] The lung grows by both the formation of new alveoli and the expansion of existing alveoli (Chapter 2). Although not known with certainty, the enlargement of the lung from birth to maturity is probably associated with increases in both surface and tissue forces, the former from simple expansion of the surface of individual alveoli and the latter from changing tissue composition; in this context, it is generally agreed that the elastic fiber system of the lung is incompletely formed at birth and continues to develop up to young adulthood.[11] It is possible that changes in the collagen framework of the lung may also contribute to an increase in tissue forces during growth.

The diminution in static elastic recoil of the lung that occurs during senescence is more difficult to account for on a structural basis than the increase that occurs during growth, although connective tissue elements have also been implicated. It was originally believed that there was a progressive increase in elastin content of the lung with age after maturity[12]; more recent data indicate that the elastin content of the pleura increases whereas that of the parenchyma remains constant.[13] However, neither report provides a satisfactory explanation for the consistent reduction in elastic recoil of the lung during senescence. One possible reason for the discrepancy is that neither the total amount of elastin present nor the elastic modulus of the individual fibers is important and that the *location* of the fibers within the lung determines the elastic recoil.[7] It can be inferred from all these observations that remodeling of the elastic tissue architecture of the lung must occur during advancing age. In this context, Wright's[14] observation of a uniform reduction in the number and thickness of the elastic fibers forming the alveolar ducts and the mouths of alveoli provides a tentative anatomic explanation for decreasing lung recoil with age.

Studies in newborns and young infants demonstrated that the compliance of the lung and chest wall combined[15] is nearly the same as that of the lung alone.[16] This means that compliance of the chest wall must be high in the neonatal period. Similar conclusions from direct measurements were reported for dogs[17] and for goats.[18] The similarities of chest wall mechanics among newborns of several mammalian species probably relate to the requirements of passage through the birth canal.

Chest wall compliance presumably decreases during childhood to the values found in young adults, although the sequence of changes has not been documented. In adulthood, a progressive reduction was demonstrated in men 24 to 78 years of age.[19] The stiffening of the chest wall is presumably related to the ossification and other structural changes within the rib cage and its articulations.

Data on both chest wall compliance and lung elastic recoil have been coupled in Figure 12–2 to depict the volume-pressure diagrams for an "ideal" newborn and 20- and 60-year-old persons. (For further discussion of how these diagrams are constructed, see Chapter 4, Figure 4–7.) The curves were compiled using data from studies previously cited.[7,10,15,19] However, these do not provide all the necessary information and so parts of the curves are conjectural, particularly the lowermost 50 per cent of the three lung curves and the chest wall curves in the newborn and 20-year-old.

LUNG VOLUMES

After the first few breaths, during which the lung liquid is absorbed and an air-liquid interface established, the pressure-volume relations of the lung and chest wall determine that the newborn's lung volumes will be approximately as shown in the left-hand panel of Figure 12–2. Owing to the high compliance and lack of recoil of the chest wall, intrapleural pressure in babies is closer to atmospheric pressure than in the adult, and the ratios of FRC and RV to TLC are low. Because transpulmonary pressure is low in the normal tidal breathing range, a precarious situation is present in which some airways must be on the verge of closing. In fact, some measurements have revealed that thoracic gas volume (measured by plethysmography) is higher than FRC (measured by equilibration), an indication that gas is trapped distal to closed airways.[10]

At 20 years of age when growth is completed, the compliance of the chest wall has decreased compared with values at birth, but that of the lung has increased. These changes result in the relationships between lung volumes depicted in the middle panel of Figure 12–2.

With increasing senescence after maturity, the chest wall becomes even stiffer and the lungs more distensible.

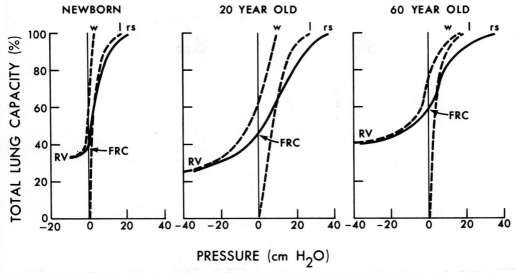

Figure 12-2 Static volume-pressure relationships of lungs (1), chest wall (w), and total respiratory system (rs) for a normal newborn and 20- and 60-year-old adults. RV = residual volume; FRC = functional residual capacity. (From data of Turner, Mead, and Wohl[7]; Nelson[10]; Richards and Bachman[15]; and Mittman, Edelman, Norris, and Shock.[19])

Thus, the lung volumes of a 60-year-old man are approximately those shown in the right-hand panel of Figure 12-2.

The relationships between RV, FRC, vital capacity, and TLC and age from birth to 80 years are shown in Figure 12-3. The increase in lung volumes from birth until somatic growth stops (depicted as occurring at age 17 in Figure 12-3) is closely correlated with increasing body height. After growth ceases, the continuing changes in lung and chest wall mechanics cause vital capacity to decrease to about 75 per cent of its value at 70 compared with 17 years of age and RV to increase nearly 50 per cent during the same period. Total lung capacity, therefore, remains virtually constant, especially when related to height; but as shown in Figure 12-3, TLC actually decreases slightly because body height decreases a few centimeters owing to flattening of the intervertebral disks.

DYNAMIC PROPERTIES

AIRFLOW RATES

Growth is associated with an increase in forced expiratory volume in 1 sec, peak expiratory flow rate, maximal midexpiratory flow rate, and specific airway conductance.[20] Expired airflow velocity increases during growth because the lung enlarges and also its elastic recoil increases (Figure 12-1). It will be recalled from Chapter 4 that elastic recoil of the lung is one of the two principal determinants of effort-independent airflow velocity; the geometry (i.e., cross-sectional area) of the airways on the alveolar side of the equal pressure point is the other.

After maturity, a consistent decline with age has been demonstrated for several indexes of expired airflow velocity: maximal expiratory flow rate, maximal midexpiratory flow,

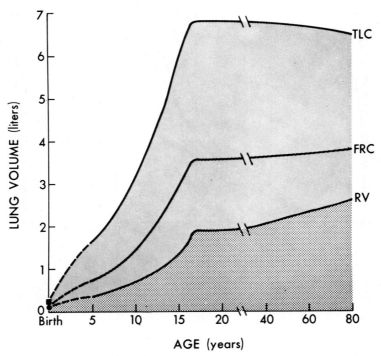

Figure 12–3 Total lung capacity (TLC), functional residual capacity (FRC), and residual volume (RV) as a function of age from birth to 80 years for a male of "average" body build.

forced expiratory volume in 1 sec, and maximal expiratory flow volume curves. Studies of normal healthy adult men in both Europe and the United States revealed a steady decline in forced expiratory volume in 1 sec of about 30 ml/year.[21]

Several studies of the effects of age on maximum expiratory flow volume relations have revealed a decrease in mean maximal flow rates within the effort-independent range of the forced vital capacity maneuver (i.e., <70 per cent of total vital capacity).[22] However, the results of one recent study (Figure 12–4) underscored the considerable variability that can occur between persons within a similar age group; furthermore, the variability was practically the same whether maximal flow was expressed in liters per sec (upper panel) or in vital capac-

ities per sec (lower panel) to compensate for differences in lung size among the subjects.[23] The largest component of the observed variability was attributed to between-individual differences in the resistance to airflow offered by large airways at high lung volumes and small airways at low lung volumes.[23] Thus, the effects of age on elastic recoil, which should result in a progressive reduction of maximal expired airflow in normal subjects, may be obscured by other nonage-related factors that affect airway geometry and resistance.

DISTRIBUTION OF VENTILATION

Newborn infants may exhibit uniform ventilation when tested by the usual relatively insensitive multiple breath N_2 washout test.[24] However,

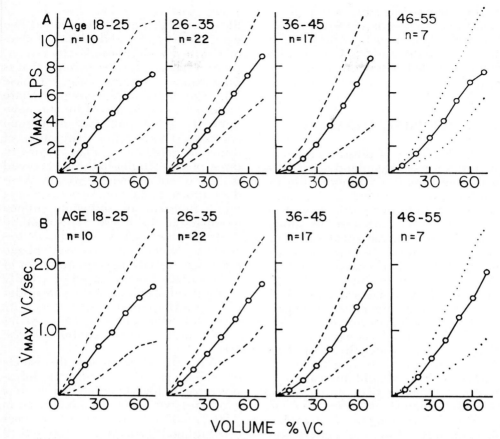

Figure 12–4 Mean values and ranges of maximal expiratory flow-volume curves in different age groups. Maximal flow (Vmax) expressed in liters per second (LPS, upper panels) or vital capacities per second (VC/sec, lower panels) is plotted against lung volume as per cent of vital capacity (% VC). (From Green, Mead, and Turner.[23] Reprinted by permission from the authors and publisher.)

the plethysmographic evidence of air trapping is convincing evidence that inspired air is distributed unevenly. Furthermore, recent studies of closing volume in children demonstrated regional inequalities that are similar to those of aged adults, and presumably the disturbances in both age groups can be related to changes in pulmonary elastic recoil.[6, 25] The low elastic recoil that characterizes childhood and aged lungs (Figure 12–1) means that airways in the dependent regions, where transpulmonary distending pressure is normally lower than in the uppermost regions, will

close at higher lung volumes than when elastic recoil is increased (Chapter 4). Gas distal to the sites of closure will be either trapped or poorly communicating, and thus nonuniformity of the mixing of inspired air must result. In normal infants and aged subjects, closing volume is larger than FRC, which means that some airways are closed and the terminal respiratory units they supply are not being ventilated continuously during normal tidal breathing. Under these conditions, the abnormalities in the distribution of ventilation should be corrected by breathing with a large tidal volume so that FRC plus tidal volume greatly exceeds closing volume; in a study of old men, breathing deeply did improve the uniformity of ventilation compared with breathing normally.[26]

DIFFUSING CAPACITY

Most studies of diffusing capacity in children have examined the 5 to 15 years age range and ignored the infancy to preschool period. The interval from birth to five years of age is of particular interest because, as shown in Table 12–1, the ratio of alveolar surface area to body surface area increases during the first four years of life from 13:3 to 33:1; thereafter, the changes are much less remarkable, the adult values reaching only 39:5.[27] As emphasized in Chapter 2, during the first few years of life there is an explosive proliferation of new alveoli and pulmonary capillaries; accordingly, the diffusing capacity should increase proportionately more than lung volume or body dimensions. After the age when the development of new alveoli probably slows or ceases and growth occurs by enlargement, the increase in diffusing capacity should keep pace with the increase in lung volume.

Detailed morphometric studies in growing rats by Weibel[28] revealed a steady increase of all variables that characterize pulmonary diffusing capacity during the first five days of life (Phase I); during the second five days, there is a rapid doubling of alveolar surface area (Phase II); thereafter, there is again a steady increase that is proportional to lung volume (Phase III). The diffusing capacity per square meter of body surface of human newborns is about half that of normal adults.[10] Whether the maturation of diffusing capacity in man occurs in three phases similar to those observed in rats is not known; however, there does appear to be a phase of extremely rapid increase in diffusion surface (comparable to Phase II) sometime during infancy-early childhood because by about five to six years of age diffusing capacity per square meter of body surface has increased practically to adult values. During the remainder of the growth period, diffusing capacity increases nearly in proportion to increases in height (comparable to Phase III).

Virtually all studies of the effects of senescence on single breath-diffusing capacity for CO agree that there is a progressive reduction ranging from 0.20 to 0.32 ml/min/mm Hg per year of adulthood for men and 0.06 to 0.18 ml/min/mm Hg per year for women.[21] These changes are caused by the loss of lung tissue with advancing age, a loss that is associated with a reduction in alveolar-capillary surface area and no discernible decrease in pulmonary capillary blood volume (Figure 12–5).[29]

Table 12–1   Postnatal Changes in Number of Alveoli, Alveolar Surface Area (S_A), Body Surface Area (S_B), and Ratio Alveolar Surface:Body Surface*

AGE	NUMBER OF ALVEOLI, $\times 10^6$	ALVEOLAR SURFACE AREA, M^2	BODY SURFACE AREA, M^2	S_A/S_B
Newborn	24	2.8	0.21	13.3
3 months	77	7.2	0.29	24.8
7 months	112	8.4	0.38	22.1
13 months	129	12.2	0.45	27.1
4 years	257	22.2	0.67	33.1
8 years	280	32.0	0.92	34.8
Adult	296	75.0	1.90	39.5

*Data from Dunnill.[27]

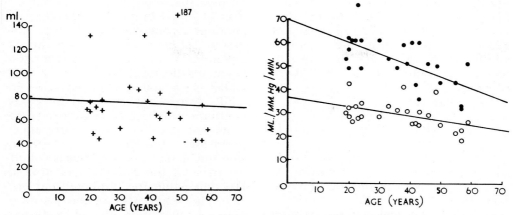

Figure 12-5 Relation between pulmonary diffusing capacity (DL = ○), membrane diffusing capacity (Dm = ●), and pulmonary capillary blood volume (Vc = +), and age. DL and DM decrease with age but Vc does not. (From Hamer.[29] Reprinted by permission from the author and publisher.)

ARTERIAL BLOOD GASES

ARTERIAL OXYGEN TENSION

Sequential changes in arterial PO_2 from birth to old age have been reasonably well documented, and values from several studies are summarized in Figure 12-6.[6,10,30] The pattern of a rise in arterial PO_2 from birth to maturity followed by a gradual decline with advancing age is exactly the same as that of changes in elastic recoil during growth and senescence (Figure 12-1). Moreover, these two variables are believed to be related through the

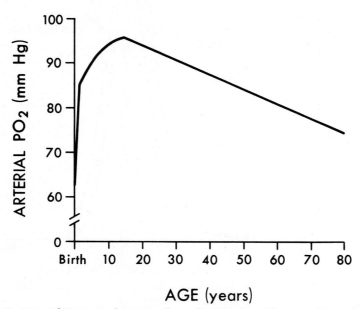

Figure 12-6 Arterial PO_2 as a function of age from birth to 80 years. (From data of Mansell, Bryan, and Levison[6]; Nelson[10]; and Sorbini, Brassi, Solinas, and Muiesan.[30])

effects of elastic recoil on airway caliber and hence on the distribution of ventilation. Computer analysis of 2233 studies of presumed normal adults (20 years of age or older) in which age and arterial PO_2 were reported yielded the following regression equation[31]:

$$Pa_{O_2} = 100.1 - 0.323 \text{ (age)}. \quad (1)$$

As indicated earlier and also in Chapter 4, dependent airways are exposed to a lower distending pressure than those located more superiorly, owing to the vertical gradient of pleural pressure (more negative at the top than at the bottom). Accordingly, dependent airways tend to close or narrow as elastic recoil decreases during deflation; this effect is exaggerated when elastic recoil is low, as it normally is in young children and old adults. Narrowing of airways decreases ventilation to their distal gas exchange units but does not necessarily affect perfusion. Thus, a ventilation-perfusion imbalance is created that accounts for most of the reduction of arterial PO_2 detectable in childhood and old age. The differences in the distributions of ventilation and of perfusion

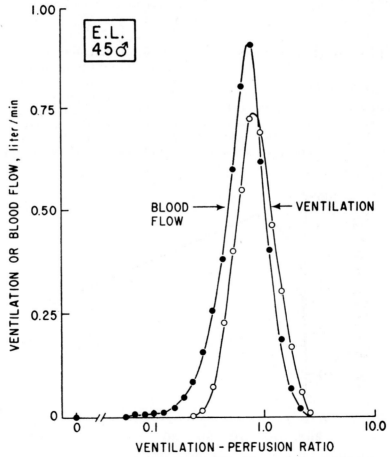

Figure 12–7 The distributions of ventilation and blood flow in a 45-year-old man and a 44-year-old man (opposite page). Compared with a younger subject (Figure 7–6), there is more dispersion and less symmetry in ventilation and perfusion curves. Both subjects demonstrate blood flow to low ventilation-perfusion regions, but the effect is greater in W. C. than in E. L. (From Wagner, Laravuso, Uhl, and West.[32] Reprinted by permission from authors and publishers.)

between a normal 44- and 45-year-old man are demonstrated in Figure 12–7 (compare also a normal 22-year-old man, Figure 7–6).

The effect of ventilation-perfusion imbalances in elderly persons is compounded by the age-related reduction in cardiac output and mixed venous O_2 content. When the O_2 content of blood perfusing poorly ventilated spaces is lowered, the effect of a given ventilation-perfusion inequality on arterial PO_2 is magnified.

ALVEOLAR-ARTERIAL OXYGEN TENSION DIFFERENCE

The causes of the reduced arterial PO_2 in infants, children, and old adults compared with young adults are re-flected by an increased alveolar-arterial PO_2 difference. Most, but not all, the PO_2 difference is attributable to the presence of ventilation-perfusion abnormalities. The other contribution is due to right-to-left shunting of blood. In infants, the usual right-to-left shunt through the foramen ovale ceases almost immediately after birth (although the foramen may remain patent for many years); the right-to-left shunt through the ductus arteriosus ordinarily reverses after birth and the new shunt becomes functionally unimportant within 24 hours.

With senescence, in addition to widening of the alveolar-arterial PO_2 difference from ventilation-perfusion inequalities, there is evidence of an increased right-to-left shunt of blood[33];

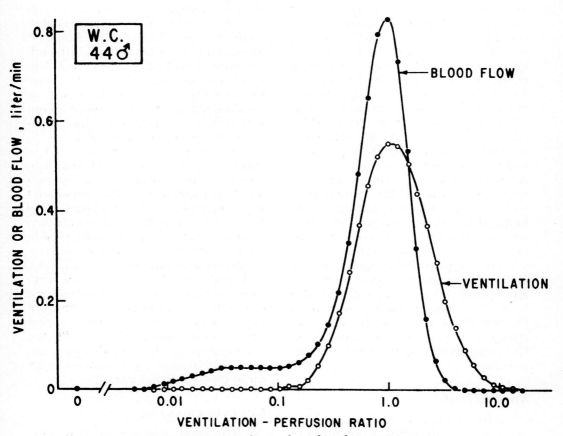

Figure 12–7 (Continued)   See legend on the opposite page.

this most likely reflects the effect of a reduction in mixed venous O_2 content, attributable to the age-related decrease in cardiac output; another possible cause is an increase in post-pulmonary shunting (e.g., through thebesian or bronchial veins). It should be mentioned that even though diffusing capacity decreases with old age and may be relatively low during infancy, the reduction does not contribute measurably to the observed alveolar-arterial P_{O_2} differences at rest.

ARTERIAL CARBON DIOXIDE TENSION

Within one to four hours, normal newborn infants lower their arterial P_{CO_2} values from about 76 mm Hg at birth to about 38 mm Hg, and by 24 hours to about 33 mm Hg (for serial measurements see *Respiration and Circulation*[34]). No one knows why arterial P_{CO_2} values are "low" in infants, but because they are similar to those found in pregnant women at the time of delivery it is possible that the maternal environment "sets" the buffering capacity of the newborn's body. After birth, increases in arterial P_{CO_2} cannot take place until the infant has developed its own HCO_3^--generating and conserving systems; any increase in P_{CO_2} evokes a brisk ventilatory response owing to the presence of well-developed CO_2 sensitivity in infants. It is not known precisely how long these adjustments take, but one review cites "several months."[10]

Once arterial P_{CO_2} reaches 40 mm Hg in the newborn period (or values appropriate for residence at high altitude), it remains virtually constant for the rest of the person's life. This constancy occurs despite the reduction in CO_2 sensitivity that occurs during senescence.

ARTERIAL pH

Arterial pH reaches its normal value of about 7.40 within a few hours of birth and tends to remain constant thereafter.[10] The stability of arterial pH while P_{CO_2} and plasma HCO_3^- are changing in the newborn period signifies that the two variables are changing proportionately to maintain the $HCO_3^-:H_2CO_3$ ratio (see Chapter 8).

CONTROL OF RESPIRATION

PERIPHERAL CHEMORECEPTORS

There is surprisingly little information about the effects of age on both peripheral and central chemoreceptor control of breathing. It is now widely accepted, after many years of uncertainty, that the peripheral chemoreceptors of newborn infants respond to changes in arterial P_{O_2}.[35] Furthermore, studies in experimental animals showed ventilatory responses to oscillations of arterial P_{CO_2} presumably mediated by the carotid bodies.[36] Thus, it is generally assumed, although not proved, that from infancy to adulthood peripheral chemoreceptor function is fully developed. However, as emphasized in Chapter 9, there is considerable variation in the range of responses among normal subjects.

A recent study demonstrated a substantial attenuation in the heart rate and ventilatory responses to hypoxia and hypercapnia in healthy persons 64 to 73 years of age compared with those in subjects 22 to 30 years of age; data from this study are presented in Table 12-2.[37] Although the reasons for the suppression of breathing are unknown and undoubtedly complex, the data indicate that aging is associated with diminution of an important protective mechanism. Moreover, elderly persons, who are most likely to be afflicted with chronic pulmonary diseases, are least able to respond to changes in arterial blood P_{O_2} and P_{CO_2}.[37]

CENTRAL CHEMORECEPTORS

The ventilatory sensitivity of newborn infants to inhaled CO_2 is slightly

Table 12–2 Heart Rate and Ventilatory Responses to Hypoxia and Hypercapnia in Young and Old Normal Subjects *

AGE RANGE † (YEARS)	YOUNG SUBJECTS 22–30 YEARS		OLD SUBJECTS 64–73 YEARS		P VALUE
	MEAN	SEM	MEAN	SEM	
Ventilatory response					
Hypoxia ($\Delta\dot{V}40$, L/min)	40.1	4.7	10.2	1.2	<0.001
Hypercapnia (L/min/mm Hg)	3.4	0.5	2.0	0.2	<0.025
Heart rate response					
Hypoxia (% change control to $P_{A_{O_2}}$ 40 mm Hg)	34.1	5.2	11.5	2.2	<0.005
Hypercapnia (% change control to $P_{A_{CO_2}}$ 55 mm Hg)	15.0	2.8	−0.9	1.0	<0.001

* Data from Kronenberg and Drage.[37]

† $\Delta\dot{V}40$ = change in ventilation (L/min) from initial value breathing room air to that during hypoxia when alveolar P_{O_2} = 40 mm Hg; $P_{A_{O_2}}$ = alveolar P_{O_2}; $P_{A_{CO_2}}$ = alveolar P_{CO_2}.

greater than that of adults.[10] Presumably, this is largely dependent upon the reduced $[HCO_3^-]$ in the baby's plasma and CSF. Thus, for any incremental increase in P_{CO_2}, a greater pH change will occur with consequent stimulation of both central and peripheral chemoreceptors. The contributions of these two sites have not been differentiated, although the central effect is undoubtedly the more profound, owing to the lower buffering capacity of CSF compared with that of plasma (see Chapter 9).

The data shown in Table 12–2 indicate that the ventilatory response to CO_2 is diminished in old compared with young healthy adult men.[37] Whether this is caused by suppression of central or peripheral receptor systems, or both, has not been established. However, because the amount of reduction of CO_2 sensitivity in the old men (41 per cent) was greater than the demonstrable total contribution of carotid chemoreceptors to the normal hypercapneic response (30 per cent), central mechanisms were probably involved.

EXERCISE CAPACITY

The complex interrelations among the factors that govern maximal O_2 up-take are discussed in Chapter 10. It is generally agreed that genetic influences are the chief determinants of the physical dimensions of the O_2 transport system, including blood volume, red blood cell mass, heart volume, vital capacity, pulmonary diffusing capacity, and skeletal muscle mass. Physical training is decisive in developing the functional capabilities inherent in the respiratory and circulatory systems. Moreover, it appears that training during youth is essential in order for persons to develop fully the potential capabilities for "maximal" maximal O_2 uptake.[38]

Figure 12–8 shows the relationship between maximal O_2 uptake and age in normal Swedish men who were in good physical condition. It is clear that in groups with comparable amounts of athletic conditioning, age is a significant factor in defining maximal O_2 uptake. In a study of many of the principal components of the O_2 transport system, it was demonstrated that significant age-related decreases occurred only in forced vital capacity and maximal heart rate; the effect of age on maximal O_2 uptake, therefore, was a loss of functional capabilities despite maintenance of the dimensional capacity of youth.[39]

This conclusion is supported by serial studies of young women who

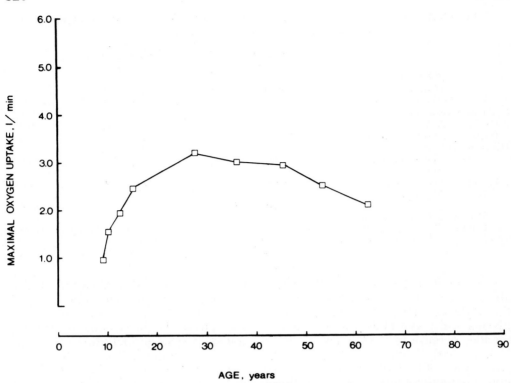

Figure 12-8   Maximal O₂ uptake as a function of age in Swedish men. (Adapted from Grimby and Saltin.[38] Reprinted by permission from the authors and publisher.)

were highly trained competitive swimmers. Follow-up measurements several years after they had ceased training (average five years) revealed no change in their dimensional characteristics but a striking decrease in maximal O_2 uptake.[40] Similar effects were noted when former successful cross-country runners and skiers were examined 10 to 30 years after they had given up competition and training.[41] However, the athletically inclined can be reassured by the evidence that regular physical training markedly retards the rate of decrease in maximal O_2 uptake with age.

DEFENSE MECHANISMS

CLEARANCE MECHANISMS

No systematic studies have been carried out to determine whether age affects either alveolar macrophage activity or mucociliary clearance. Accordingly, possible age-dependent influences on macrophage motility, phagocytosis, and bactericidal capabilities are unknown. Similarly, information is lacking about the effects of age on mucus composition and physical properties and on the number and mechanical behavior of cilia. As a first assumption, it is likely that the nonspecific components of host defenses share the age-related pattern of attrition of function demonstrated by many other organ systems and their components. Thus, the effectiveness of the clearance system probably increases during growth and then wanes during senescence. Studies are obviously needed to examine this hypothesis.

HUMORAL IMMUNITY

It is well accepted that human fetuses produce selective immunoglobulins, especially during the last half of gestation.[42] The various immuno-globulin fractions vary considerably in their concentrations at birth, in the duration required to attain peak values, and in the variations that occur with age after maximum production is reached. In general, these changes can be correlated with the proliferation and subsequent atrophy of different components of the lymphatic system.

The major immunoglobulin fraction of newborns, like adults, is IgG. Levels of IgG vary during the human lifetime,[43,44] as shown in Table 12–3. Most of the IgG present at birth is derived from maternal sources, and hence the newborn is briefly protected against the same diseases as its mother. During the first few months of infancy, the passively transferred IgG is catabolized, and by the third month the baby's own supply becomes dominant.[42] The quantity increases rapidly during childhood to a plateau in adolescence or early adulthood; thereafter, the serum levels gradually increase. Despite the increased IgG concentrations, the antibody response to extrinsic antigens, such as pneumococcal constituents, is reduced considerably in old age; presumably, the increased immunoglobulin values reflect production of antibody to various intrinsic antigens, including those from nuclear, gastric, and thyroid sources.[45]

The IgM, which does not cross the placental barrier, is normally synthesized by the fetus after the fourteenth week, and small amounts are measurable at birth (11 ± 5 mg/100 ml); in cases of antenatal infection, larger amounts may be demonstrable and, if present, serve as a guide to the detection of intrauterine complications.[42] Levels of IgM in the serum increase rapidly during infancy and childhood, although the exact sequence has not been agreed upon. During senescence, serum values of IgM tend to decrease dramatically.

There is virtually no IgA in the serum of human infants at birth, but small amounts are detectable shortly afterward, and the concentration increases steadily, reaching adult levels after puberty. In contrast, the secretory IgA system reaches maturity within one or two months of age, at least in judging from the quantities of IgA present in saliva.[46]

CELLULAR IMMUNITY

The effects of age on humoral immunity have received more intensive study than the effects on cellular immunity. Recently, attention has been directed toward the development of various cellular aspects of immunity during growth and their attenuation

Table 12–3   Levels of Immunoglobulins in Serum of Normal Subjects at Different Ages*

AGE GROUPS	IgG MEAN	IgG SD	IgM MEAN	IgM SD	IgA MEAN	IgA SD
Newborn	1031	200	11	5	2	3
1-3 months	430	119	30	11	21	13
7-12 months	661	219	54	23	37	18
3-5 years	929	228	56	18	93	27
12-16 years	946	124	59	20	148	63
20-29 years	865	459	–	–	–	–
40-49 years	979	739	–	–	–	–
60-69 years	1393	541	–	–	–	–
Adults, all ages	1158	305	99	27	200	61

*Data from Stiehm and Fudenberg;[43] and Das and Bhattacharya.[44]

during senescence. It has been recognized for many years that normal newborn experimental animals are capable of expressing the presence of cellular immunity by rejecting transplants of foreign tissues. In addition, it is now known that three cellular immune functions are well developed in human fetuses and newborns: (1) the blastogenic response of lymphocytes to phytohemagglutinin, (2) the nonspecific ability of cord lymphocytes to destroy target cells (chicken erythrocytes), and (3) the development of rosette-forming cells in several different human fetal lymphoid organs.[47] Although it is difficult to compare the results of these experiments with comparable studies in the adult, it can be concluded that many important aspects of cellular immunity are fully developed in human beings at birth. The blastogenic response to plant mitogens (phytohemagglutinin and pokeweed mitogen) has also been used to demonstrate a functional depression in the lymphocytes from elderly (75 to 96 years) compared with young (25 to 40 years) adults.[48] Similarly, the number of positive delayed hypersensitivity skin reactions to five common antigens was significantly lower in the aged than in the young; furthermore, the mortality rate of old persons (>80 years of age) who were hyporesponsive to the battery of skin tests was significantly higher than that of old persons who were responsive.[49]

SUMMARY

The effects of age on the nonspecific and particularly on the specific defense systems are responsible for the familiar clinical observations concerning vulnerability to infections; very young and very old persons are most susceptible. Although less appreciated, the age-related incidence of malignancy is similar: 20/100,000 in the first year of life, 10/100,000 between 10 and 14 years of age when immunologic capabilities are maxi-

mum, and 2140/100,000 at greater than 85 years of age.[50] The poorly protected host has increasing difficulty withstanding both the continuous onslaught of hostile microorganisms and other noxious agents from the external environment, and the cellular mischief constantly taking place in his own body; it is also possible that immunologic failure may accelerate the ravages of degenerative diseases. Thus, attrition of defense mechanisms, including impairment of immune surveillance, sets the stage for the clinical consequences that inevitably terminate in death.

REFERENCES

1. Comfort, A.: Ageing: The Biology of Senescence. New York, Holt, Rinehart and Winston, 1964, p. 5.
2. Hayflick, L.: The biology of human aging. Am. J. Med. Sci., 265:432-445, 1973.
3. Goldstein, S.: The biology of aging. New Eng. J. Med., 285:1120-1129, 1971.
4. Polgar, G., and Promadhat, V.: Pulmonary Function Testing in Children: Techniques and Standards. Philadelphia, W. B. Saunders Company, 1971, 273 pp.
5. Cook, C. D., Mead, J., and Orzalesi, M. M.: Static volume-pressure characteristics of the respiratory system during maximal efforts. J. Appl. Physiol., 19:1016-1022, 1964.
6. Mansell, A., Bryan, C., and Levison, H.: Airway closure in children. J. Appl. Physiol., 33:711-714, 1972.
7. Turner, J. M., Mead, J., and Wohl, M. E.: Elasticity of human lungs in relation to age. J. Appl. Physiol., 25:664-671, 1968.
8. Zapletal, A., Misur, M., and Samanek, M.: Static recoil pressure of the lungs in children. Bull. Physiopathol. Resp., 7:139-143, 1971.
9. Gribetz, I., Frank, N. R., and Avery, M. E.: Static volume-pressure relations of excised lungs of infants with hyaline membrane disease, newborn and stillborn infants. J. Clin. Invest., 38:2168-2175, 1959.
10. Nelson, N. M.: Neonatal pulmonary function. Pediat. Clin. N. America 13:769-799, 1966.
11. Loosli, C. G., and Potter, E. L.: Pre- and postnatal development of the respiratory portion of the human lung. With special reference to the elastic fibers. Am. Rev. Resp. Dis., 80(Suppl. 1):5-20, 1959.

12. Pierce, J. A.: Age related changes in the fibrous proteins in the lungs. Arch. Environ. Health, 6:50-54, 1963.

13. John, R., and Thomas, J.: Chemical compositions of elastins isolated from aortas and pulmonary tissues of humans of different ages. Biochem. J., 127:261-269, 1972.

14. Wright, R. R.: Elastic tissue of normal and emphysematous lungs. A tridimensional histologic study. Am. J. Pathol., 39:355-367, 1961.

15. Richards, C. C., and Bachman, L.: Lung and chest wall compliance of apneic paralyzed infants. J. Clin. Invest., 40:273-278, 1961.

16. Cook, C. D., Sutherland, J. M., Segal, S., Cherry, R. B., Mead, J., McIlroy, M. B., and Smith, C. A.: Studies of respiratory physiology in the newborn infant. III. Measurements of mechanics of respiration. J. Clin. Invest., 36:440-448, 1957.

17. Agostoni, E.: Volume-pressure relationships of the thorax and lung in the newborn. J. Appl. Physiol., 14:909-913, 1959.

18. Avery, M. E., and Cook, C. D.: Volume-pressure relationships of lungs and thorax in fetal, newborn, and adult goats. J. Appl. Physiol., 16:1034-1038, 1961.

19. Mittman, C., Edelman, N. H., Norris, A. H., and Shock, N. W.: Relationship between chest wall and pulmonary compliance and age. J. Appl. Physiol., 20:1211-1216, 1965.

20. Weng, T.-R., and Levison, H.: Standards of pulmonary function in children. Am. Rev. Resp. Dis., 99:879-894, 1969.

21. Muiesan, G., Sorbini, C. A., and Grassi, V.: Respiratory function in the aged. Bull. Physiopathol. Resp., 7:973-1009, 1971.

22. Black, L. F., Offord, K., and Hyatt, R. E.: Variability in the maximal expiratory flow volume curve in asymptomatic smokers and in nonsmokers. Am. Rev. Resp. Dis. 110:282-292, 1974.

23. Green, M., Mead, J., and Turner, J. M.: Variability of maximum expiratory flow-volume curves. J. Appl. Physiol. 37:67-74, 1974.

24. Strang, L. B., and McGrath, M. W.: Alveolar ventilation in normal newborn infants studied by air wash-in after oxygen breathing. Clin. Sci., 23:129-139, 1962.

25. Holland, J., Milic-Emili, J., Macklem, P. T., and Bates, D. V.: Regional distribution of pulmonary ventilation and perfusion in elderly subjects. J. Clin. Invest., 47:81-92, 1968.

26. Edelman, N. H., Mittman, C., Norris, A. H., and Shock, N. W.: Effects of respiratory pattern on age differences in ventilation uniformity. J. Appl. Physiol., 24:49-53, 1968.

27. Dunnill, M. S.: Postnatal growth of the lung. Thorax, 17:329-333, 1962.

28. Weibel, E. R.: Morphological basis of alveolar-capillary gas exchange. Physiol. Rev., 53:419-495, 1973.

29. Hamer, N. A. J.: The effect of age on the components of the pulmonary diffusing capacity. Clin. Sci., 23:85-93, 1962.

30. Sorbini, C. A., Brassi, V., Solinas, E., and Muiesan, G.: Arterial oxygen tension in relation to age in healthy subjects. Respiration, 25:3-13, 1968.

31. Mays, E. E.: Unpublished observations, 1974.

32. Wagner, P. D., Laravuso, R. B., Uhl, R. R., and West, J. B.: Continuous distributions of ventilation-perfusion ratios in normal subjects breathing air and 100% O_2. J. Clin. Invest., 54:54–68, 1974.

33. Kanber, G. J., King, F. W., Eshchar, Y. R., and Sharp, J. T.: The alveolar-arterial oxygen gradient in young and elderly men during air and oxygen breathing. Am. Rev. Resp. Dis., 97:376-381, 1968.

34. Senior, R. M., and Fishman, A. P.: Carbon dioxide pressures in alveolar air and arterial blood: man. In Altman, P. L., and Dittmer, D. S. (eds.): Respiration and Circulation. Bethesda, Md., Federation of American Societies for Experimental Biology, 1971, pp. 129-130.

35. Brady, J. P., Cotton, E. C., and Tooley, W. H.: Chemoreflexes in the new-born infant: effects of 100% oxygen on heart rate and ventilation. J. Physiol. (Lond.), 172:332–341, 1964.

36. Avery, M. E., Chernick, V., and Young, M.: Fetal respiratory movements in response to rapid changes of CO_2 in carotid artery. J. Appl. Physiol., 20:225-227, 1965.

37. Kronenberg, R. S., and Drage, C. W.: Attenuation of the ventilatory and heart rate responses to hypoxia and hypercapnia with aging in normal men. J. Clin. Invest., 52:1812-1819, 1973.

38. Grimby, G., and Saltin, B.: Physiological effects of physical training. Scand. J. Rehab. Med., 3:6-14, 1971.

39. Davies, C. T. M.: The oxygen-transporting system in relation to age. Clin. Sci., 42:1-13, 1972.

40. Eriksson, B. O., Engström, I., Karlberg, P., Saltin, B., and Thorén, C.: A physiological analysis of former girl swimmers. Acta Paediat. Scand. [Suppl.], 217:68-72, 1971.

41. Saltin, B., and Grimby, G.: Physiological analysis of middle-aged and old former athletes: comparison with still active athletes of the same ages. Circulation, 38:1104-1115, 1968.

42. Frommel, D., and Good, R. A.: Immunological mechanisms. In Gairdner, D., and Hull, D. (eds.): Recent Advances in Paediatrics, 4th Ed. London, J. & A. Churchill, 1971, pp. 401-427.

43. Stiehm, E. R., and Fudenberg, H. H.: Serum levels of immune globulins in health and disease: a survey. Pediatrics, 37:715-727, 1966.

44. Das, B. C., and Bhattacharya, S. K.: Changes in human serum protein fractions with age and weight. Canad. J. Biochem. Physiol., 39:569-579, 1961.

45. Rowley, M., Buchanan, H., and Mackay, I. R.: Reciprocal change with age in antibody to extrinsic and intrinsic antigens. Lancet, 2:24-26, 1968.

46. Selner, J. C., Merrill, D. A., and Claman, H. N.: Salivary immunoglobulin and albumin: development during the newborn period. J. Pediat., 72:685-689, 1968.

47. Stites, D. P., Wybran, J., Carr, M. C., and Fudenberg, H. H.: Development of cellular immunocompetence in man. In Ontogeny of Acquired Immunity. New York, Associated Scientific Publishers, 1972, pp. 113-132.

48. Weksler, M. E., and Hütteroth, T. H.: Impaired lymphocyte function in aged humans. J. Clin. Invest., 53:99-104, 1974.

49. Roberts-Thomson, I. C., Whittingham, S., Youngchaiyud, U., and Mackay, I. R.: Ageing, immune response and mortality. Lancet, 2:368-370, 1974.

50. California Tumor Registry, Cancer Incidence System, 1972-73 data, unpublished observations.

Index

Note: Page numbers in *italic* type refer to illustrations.